COMPLICATIONS

ANALYSIS AND MANAGEMENT IN AESTHETIC MEDICINE

169 Photos
66 Illustrations
12 Videos

Browse Acta Medica books catalogue
on www.griffineditore.it in the aesthetic medicine
category or scan the QR code

COMPLICATIONS
Analysis and management in aesthetic medicine
ISBN 978-88-97438-76-2

Publishing coordination: Giuseppe Roccucci
Editing: Rachele Villa
English translation: Annette Fowles
Design and layout: Massimo D'Onofrio
Illustrations: Massimiliano Crespi

Printing: Starprint srl
First edition: March 2023

PUBLISHER
Griffin srl unipersonale
Via Don Luigi Meroni 58 - 22060 Figino Serenza (Como) - Italy
Tel. + 39 031.789085
customerservice@griffineditore.it
www.griffineditore.it

QR Code VIDEO System

To watch the videos scan the QR codes using the camera on your
device or download a QR reader app

PREFACE

The problems relating to the management of complications and side effects of medical practice are becoming the subject of epidemiological study and legislative production within the framework of the set of guidelines and procedures gathered under the name of "Risk Management". The complexity of the subject is demonstrated by the fact that simple and complex Risk Management structures are springing up and becoming increasingly prominent in all healthcare facilities. Added to this are the economic problems associated with litigation: many healthcare facilities are unable to find insurance companies that will take on the economic risk of litigation and it is also hard to find facilities that have implemented risk management activities as part of their medico-legal competencies before automatically transferring the management of risk to the insurance company. The role of the patient is also significant. Patients read about miraculous treatments on the internet and on social networks and completely disregard the possibility that a treatment or procedure may generate complications and side effects. The situation is therefore extremely complex and, in the practice of aesthetic medicine, these contradictions are even more evident. The patients of aesthetic medicine are usually healthy individuals who want to improve the way they look, making them even less willing to accept the possibility that a problem may occur as a result of a medical practice. The role of training is key in this issue: doctors and health professionals lack adequate training in clinical risk and its prevention and management. Even the General Managers of healthcare facilities have difficulty in creating the structures within the Corporate Acts capable of handling litigation.

I have repeatedly pointed out the need for those entering the aesthetic medical profession to be adequately trained, with an appropriate pre-graduate programme and subsequent specialisation. As yet, no response has been forthcoming in relation to the need to regulate access to aesthetic medicine.

This book tackles the subject for every angle, starting with the medical-legal aspects and then investigating the causes and management of complications in every area of the world of aesthetic medicine. Consequently, besides being useful to those who practice this profession, the book may also be of interest to those who are interested in Health Management, Health Legislation and Risk Management from various perspectives.

Professor Maria Triassi
President of the School of Medicine and Surgery
Università Federico II di Napoli

PREFACE

Sapiens nihil affirmat quod non probet.

It is an honour for me to write the preface for this new book about aesthetic complications by Professor Giuseppe Sito and his team, for two reasons. Not only is Giuseppe Sito a friend and a globally renowned expert in the aesthetic arena, but this is also one of my favourite topics with the Expert2expert group [1].

It is a well-known fact that there is no medicine without complications, and a good captain is always recognized by his behaviour in a storm.

With this in mind, for those readers who are convinced they will never have to deal with complications at their clinic, this book provides the solutions suggested by experts when they are in the eye of the storm.

The management of clinical complications is based on three actions: Prevent, Recognize and Treat. The first thing we must do in aesthetic medicine is Prevent complications and to do so, and thereby ensure safety, we must apply all our technical expertise. Recognize that the sooner a complication is identified, the sooner the patient will recover from it, and, last but not least, Treat it with the correct medication to avoid further consequences.

Unfortunately, and for multiple reasons, the analysis and management of complications in the aesthetic field rarely follow evidence-based medicine but tend to be based more on "impression and philosophy". The main reason is the absence of sufficient peer-reviewed data to achieve the statistical level of evidence needed to draw up strong guidelines.

We need to convince our colleagues that they must unashamedly declare their adverse events as this is the only way to enable national health authorities to develop working groups and issue publications to recommend the best practice.

This book is a new step forward to help all health practitioners analyse and manage complications in aesthetic medicine

Enjoy!

Patrick Trevidic
Reconstructive and Aesthetic Plastic Surgeon

1. Criollo-Lamilla G, DeLorenzi C, Karpova E, et al. Anatomy & filler complications. Paris: Expert2Expert Medical publishing; 2017.

PRESENTATION

Complications exist. Yes, they do, and they occur precisely when we feel most confident, when our movements become steadier and our hands move in unison, almost automatically.

That is when persistent oedema, ischaemia or perhaps even something worse and more challenging happens. And the idea that we failed to take every possible precaution, that we didn't cleanse the skin, or that we injected too deeply or too superficially starts to form in our minds, and we look for help. Sooner or later it happens to everyone, and we all always need to double check. And so begins the process of self-criticism and the search for something or someone to clarify our ideas.

This book intends (perhaps a little presumptuously) to be that something or someone that can provide an explanation and, consequently, the help we need.

In this publication, which I have been lucky enough to share with those whom I consider to be the leading Italian experts in the field of Aesthetic Medicine, we wanted to examine the most well-known but also the most unusual complications described in international literature, which have happened to more renowned colleagues but also to beginners. The genesis, description and then the solution have been reported for every one of them, together with how to diagnose and then deal with them. The leading techniques of Aesthetic Medicine have been analysed individually and framed with stringent criteria of knowledge.

What does this book expect?

Definitely to be purchased and consulted, it expects to be considered as a sort of *port bonheur* to keep in your library (because you never know). And it definitely expects to be browsed through because every book is always a source of knowledge and we, the authors, have worked with this spirit: knowledge as a means of avoiding or ultimately healing, exactly as our profession teaches us.

So our hope is that you keep it, but never have to use it!

Professor Giuseppe Sito
Aesthetic Surgeon and Physician

EDITOR

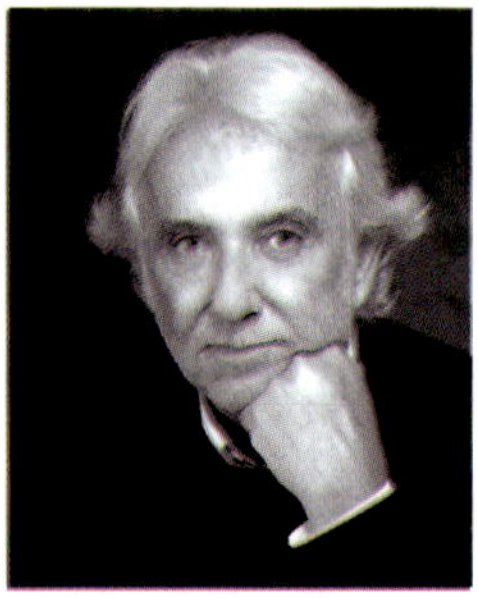

Giuseppe Sito

Born in Naples, he graduated with honours from the University of Naples. He then obtained diplomas as a specialist in General and Endocrine Surgery at the same university, and in Urology at Rome's Università Cattolica del Sacro Cuore. He attended courses in Aesthetic Surgery at the Société de Chirurgie Esthétique in Paris, obtaining the relevant diploma.

He is scientific director of Università Pegaso for the 1st and 2nd level master's degrees in Aesthetic Medicine and the Advanced Training Course in Aesthetic Medicine.

He is a member of the Società Italiana di Chirurgia Plastica Estetica.

He teaches at Agorà Postgraduate School of Medicine specialising in Aesthetic Medicine in Milan and at School of Aesthetic Medicine of Fondazione Fatebenefratelli in Rome. He has taught at the Scuola di Perfezionamento Universitario in Chirurgia Plastica ed Estetica of the University of Pavia.

He was one of the founders of the Associazione Italiana Terapia Estetica Botulino and held office at its Deputy President for several years.

He is reviewer for journals of Plastic Surgery and Aesthetic Medicine with a high impact factor in the United States. He is Editor-in-Chief of the *Journal of Plastic and Aesthetic Surgery*.

He is the author of over 100 publications and consultant to numerous publications in the field of Aesthetic Medicine. He published with Griffin-Acta Medica: *Filler - Illustrative manual of injection techniques* and *Botulinum Toxin - Illustrative manual of injection techniques*.

He is legal medical consultant, specialised in Aesthetic Medicine, for the Court of Naples.

AUTHORS

Lucia Calvisi

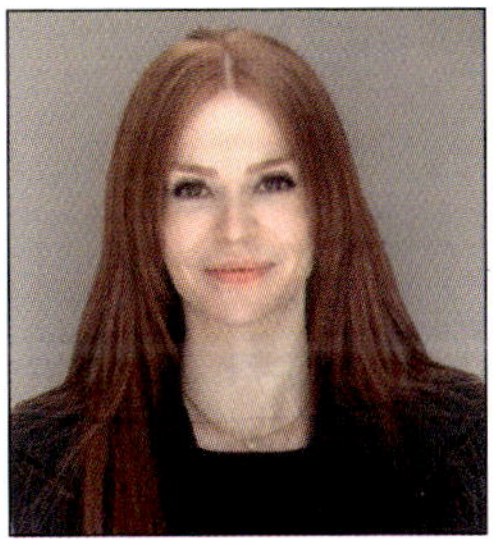

A surgeon, she specialised in Dermatology at the University of Cagliari. Since then, she has perfected her professional training, concentrating mainly on the field of aesthetics, actively participating in the most prestigious national and international congresses and maintaining an active collaboration with the University of Brooklyn, New York.

She currently lectures at the Pegaso Online University, works as an opinion leader for major companies and is the author of numerous national and international publications.

Alberto Diaspro

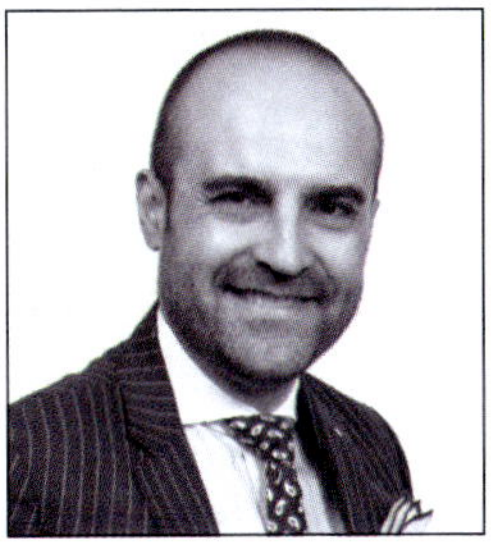

Surgeon specialised in maxillo-facial surgery at the University of Turin. He obtained a master's degree in Facial Plastic Surgery at Rome's "Tor Vergata" University, a master's degree in Aesthetic Medicine and Therapy at the University of Camerino and a Diploma as Expert and Consultant in Aesthetic Medicine at the Agorà Postgraduate School of Milan.

He is a member of Aicpe (Associazione Italiana Chirurgia Plastica ed Estetica), Eafps (European Academy of Facial Plastic Surgery), Aiceff (Associazione Italiana Chirurgia Estetica e Funzionale della Faccia) and Sicmf (Società Italiana di Chirurgia Maxillo-facciale).

He is currently Medical Director at Rigeneralab - Centro di Medicina Rigenerativa in Turin.

Luigi Emanuelli

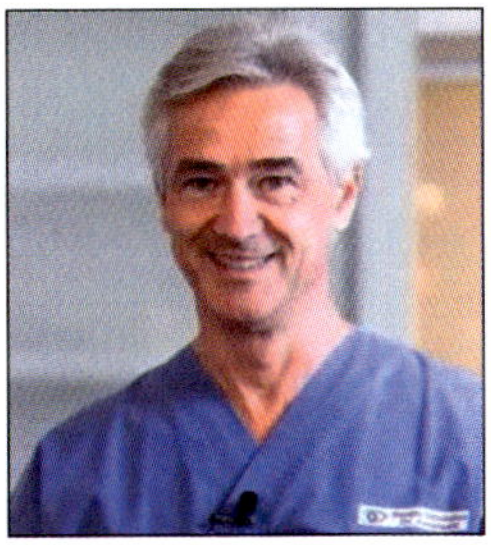

Born in Rome, he graduated from the University of Turin with an honours Degree in Medicine and Surgery in 1992. In that same year, he received his licence to practise as a Surgeon and was enrolled in the professional register of the Order of Surgeons of Turin. In 1996, he completed his Postgraduate Diploma in Ophthalmology at the University of Turin.

After 14 years of hospital experience as Medical Director at the Ospedale Mauriziano in Turin, the Ospedale Oftalmico and the Ospedale Maria Vittoria, he decided to concentrate exclusively on private practice at his own surgeries in Turin and Ciriè.

Maria Vittoria Giatti

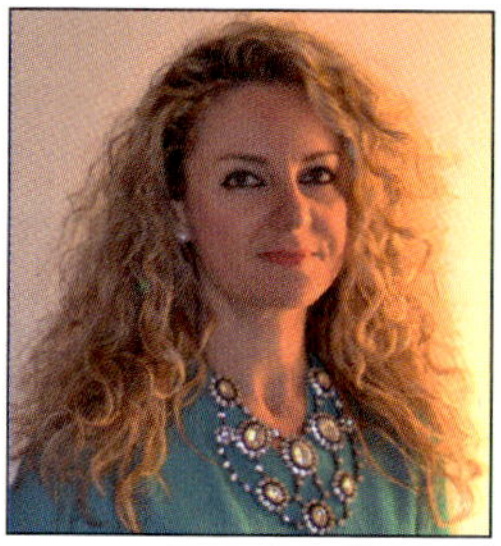

Surgeon specialised in Plastic and Reconstructive Surgery.
She is a member of the Società Italiana di Chirurgia Plastica Ricostruttiva ed Estetica (Sicpre), the Aesthetic Multispecialty Society (Ams) and the American Society of Plastic Surgeons (Asps), and was formerly a member of the International Society of Plastic & Regenerative Surgeons (Ispres).
She has worked with internationally renowned plastic surgeons and lecturers in various theoretical and practical courses for doctors and specialists in the field. She has taken part in numerous national and international master's degree courses and scientific congresses and has produced several communications and scientific publications. Beauty coach and scientific consultant for innovative pharmaceutical and medical companies. She has worked in prestigious clinics in Paris, Florence, Bologna, Verona, Rovigo and Ferrara. She currently works in her own practice in Bologna, where she also runs the Medical Academy for the training of medical specialists in advanced plastic surgery and aesthetic medicine techniques.

Giuseppe Maria Izzo

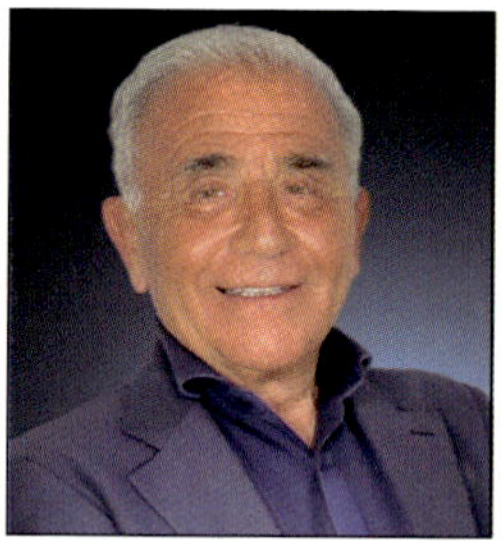

After graduating in Medicine and Surgery, he specialised in Dermatology and Venereology at the Federico II University of Naples in 1979. From 1979 to 1987, he was director of the Centre for Dermatological Photochemotherapy.
In 1990, he completed a master's degree in Aesthetic Medicine at the CPMA School of Aesthetic Medicine in Bologna (Valet), where he was a lecturer until 2017. He was an Isplad lecturer in the Master's Degree Course at Rome's Tor Vergata University, lecturer in the Master's Degree Course in Aesthetic Medicine at the Federico II University of Naples and at the University of Valencia.
He currently lectures at the Pegaso Online University for the postgraduate course in Aesthetic Medicine.

Teresa Lacava

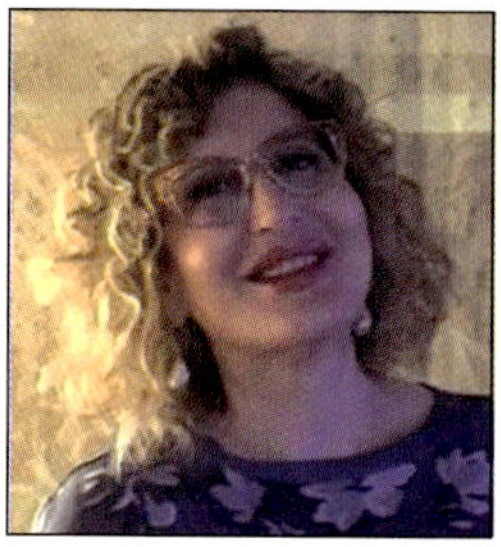

After graduating in Medicine and Surgery in 1988, she qualified as a surgeon in the same year. She holds a master's degree in Aesthetic Medicine, Homoeopathy and Acupuncture. She has attended numerous specialised refresher courses over the years.

Leonardo Longo

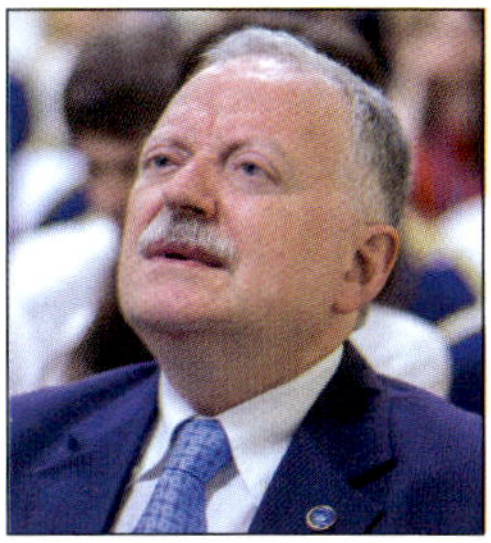

A Surgical Endocrinologist, he has taught Laser Surgery and Medicine at the Universities of Siena, San Marino and eCampus of Milan. He has been Visiting Professor at the Bethesda and Vanderbilt University (USA); Czeske Budejovice, Kladno Prague (Czech Republic); Vilnius (Lithuania); Chennai (India); São Paulo (Brazil).
He is director of the Institute of Laser Medicine in Florence (Ilm), founding president of the International Academy Laser Medicine and Surgery (Ialms), fellow of 28 scientific societies, honorary member of five. He is Editor-in-chief of the international scientific journal *Laser Therapy* and is on the editorial board of seven other international journals. He has been President of the annual International Laser Florence Congress since 1997. Author of monographs and various texts on lasers in medicine, more than 100 scientific articles and 350 international congress papers.

Ruben Oddenino

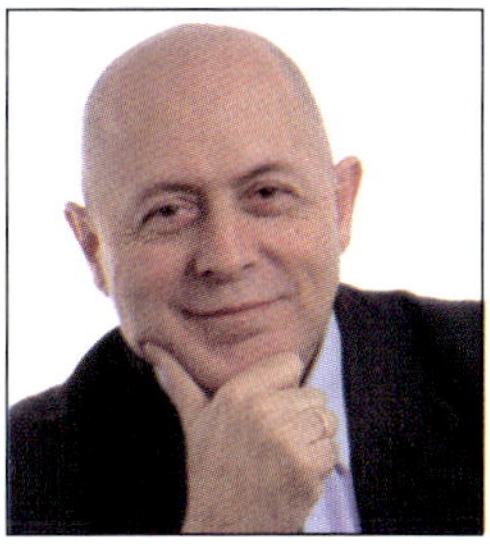

Plastic Surgeon, lecturer at the School of Specialisation in Reconstructive and Aesthetic Plastic Surgery at the University of Milan and former lecturer in the master's degree courses in Aesthetic Surgery at the Universities of Milan, Pavia, Genoa and Turin. A member of Sicpre (Italian Society of Reconstructive-Regenerative and Aesthetic Plastic Surgery), he founded the humanitarian movement "Medici Ovunque" in 2001. A graduate in Legal Sciences, he served for three years as an honorary judge at the Milan Court of Surveillance.

Patrizia Piersini

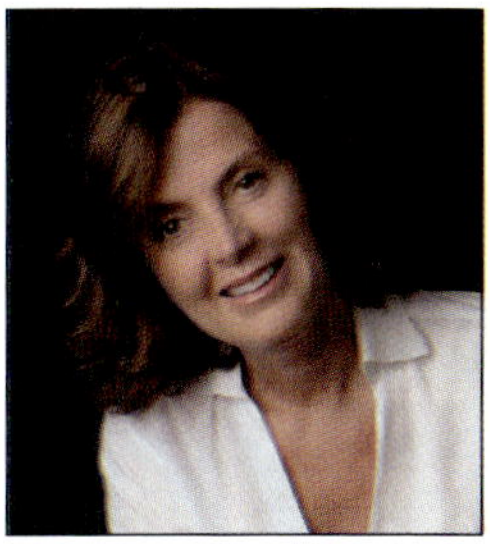

A surgeon, she graduated from the Agorà Post-University School of Aesthetic Medicine in Milan. She has attended numerous refresher courses, including the laser course of the American Academy of Facial Plastic and Reconstructive Surgery in Scottsdale (USA) and the peeling course at Princeton University (USA). She has been head of the Aesthetic Medicine Service at the Koelliker Hospital in Turin.
She has taken part as speaker, moderator and session chair in numerous congresses on Aesthetic Medicine, Aesthetic Surgery, Dermatology and Cosmetological Chemistry, in Italy and abroad. She collaborates as lecturer with the Agorà School of Aesthetic Medicine in Milan and is a member of the scientific-organisational committee of the Agorà Congress of Aesthetic Medicine. She has lectured for the postgraduate course in "Aesthetic Surgery and Aesthetic Medicine" at the University of Turin. She has collaborated with numerous publications in the field of Aesthetic Medicine

Francesco Romeo

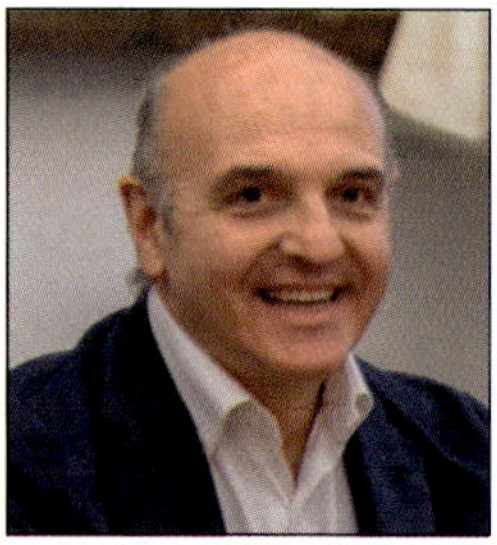

He completed a degree in Medicine and Surgery and a specialisation in General Surgery, both cum laude, at the Faculty of Medicine of "La Sapienza", University of Rome.
He obtained a Level II Master's Degree in Aesthetic Plastic Surgery from the School of Specialisation in Reconstructive and Aesthetic Plastic Surgery at the University of Padua, with distinction.
Since 2014, he has been Sole Consultant in Oncoplastic Surgery at the Regina Apostolorum Classified Hospital in Albano Laziale. He is Adjunct Professor at "La Sapienza" University of Rome, and lecturer in the Level II Master in Aesthetic and Regenerative Medicine.
He has been a full member of the Italian Association of Plastic and Aesthetic Surgery (Aicpe) since its foundation.
He is the author of original papers published in international scientific journals with impact factor and referee for major scientific journals. In 2023, he published *Lo Sguardo. Advanced Multidisciplinary Experiences*, with Griffin-Acta Medica.

Cristina Sartorio

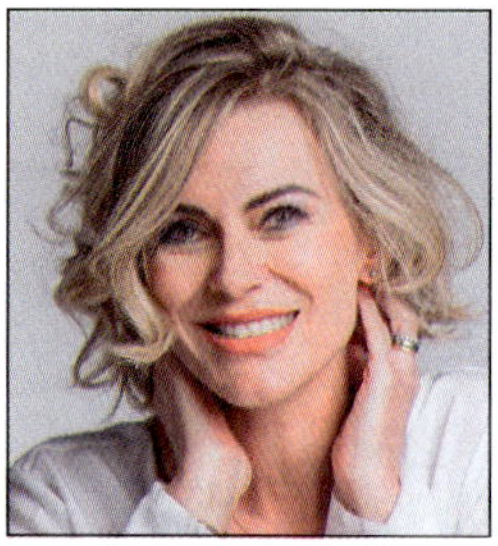

Having graduated in Medicine and Surgery from the University of Turin, she attained her post-graduate diploma in Aesthetic Medicine at the Agorà Post-University School of Aesthetic Medicine in Milan, also specialising in Laser Therapy and Laser Surgery at the same institution.
She focuses on the in-depth study of Aesthetic Medicine and all its psychological and social implications. This ongoing research has led her to train as a Senior Health Coach to help people achieve superior results, not only in the field of aesthetics. She has worked in the field of nutrition for over 20 years.
She is a member of the American Academy of Aesthetic Medicine, of Aiteb (Associazione italiana terapia estetica botulino), Fime (Federazione italiana medici estetici), Agorà and Sime (Società italiana di medicina estetica) and the Piedmont representative of Sies (Società italiana di medicina e chirurgia estetica). She lectures at the the Agorà Post-University School of Aesthetic Medicine in Milan, where she teaches both theory and practical aspects. She is a member of the Teoxane Academy Italia.
She participates as a speaker at numerous national and international congresses specialising in Aesthetic and Anti-Aging Medicine. She is Key Opinion Leader for some of the most reputable companies in the sector, for which she holds training courses for doctors.

Silvia Silenzi

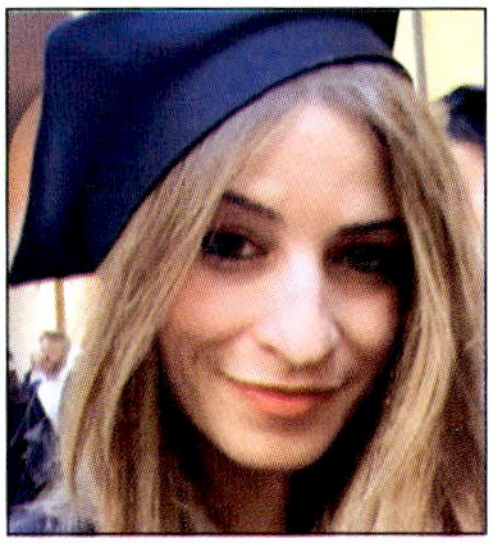

A specialised biologist, she works at the Microbiology Operating Unit of the IRCCS Azienda Ospedaliero-Universitaria-Policlinico di S. Orsola in Bologna.
Her educational background includes a Specialisation in Microbiology and Virology from the University of Turin in 2021 and a PhD in Biomedical Sciences and a MSc in Molecular and Cellular Biology from the Alma Mater Studiorum of the University of Bologna, in 2015 and 2011, respectively. Her interest in research and microbiology has led her to collaborate, since 2010, with the CRREM (Centro Regionale di Riferimento per la Microbiologia Emergenze) laboratory of the Microbiology Department of the S. Orsola Hospital in Bologna and to participate as speaker at several national and international congresses.
Since 2017, she has focused on the field of Aesthetic Medicine, working as Clinical and Regulatory Manager for a leading company in the sector and collaborating on the writing and reviewing of several scientific papers.

Raffaella Sommariva

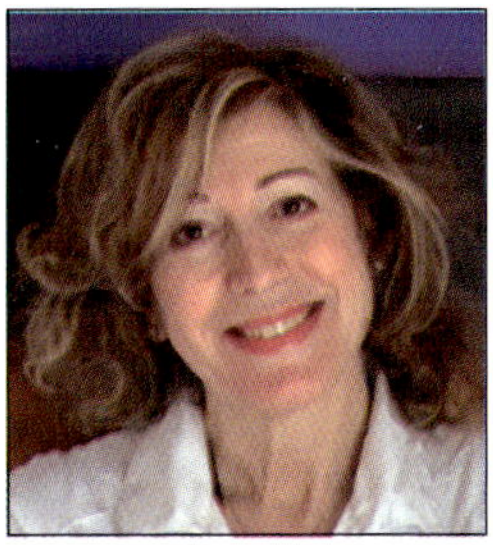

After graduating in Medicine and Surgery from the University of Genoa, she specialised in Reconstructive and Aesthetic Plastic Surgery. In 2000, she completed her training diploma at the International School of Aesthetic Medicine in Rome. From 1991 to 2010 she was a 1st level Medical Director in the Plastic Surgery Division of the "Villa Scassi" Hospital in Genoa Sampierdarena. She is a lecturer and member of the scientific committee of the Agorà Post-University School of Aesthetic Medicine in Milan, where she has held refresher courses on basic surgical techniques for aesthetic doctors and holds single-topic courses on injection techniques. She has published numerous works on Plastic Surgery in scientific journals; she collaborates with numerous publications in the field of Aesthetic Medicine and Surgery and has been present for several years as a speaker and/or moderator at medical congresses in the sector. Since 1995, she has operated as a private practitioner in Genoa and Acqui Terme.

CONTENTS

To Alessandra, Lorenzo, Sissi and my first grandchild, who will be delighted to know that Grandad was thinking about him even before he was born.

G. Sito

1

GENERAL CHARACTERISTICS OF COMPLICATIONS IN AESTHETIC MEDICINE

COMPLICATIONS AND ADVERSE EVENTS: DIFFERENCES, CLASSIFICATION AND TREATMENT

Giuseppe Sito, Silvia Silenzi

The popularity of aesthetic medical procedures has grown rapidly in recent years because they offer aesthetic rejuvenation and enhancement treatments that were previously only achievable with plastic surgery, at a lower cost and with little or no recovery time. According to data from the International Society of Aesthetic Plastic Surgery (ISAPS), more than 14 million non-surgical aesthetic procedures were performed in 2020. Botulinum toxin and hyaluronic acid fillers accounted for 43.2 and 28.1% of these respectively [1]. As public awareness and acceptance of fillers and neuromodulators has grown, so has the size of the market. As far as hyaluronic acid is concerned, there are currently around 160 fillers, produced by more than 50 companies, available worldwide [2]. Hyaluronic acid fillers are used mainly to fill wrinkles and folds, to correct loss of soft tissue due to illness or age and also to enhance the volume of the middle third and of the lips, to rejuvenate the hands and to correct facial asymmetries [2,3]. Treatment with botulinum toxin, often in conjunction with hyaluronic acid injections, is performed to diminish dynamic facial expression lines. In fact, its neuromodulatory nature is exploited to temporarily inhibit the action of the mimic muscles of the upper (forehead, glabella and periocular region) and lower (perioral region) parts of the face. There are seven types of botulinum neurotoxin (A, B, C1, D, E, F and G) all derived from highly selected and laboratory-controlled strains of the *Clostridium Botulinum* bacterium. The toxins that can be used in humans, and which are currently commercially available, are Type A and Type B, and these are produced and distributed by several companies.

The increase in the number of applications, products available and procedures performed inevitably has led to an increase in the occurrence of complications. Although the products offered on the market today are subject to strict controls and specifically enacted laws, a large number of adverse events still occur. Injectable products, such as hyaluronic acid fillers, can, due to their nature, theoretically be used in all areas of the body. However, as mentioned above, they are used mainly in aesthetic facial treatments. This happens mainly for two reasons:

- the new Medical Device Regulation (MDR) 2017/745, which came into force on 26 May 2021, obliges manufacturers, authorised representatives, importers and distributors of medical devices released onto the European Union (EU) market to indicate the intended use. This exposes the injecting practitioner to the consequences of any changes to that intended use;
- the second reason is definitely the cost. The price of a single vial, which usually contains 1 ml, does not allow use for larger regions, assuming

there is a need, for purely economic reasons. An attempt was made several years ago to market a filler with larger particles, suitable for the correction of macro areas, but it was very short lived.

In general, understanding the different characteristics, capabilities, techniques of use, risks and limitations of the various medical devices available for the performance of aesthetic medical procedures is essential in order to reduce the risk of complications, improve results, and care for patients who have suffered any adverse events. This requires a thorough knowledge of the properties and potential complications of a wide range of medical devices, including those that are not available in the practitioner's country of practice, as patients may experience adverse reactions following treatments carried out abroad. This has made it necessary for experts in aesthetic medicine to draw up guidelines on complications in order to support practitioners in recognising them and to provide clear guidance on the protocol to be adopted for their management and resolution.

Definition of complication and adverse event

The term "complication" is mostly used in pharmacology but can also be used with the same meaning in aesthetic medicine. In health science literature, the complication indicates a harmful event that manifests itself at any time during the course of treatment and which, although abstractly foreseeable, is not inevitable. An example would be the occurrence of post-traumatic thrombosis despite the adoption of adequate heparin coverage. An "adverse event", on the other hand, represents an unwanted effect secondary to a therapeutic action such as a failure to heal, the onset of disease or even death. Although the two terms may seem synonymous, it is not always easy to discern whether an adverse event was caused by individual responsibility or unavoidable fate. Consider a patient being treated with a filler to restore facial volume due to the atrophy of subcutaneous fatty tissue. The aesthetic treatment is perfectly successful when the patient is found to have contracted a dental treatment-related infection sustained by bacteria that are highly resistant to antibiotics, which could have a lethal outcome. We can therefore define an "adverse event" as an undesirable occurrence, secondary to a therapeutic action; while the term "complication" refers to a longer-lasting side effect which is hard or impossible to remedy.

Based on a statistical survey, adverse effects of medical treatment caused 142,000 deaths globally in 2013 compared to 94,000 in 1990. Every country in the world has its own system for reporting complications, from which doctors cannot escape. In Italy, for example, the reporting of a suspected adverse reaction linked to the use of a medical device for an aesthetic medical treatment can be reported in one of the following ways:

- by filling in the adverse event report form (downloadable from the website of AIFA - the Italian Medicines Agency) and sending it by e-mail

to the head of pharmacovigilance at your facility or to the Marketing Authorisation Holder (MAH) of the medicine suspected of causing the adverse reaction;
- by sending the report directly online to the AIFA website [4].

However, in addition to the necessary reporting of the complication to AIFA, it seems more appropriate than ever to have a classification that can assist the doctor in the recognition, prevention and treatment of adverse events or complications.

Classification of complications

No aesthetic procedure is exempt from risk. The extension of indications and the increase in the number of treatments performed will lead to an increase in the number and spectrum of adverse events. Some complications occur during or immediately after treatment, while others have a delayed onset. Currently, the most frequently described complications are those related to treatments with hyaluronic acid, which can be overlaid on other aesthetic medical procedures. In literature, complications are classified according to severity (mild, moderate and severe); the nature of the adverse event (ischaemic or non-ischaemic) or the time of onset (immediate, early or delayed) [2,6,7]. Adverse events are usually classified by time of onset as: immediate (within 24 hours post-treatment), early (24 hours to 4 weeks post-treatment) or delayed (more than 4 weeks post-treatment) [2,5-9]. However, it is considered more appropriate and easier to propose a classification based on the severity of the complication rather than the time of onset.

While most adverse reactions are mild and transient, more serious adverse events can occur, leaving patients with long-lasting or even permanent functional and aesthetic deficits. Mild, moderate and severe complications are divided into three classes (table 1), described below.

Class I. Mild complications, generally of immediate onset, which resolve spontaneously within 24-48 hours. Complications belonging to this class occur mainly at the site of treatment and include bruising, oedema, rash, swelling, redness, pain, bleeding and itching. These complications do not require immediate control or medical intervention.

Class II. Moderate complications, either early or delayed, include haematomas, early non-inflammatory nodules, malpositioning or dislocation of the product, hypercorrection, Tyndall effect, reactivation of a herpes infection, bacterial infection by biofilm or atypical mycobacteria, type I and IV hypersensitivity, paraesthesia and discolouration. Resolution of these complications requires monitoring by a specialist and sometimes therapeutic intervention. Adverse events belonging to this class usually clear up without consequences.

Class III. Severe complications can be either early or delayed and mainly occur in the form of single or multifocal inflammatory nodules (including granulomas), delayed inflammatory oedemas and vascular impairment which manifests itself as an immediate skin

TABLE 1 - CLASSIFICATION OF COMPLICATIONS. LIST OF COMPLICATIONS COMMONLY RECORDED IN AESTHETIC MEDICINE DIVIDED INTO THREE CLASSES ACCORDING TO THEIR DEGREE OF SEVERITY

Class I Mild complications	Class II Moderate complications	Class III Severe complications
Reactions in the injection/treatment site	Skin discolouration (Tyndall effect, hyperpigmentation, neovascularisation)	Vascular complications
Bruising Oedema Rash Redness/pain Stinging Bleeding Itching	Infections (bacterial, fungal, viral, e.g.: reactivation of herpetic infection)	Delayed inflammatory nodules (biofilms, granulomas)
	Non-antibody-mediated or non-mediated oedema (type I and IV hypersensitivity)	Infections
	Non-inflammatory nodules	

discolouration or whitening in the injection site, followed by *livedo reticularis* and the formation of pustules and blisters over the following days.

These complications always require prompt control by the specialist and appropriate therapeutic intervention. If not managed properly they can lead to long-lasting functional and aesthetic deficits and leave permanent damage such as blindness, necrosis and scarring.

Complications in aesthetic medicine: how to avoid and manage them

Based on the above classification, the following are recommendations for the prevention, diagnosis and treatment of the main aesthetic medical complications in each class.

Class I: mild complications

Bruising

Bruising is one of the most common complications of aesthetic medical procedures and one which patients do not like very much (fig. 1). Bruising is most frequently observed after dermal and subcutaneous injections using fan and retrograde techniques [10]. Bruising is less evident when the product is injected at pre-periosteal level [2].

It is possible to reduce bruising by applying cold compresses after the procedure and soothing creams containing arnica, aloe vera or vitamin K [2,11,12]. For patients who report fragile blood vessels, injection of a vial of injectable arnica twice a day for five days prior to the procedure seems to be useful. Bruising is a mild complication that

usually resolves spontaneously within a few days, but where it persists, treatment with pulsed light or potassium-titanyl-phosphate (KTP) laser is possible. The light emitted by these lasers is selectively absorbed by haemoglobin with a maximum penetration depth of 0.5 mm. This makes them suitable for treating superficial vascular lesions due to their efficiency, precision and high level of safety.
The risk of bruising can be minimised by taking precautions such as injecting the product slowly and having the patient stop taking all anticoagulant drugs (non-steroidal anti-inflammatory drugs, various vitamin/herbal supplements and anti-platelet agents) 7-10 days before treatment [2,7,8,13], after consultation with the practitioner. Although not forbidden, as long as bruising persists it is advisable to avoid exposure to the sun and strenuous exercise for the first 24 hours, so as not to increase blood pressure [7].
Therefore, with regard to bruising following aesthetic medical treatments, experts recommend preventive use of arnica creams containing vitamin K for 3-4 days before the procedure and treatment with creams containing arnica, vitamin K, lactoferrin and sunscreen [6].

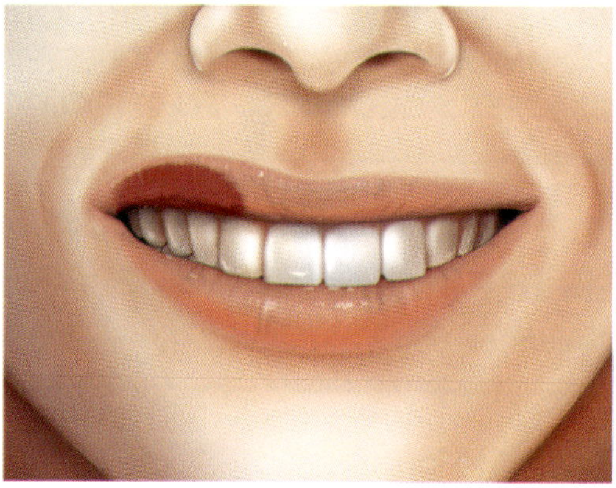

Figure 1 Patient with bruising at the level of the right upper hemilip with slight asymmetry

Oedema
Mild oedema is short-term post-traumatic oedema. Temporary swelling is a normal occurrence with certain aesthetic treatments such as injections. This type of oedema occurs immediately following the procedure and it is important not to confuse it with antibody-mediated oedema (angioedema), which is extremely rare and falls under class II complications [2,6,12]. In the case of injectable treatments, the areas commonly affected by temporary oedema are the lips and periorbital region (fig. 2). The extent of the swelling depends on the nature and the volume of the product, the injection technique and also patient factors such as dermographism. In most cases, oedema related to post-procedure trauma clears up within a week. Advice on how to avoid or treat it is the same as that given for cases of bruising [2].

Rash
A reddening of the skin immediately after treatment is normal and clears up spontaneously within a few days. However, if the rash persists, it could be a hyper-sensitivity reaction and these will be described in the section dedicated to class II complications. Although this is a mild complication, it can be a source of discomfort for the patient. The application of a topical soothing

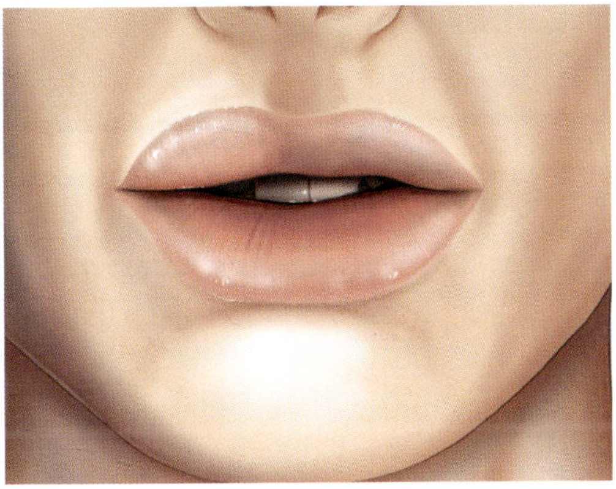

Figure 2 Patient with oedema of the lips some days after infiltration

vitamin K cream may help speed up the healing of a rash [14].

Pain

Pain is one of the most common adverse events associated with aesthetic procedures and is a major cause of concern for patients. It is usually mild and temporary, and persistent pain could be related to a moderate and/or severe complication (described below). Pain associated with an aesthetic treatment can be minimised by adopting certain precautions, including the application of local anaesthetic and ice prior to the procedure. In the case of injectable treatment, pain can be reduced by the use of a small-calibre needle or bevelled cannulae, and reducing the injection speed.

Class II: moderate complications

Infections

Bacterial infection

Any procedure that causes a break in the skin surface continuum carries a risk of infection. Acute infections are usually caused by pathogens that are commonly found on the skin such as *Staphylococcus aureus*, *Staphylococcus epidermidis* or *Streptococcus pyogenes*. These occur in the form of acute inflammation or abscesses in the area treated. Mild forms can be treated with oral antibiotics, while more severe forms require intravenous antibiotics and hospitalisation. If not treated adequately, these infections can lead to sepsis, especially in elderly or immunocompromised patients [2,6,16].

To minimise the risk of infection, it is necessary to thoroughly disinfect the treatment site with an effective topical disinfectant before the procedure. Always wear gloves and ensure that the devices used are sterile and not contaminated during treatment [13].

Although uncommon, the infections reported in aesthetic medicine usually occur following injectable treatments and are bacterial. Nevertheless, fungal or viral infections can also occur, in addition to delayed bacterial infections due to the formation of biofilms (described below).

With regard to the treatment of the main infections caused by bacteria residing on the skin, experts recommend the following antibiotic treatment:

- amoxicillin/clavulanic acid: 4 g every 24 h for 15 days;
- ciprofloxacin 500–750 mg BID for 2–4 weeks.

The complete list of antibiotics for the treatment of bacterial infections, along with their dosage, is given in table 2 (treatments recommended by experts).

TABLE 2 - LIST OF DIFFERENT ANTIBIOTIC TREATMENTS RECOMMENDED BY EXPERTS [6].

Antibiotic	Dose	Duration of treatment
Amoxicillin/clavulanic acid	4 g/24 h	For 10-15 days
Cloxacillin	3 g/24 h	For 10-15 days
	500 mg/8 h	For 30 days
Ciprofloxacin	500 mg/8 h	For 3-6 weeks
Azitromicin	500 mg/24 h	For 3 days
Minociclin	500 mg/12 h	For 30 days
Flucloxacillin	500 mg/8 h	For 7 days

Herpetic reactivation

Injection procedures can lead to the reactivation of viral herpes simplex infections. Most herpetic reactivations occur in the initial site of infection, such as the perioral area, nasal mucosa and mucosa of the hard palate [2,7,8,12].
When treating critical areas, in patients with a history of severe cold sores (more than three episodes), preventive treatment is recommended to minimise the risk of herpes reactivation. In these patients, experts recommend valacyclovir 1 g/24 h one day before treatment and 1 g/24 h for three to five days post injection [2,6]. If the patient has received no treatment but the infection is detected early, the practitioner should prescribe valacyclovir 2 g/24 h for one day. Herpetic reactivation following injectable treatment is rare but not impossible. When a blistering reaction is observed outside the critical areas of herpes simplex infection, possible vascular compromise must be considered. In patients with active herpetic lesions, injectable treatments should be delayed until their complete resolution.

Non-inflammatory nodules

Nodules represent one of the most common complications associated with soft tissue augmentation and are particularly visible in areas where the skin is thinner [2,12]. As they can result from various causes, investigation may be necessary to establish a diagnosis. As a general rule, first of all it is important to establish whether the nodule is inflammatory or non-inflammatory. This section looks at non-inflammatory nodules, as they represent a moderate complication, while inflammatory nodules will be treated as a severe complication.
Non-inflammatory nodules usually appear within a few days or weeks following the injectable treatment and tend to be painless, palpable, visible, isolated and well-defined from the surrounding tissue. Implant nodules are one of the most common adverse events following injection procedures and are the result of sub-optimal technique, overcorrection, excessively superficial placement or incorrect indication of the product (e.g. a product with

high G' used improperly for superficial corrections). Their incidence can be reduced by taking care to avoid placement too close to the surface, selecting the appropriate product for the site to be treated, massaging the area after injection to ensure even distribution and avoiding intramuscular injection [2].

Nodules that appear soon after treatment may respond to vigorous massage or be treated according to the material used as follows:

- hyaluronic acid fillers: hyaluronidase, paying attention to possible allergic reactions (preparation, dilution and doses are given in tab. 3);
- fillers other than hyaluronic acid: vigorous massage, destruction with lidocaine or saline solution, extrusion of the material via aspiration with a high calibre needle (e.g. 21 G or higher) or by incision.

However, nodules may also have a delayed onset or be persistent; in these cases, treatment as follows is recommended:

- with intralesional steroids, in small amounts to avoid skin atrophy;
- injection (a series of three or more injections with 0.1-0.5 ml per nodule depending on location) with:
  - 5-fluorouracil (5-FU), 0.5 ml [50 mg/ml];
  - 0.3 ml each of triamcinolone and lidocaine (or 40 mg/ml depending on localisation and degree of inflammation) [10 mg/ml] and 0.2 ml of 2% lidocaine with adrenaline;
  - 0.5 ml [50 mg/ml] of 5-FU and lidocaine and 0.2 ml of 2% lidocaine with adrenaline;
- fractional lasers, used after reabsorption of the material in the eyelids and lips [31,32];
- excision of the implanted material as a last resort. Chronic, intractable nodules that persist for months despite discontinuation and become increasingly fibrotic are most probably foreign body granulomas and require excision.

Skin discolouration

Rash

A rash is classed as a moderate compli-

TABLE 3 - PREPARATION, DILUTION AND DOSES OF HYALURONIDASE RECOMMENDED BY EXPERTS FOR THE RESOLUTION OF COMPLICATIONS CAUSED BY HYALURONIC ACID FILLERS [3]

Dilution	Dose
150 IU/ml (saline solution)	150 UI/ml
1 x 104 μg in 3 ml (saline solution)	0.3-0.5 ml per injection point
1 x 103 UI in 2- 4 ml (saline solution)	50-200 UI into nodules
1.5 x 103 UI in 10 ml (saline solution)	500-1000 UI in patients at risk of necrosis
	100-200 UI 3-4 mm deep*

*This strategy refers to the injection of hyaluronidase in the entire area around the point of vascular occlusion in order to favour its intravascular penetration and facilitate the removal of the hyaluronic acid that is obstructing the vessel.

cation if it does not clear up spontaneously within a few days of the aesthetic treatment. A persistent change in colour of the skin or mucous membranes could indicate an erythema due to a hypersensitivity reaction. In this case the same treatments as those used for rosacea, including oral tetracycline or isotretinoin, may be effective [2]. The use of a medium strength topical steroid is recommended for a persistent rash, although long-term use of high potency steroids should be avoided as they can cause atrophy and telangiectasias. Application of vitamin K cream as seen in the case of a mild rash can also help accelerate the clearing up of a moderate rash [14].

Hyperpigmentation

Hyperpigmentation is a possible complication following dermal filler injection procedures. This complication occurs especially in subjects with skin types IV-VI on the Fitzpatrick scale, although it has also been observed in other skin types [17,18]. Hyperpigmentation should be treated initially with topical bleaching agents such as hydroquinone (2-8%) and Restin-a (tretinoin) combined with daily application of broad-spectrum sunscreen. In cases of persistent post-inflammatory hyperpigmentation, chemical peelings can also be used. If treatment is unsuccessful, treatments with IPL (Intense Pulsed Light), a pulsed dye-laser or fractional laser can be carried out [2,6]. The Q-switched low-fluence Nd:YAG 1,064 nm laser is also effective in the treatment of hyperpigmentation. Current lasers are of limited use in the treatment of Fitzpatrick skin types IV-VI but the long wavelength Nd:YAG laser allows the treatment of darker skin without interrupting the natural skin colour, while IPL systems can be used in the treatment of Fitzpatrick skin types I-IV.
Limiting the number of skin punctures during the injection process, using the retrograde linear or fan technique as well as pre-periosteal injection, can reduce post-injection rash and thereby prevent post-inflammatory hyperpigmentation [2].

Tyndall effect

The Tyndall effect or "Raleigh scattering" describes the optical phenomenon that causes a bluish skin tone following superficial implantation of hyaluronic acid fillers. It has been shown that, if left untreated, superficially injected material can last a long time, even years [12]. Injection of the filler with the right technique at the right depth is recommended to minimise the risk of this adverse event. To correct this blemish, hyaluronic acid should be dissolved with a hyaluronidase-based treatment (for dilution and doses see table 3). In more difficult cases the Tyndall effect can be treated by removing the superficial filler by piercing the skin with a small-calibre needle or surgical scalpel. This therapeutic strategy can be applied immediately and more than 12 months after the aesthetic treatment [19].

Neovascularisation

New capillaries, arterioles and venules may appear in the area treated due to tissue trauma caused, for example, by the expansion and/or excessive sculpting of a filler. These tiny new blood vessels can appear days or weeks after treatment and should disappear within 3-12 months without further treatment. However, in the case of telangiectasias, the use of certain lasers has proven effective: KTP at 532 nm, copper vapour diode at 532 nm, pulsed dye-laser at 585 nm and intense pulsed light (IPL). Of course, the choice of laser depends on the size of the vessel and the area to be treated [2,6]. Further laser treatments have been described in the section on bruising.

Oedema

Antibody-mediated oedema (angioedema - type I hypersensitivity)

Prolonged oedema can be caused by a hypersensitivity reaction due to the presence of foreign bodies, such as threads and fillers, mediated by the immune response of immunoglobulin E (IgE) and referred to as type I hypersensitivity. While rare, angioedema occurs within hours of treatment and may last for several weeks [2,15]. This type of reaction can occur after both initial and repeated exposure to the non-self material. IgE, attached to the surface of mast cells, binds the antigen and stimulates its degranulation, resulting in the release of proteases, heparin, histamine, cytokines, prostaglandins, leukotrienes and platelet-activating factor. These mediators cause the symptoms of a classic allergic reaction, including oedema, rash, pain and itching. Angioedema typically has an early onset, within hours of exposure to the antigen, but more severe episodes lasting more than six weeks, with localised or generalised oedema, may also occur [2,6,15]. In some cases, an acute idiopathic allergic response in which it is impossible to identify the allergen that triggered the reaction may also occur [2].

The treatment of angioedema, be it of known cause or idiopathic, depends on its severity. Some cases are hard to treat and can have a variable response to drugs. In general, the therapeutic approach to angioedema should be gradual, moving to the next stage if an adequate response to treatment has not been obtained. If there is no spontaneous healing, even after treatment with cold compresses and anti-inflammatory enzymes (bromelain), oral antihistamines are recommended. However, in cases of persistent oedema or oedema that fails to respond to antihistamines, experts recommend the prescription of prednisone by mouth.

The first line of treatment recommended for the resolution of angioedema is as follows:

- anti-inflammatory enzymes (Bromelain: 300 mg/day, divided into 3 doses);
- arnica/gelsemium (4-5 tablets/24h for 3-4 days);
- cold compresses (about 5 minutes) [6].

If the oedema persists, experts recommend moving on to the second line of treatment with:

- streptokinase/streptodornase (10,000/2,500 U: 2 tablets/8h for 3-6 days);
- non-steroidal anti-inflammatory drugs (NSAIDs):

- Cox 1: ibuprofen 400-600 mg/8h;
- Cox 2: colecoxib 200-400 mg/24h.

Before prescribing NSAIDs, it is important to consider the following recommendations: use the lowest dosage and for the shortest possible time; choose the NSAID according to the drug profile and the patient's risk factors; use gastroprotective agents to minimise the gastrointestinal damage associated with the use of these drugs [6].

In cases of persistent oedema or oedema that fails to respond to antihistamines, experts recommend the prescription of the following therapy:

• prednisone (1 mg/kg/day) + pantoprazole (40 mg) for about 3 days depending on clinical progression;
• deflazacort (1- 1.5 mg/kg/day) + pantoprazole (40 mg) for about 3 days depending on clinical progression [2,6,20].

As mentioned above, angioedema usually occurs within a few hours of exposure to the foreign body and generalised oedema may be indicative of anaphylaxis; consequently the patient's vital signs should be monitored. However, more severe reactions lasting several weeks may occur [6,15]. In these cases, the patient should be carefully monitored to ensure that the oedema does not have an infectious aetiology. Rapidly progressing angioedema should be treated as a medical emergency, as there may be a risk of airway obstruction [2,7,8].

Non-antibody-mediated oedema (delayed - type IV hypersensitivity)

Delayed or type IV, non-antibody-mediated oedema is mediated by T lymphocytes rather than antibodies. These reactions are characterised by hardening, rash and oedema of the area treated and generally occur one day after treatment but may develop for up to several weeks and persist for many months [2,6,21,22]. Delayed hypersensitivity reactions may not respond to antihistamines and in these cases the best approach is to eliminate the allergen. Hyaluronidase is used in patients treated with hyaluronic acid, while for other fillers a short course of treatment with steroids until the filler is resorbed, laser treatment and/or extrusion is recommended [6,23]. Excision represents a last resort.

Class III: severe complications

Inflammatory nodules

Inflammatory nodules often have a delayed onset (from 4 weeks to 1 year and more) and are mostly caused by foreign body and/or infection-related immune responses, including the formation of biofilms [6,24,25].

Biofilm

Biofilms are common in nature and consist of aggregations of bacteria that form thin films that adhere to substrates. These surfaces can consist of organic material (e.g. animal tissue) or abiotic material (e.g. plastic, glass, etc.). When a material is placed in the skin or subcutaneous tissue, as is the case with fillers, threads and other products used in aesthetic medicine, it can be colonised by bacteria and form a biofilm. This is made up of an extracellular polymeric matrix secreted by bacteria that protects them from environmental stress and allows them to irreversibly adhere to a substrate, resulting in chronic antibiotic-resistant infection [16,26]. Many bacterial species form biofilms and become increasingly drug resistant as they progress. Biofilms caused by injection procedures can cause a local, systemic infection or a granulomatous or inflammatory response. However, it is hard to distinguish inflammation caused by the formation of a biofilm rather than a low-grade hypersensitivity reaction. If reddening and hardening of the area treated are observed at any time after treatment and regardless of duration, the formation of a biofilm should be suspected [24,27]. In some cases, it has been observed that biofilm was the cause of persistent inflammatory complications in patients treated with permanent fillers who did not respond to any therapy despite having a negative biopsy for bacteria [28]. As culture tests are sometimes negative, it is important to use molecular techniques such as polymerase chain reaction (PCR) or fluorescent in situ hybridisation (FISH) tests to confirm the infectious aetiology in cases of delayed-onset nodules where biofilm formation is suspected [24].

These infections are hard to treat, with treatment entailing removal of the implant, which is not always possible. Before excision of the nodule, even if the results of the culture examination are negative, empirical broad-spectrum antibiotic therapy with clarithromycin 500 mg plus moxifloxacin 400 mg twice daily for 10 days, or ciprofloxacin 500-750 mg twice daily for 2-4 weeks is recommended [6,12]. If there is a strong suspicion of biofilm, intralesional steroids should not be used before antibiotic therapy as these may aggravate the complication. If the nodule persists then it must be removed. In the case of hyaluronic acid fillers, hyaluronidase can be used. However, caution is required even in this case because, according to the IFU, hyaluronidase should not be used in the presence of an active infection (cellulitis) as it could facilitate the spread to adjacent tissues [29]. Another strategy for treating biofilm, if steroids have already been used, includes injection with 5-fluorouracil (5-FU) up to 50 mg/ml (0.5 cc), alone or in combination with steroids, repeated regularly every 2-4 weeks until the problem is solved. Though the reason for the therapeutic success of 5-FU remains unknown, it has been suggested that it interacts with AriR, a regulatory gene that inhibits the formation of biofilms [30].

Further treatment can be carried out with injections of platelet-rich plasma into the biofilm-infected area. There is evidence in literature to support that the injection of platelet-rich plasma into biofilm-infected areas has an antimicrobial effect, promotes the breakdown of hyaluronic acid in the inflamed tissue and destroys the biofilm [31-33]. If the hardness persists despite the various treatments mentioned above, a further option to consider is laser lysis, incision and washing of the cavity with antibiotics. Exposing the inflammatory nodule to the immune system always has advantages. Laser technology has been reported to have beneficial effects in treating infectious filler complications. The intralesional subcutaneous introduction of an optical microfibre laser and the subsequent production of heat causes a reduction in the bacterial burden at biofilm level and, at the same time, the liquefaction of filler microparticles. Radiofrequency heating has been used in the same way. These minimally invasive techniques could be an intermediate step before attempting surgical removal of an inflamed area. Surgical removal should be used as a last resort, dictated by failure to respond to antibiotics. If the nodule persists and becomes increasingly fibrotic, the differential diagnosis is foreign body granuloma.

The incidence of biofilms following aesthetic treatments is unknown and diagnosis is difficult. However, it is important to take precautions to prevent infection when performing aesthetic medical treatments with implants (e.g. fillers, threads). Strategies to reduce the risk of biofilm development include cleaning the face thoroughly before injection, avoiding injection through the oral or nasal mucosa and permanent hydrophilic materials, and not injecting over a previous implant or into traumatised tissue [2].

Foreign body granuloma

Although foreign body granuloma can occur with all implantable materials, it is a rare occurrence. With injectable fillers, the incidence is estimated to be between 0.01 and 1.0% and usually occurs after a period of latency, which can vary from several months to years after injection [34-37]. Clinically, foreign body granulomas appear as red papules, nodules or patches with or without ulceration and, over time, the lesions become more solid due to fibrosis.

These granulomas consist of cell aggregates of the immune system (macrophages and T lymphocytes) activated in response to the presence of non-self material. The nodule consists of a peculiar concentric structure made up, from the centre to the edge, of a necrotic centre that encloses the material responsible for the immune response by isolating it from the body, cells of the immune system, macrophage cells (epithelioid histiocytes) and giant multinucleated cells with a lymphocytic corona, with a fibrous halo and plasma cells on the outside. The presence of these cells is characteristic of inflammatory nodules and confirmation of a granulomatous reaction can be achieved through histological examination if a biopsy can be taken.

Various factors could influence the development of a foreign body granuloma, including the properties of the material, the volume injected or intramuscular injection in the case of a filler. In addition, certain patient characteristics could also favour the formation of granulomas, such as previous infections, allergic reactions or trauma. In injectable products, it would seem that the shape of the microspheres is an important factor in the occurrence or otherwise of granulomas: granulomatous reactions occur less frequently after implantation of a product with smooth microspheres. Particles with an irregular surface can induce more serious granulomatous reactions [38]. Furthermore, in literature granulomatous foreign body reactions have also been described after dermal filler injections in two patients with hepatitis C, treated with interferon, and in a patient with severe persistent allergic asthma, treated with omalizumab, a monoclonal antibody drug that targets circulating IgE [39].

The mechanism behind delayed inflammation or granuloma formation is still unknown and diagnosis is made difficult as practitioners sometimes have to deal with patients with an unknown or incomplete medical aesthetic treatment history.

Once infection has been ruled out as the cause of nodule formation, the initial treatment of granulomas is with steroids (triamcinolone, betamethasone or prednisone), either intralesional or by mouth. In patients with lesions that do not respond to steroids alone, 5-FU is added to corticosteroids. Besides curbing fibroblast activity, this combined treatment has the advantage of reducing the amount of steroids injected with the associated risk of adverse events such as tissue atrophy and telangiectasia [40].

Granulomas caused by hyaluronic acid fillers can be treated with hyaluronidase (150 U/ml). For more difficult cases, in which treatment has failed repeatedly, the treatment of choice for the resolution of foreign body granuloma is surgical excision [34].

Vascular complications

Vascular complications usually occur following an injectable treatment in which accidental intravascular injection causes embolisation with blockage of blood flow. It has been proven that external compression of a vessel by a filler alone cannot cause an ischaemic event [41]. Vascular compromise is a severe complication with a usually immediate onset, which can lead to severe consequences such as necrosis of the tissue supplied by the occluded vessel (fig. 3). Cases of severe loss of vision and hemiplegia following autologous fat injection for ocular and cerebral embolism have been reported in literature [42-45]. An acute fatal stroke after autologous fat injection into the glabellar area has also been reported [46]. It is possible that these adverse events can result from migration of fragments of fatty tissue to the ocular and cerebral arteries via reverse flow, causing an embolism. In the case of treatments with fillers, an intravascular injection can cause both anterograde and retrograde tissue necrosis. The product is carried through the vascular system and can cause local or distal necrosis of the irrigated tissues with disastrous consequences.

The cases of vascular complications described in literature are increasingly frequent and it is believed that the incidence of these adverse events is underestimated [9]. A global survey conducted among 52 experienced injectors reported that 62% of them had recorded one intravascular injection or more [47]. Vascular complications can occur after injection of any filler and the areas with the highest risk are those where the blood supply is dependent on a single arterial branch

(axial pattern blood supply) such as the nasolabial folds, glabellar folds, nose and lips.
Recognition of the signs of a vascular event and prompt and aggressive treatment are necessary to avoid serious, potentially irreversible complications [48-53]. The two primary diagnostic symptoms of vascular occlusion are abnormal pain during injection and rapid whitening in the vascular area (depending on the injection site), followed by *livedo reticularis* (fig. 4) and blistering over the following days. When these signs occur, with suspicion of vascular occlusion, it is necessary to stop the injection and intervene immediately. The treatment recommended by experts aims to promote blood flow. In the case of vascular occlusion caused by hyaluronic acid fillers, experts recommend the following [8,12,54]:

- application of a hot gauze, patting to promote vasodilation and massaging the area;
- use of a nitroglycerin-based topical paste (1 or 2%) 2 or 3 times a day. Sublingual nitroglycerine tablets can also be used;
- injection of high doses (200-400 IU/ 1-2 ml) of hyaluronidase, covering the entire ischaemic area and not just the original treatment site (tab. 3).

Although it has not been absolutely proven, it seems that acetylsalicylic acid (500 mg/8 h, 24-48 h) could be useful in the treatment of vascular impairment.
If there is no sign of improvement, the procedure should be repeated every hour until clinical resolution is achieved

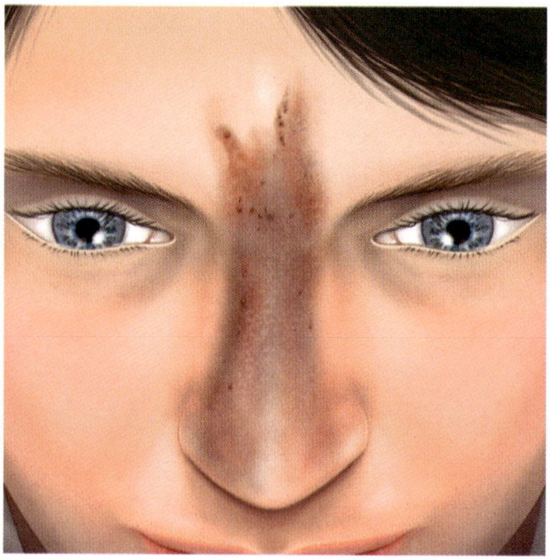

Figure 3 Patient with a large necrotic area following vascular complication from filler injection

[8]. Doses of up to 1,500 U may be required to achieve reversal of vascular impairment [8,12,54].
The risk of vascular compromise can be reduced by applying various strategies such as injecting the product slowly, in small volumes and at the right depth, paying particular attention to areas of risk. A thorough knowledge of facial anatomy on the part of all injectors is essential to avoid this type of complication.

Bibliography

1. International Society of Aesthetic Plastic Surgery (ISAPS). 2020 Global statistic. ISAPS Global Survey Results 2020. Available from: https://www.isaps.org/medical-professionals/isaps-global-statistics. Data consulted on 10 October 2022.
2. Funt D, Pavicic T. Dermal fillers in aesthetics: an overview of adverse events and treatment approach-

es. Plast Surg Nurs. 2015 Jan-Mar;35(1):13-32.
3. Rzany B et al. Expert guideline on the use of porcine collagen in aesthetic medicine. J Dtsch Dermatol Ges. 2010;8(3): 210–217.
4. Form for reporting adverse reactions. Available from: https://www.aifa.gov.it/moduli-segnalazione-reazioni-avverse.
5. Wagner RD et al. Etiology, Prevention, and Management of Infectious Complications of Dermal Fillers. Semin Plast Surg. 2016;30(2): 83-86.
6. Urdiales-Gálvez F, Delgado NE, et al. Treatment of Soft Tissue Filler Complications: Expert Consensus Recommendations. Aesthetic Plast Surg. 2018 Apr;42(2):498-510.
7. De Boulle K, Heydenrych I. Patient factors influencing dermal filler complications: prevention, assessment, and treatment. Clin Cosmet Investig Dermatol 2015;8:205-14.
8. Signorini M, Liew S, Sundaram H, et al., Global Aesthetics Consensus: Avoidance and Management of Complications from Hyaluronic Acid Fillers-Evidence and Opinion-Based Review and Consensus Recommendations. Plast Reconstr Surg 2016;137:961e–71e.
9. Trocchi G et al. Consensus report sulla classificazione, prevenzione, diagnosi e trattamento delle complicanze gravi da filler di acido ialuronico. Esperienze Dermatologiche 2019 Giugno;21(Suppl. 1 n. 2):1-8.
10. Gladstone HB, Cohen JL. Adverse effects when injecting facial fillers. Semin Cutan Med Surg. 2007;26(1):34–39.
11. Shah NS, Lazarus MC, Bugdodel R et al (2002). The effects of topical vitamin K on bruising after laser treatment. J Am Acad Dermatol 47(2):241–244.
12. Fitzgerald R, Bertucci V, Sykes JM, Duplechain JK (2016) Adverse reactions to injectable fillers. Facial Plast Surg 32(5):532–555.
13. Bailey SH, Cohen JL, Kenkel JM.

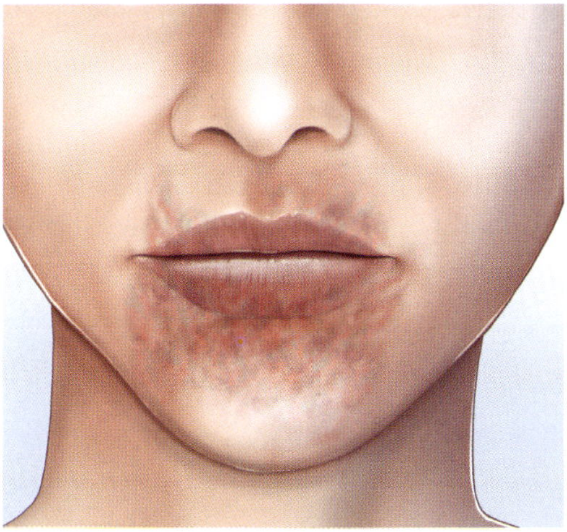

Figure 4 Patient with *livedo reticularis*, which is a prelude to an ischaemic event

VIDEO 1.1

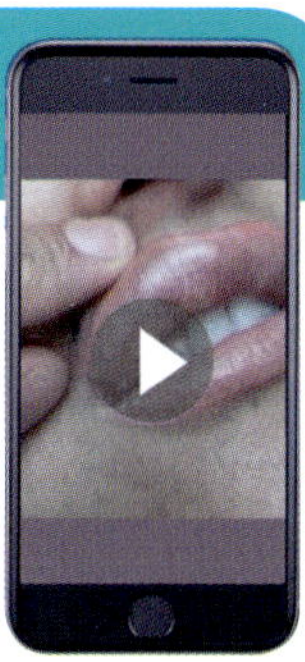

Ischemia of the right upper hemilip. Courtesy of Dr. Sergio Marlino

Etiology, prevention, and treatment of dermal filler complications. Aesthet Surg J. 2011;31(1):110–121.
14. Cohen JL, Bhatia AC (2009) The role of topical vitamin K oxide gel in the resolution of postprocedural purpura. J Drugs Dermatol 8(11):1020–1024.
15. Van Dyke S, et al. Severe Acute Local Reactions to a Hyaluronic Acid-derived Dermal Filler. J Clin Aesthet Dermatol. 2010;3(5):32–35.
16. Christensen LH (2009) Host tissue interaction, fate, and risks of degradable and non-degradable gel fillers. Dermatol Surg 35:1612–1619.
17. Taylor SC, Burgess CM, Callender VD (2009) Safety of nonanimal stabilized hyaluronic acid dermal fillers in patients with skin of color: a randomized, evaluator-blinded comparative trial. Dermatol Surg 35(Suppl 2):1653–1660.
18. Heath CR, Taylor SC (2011) Fillers in the skin of color population. J Drugs Dermatol 10(5):494–498.
19. Douse-Dean T, Jacob CI (2008) Fast and easy treatment for reduction of the Tyndall effect secondary to cosmetic use of hyaluronic acid. J Drugs Dermatol 7(3):281–283.
20. Snozzi P, van Loghem JAJ. Complication Management following Rejuvenation Procedures with Hyaluronic Acid Fillers an Algorithm based Approach. Plast Reconstr Surg Glob Open. 2018 Dec 17;6(12): e2061.
21. Arron ST, Neuhaus IM (2007) Persistent delayed type hypersensitivity reaction to injectable non-animal-stabilized hyaluronic acid. J Cosmet Dermatol 6(3):167–171.
22. Geisler D, Shumer S, Elson ML. Delayed hypersensitivity reaction to Restylane®. Cosmetic Dermatol. 2007;20(12):784–786.
23. Cassuto D, Marangoni O, De Santis G, Christensen L (2009) Advanced laser techniques for filler-induced complications. Dermatol Surg 35(Suppl 2):1689–1695.
24. Dayan SH, Arkins JP, Brindise R (2011) Soft tissue fillers and biofilm. Facial Plast Surg 27:23–28.
25. Ledon JA et al. (2013) Inflammatory nodules following soft tissue filler use: a review of causative agents, pathology and treatment options. Am J Clin Dermatol 14:401–411.
26. Monheit GD, Rohrich RJ. The nature of long-term fillers and the risk of complications. Dermatol Surg. 2009;35 Suppl 2:1598–1604.
27. Narins RS, Coleman WP, Glogau RG. Recommendations and treatment options for nodules and other filler complications. Dermatol Surg. 2009;35 Suppl 2:1667-1671.
28. Bjarnsholt T et al. (2009) Detection of bacteria by fluorescence in situ hybridization in culture-negative soft tissue filler lesions. Dermatol Surg 35(Suppl 2):1620–1624.
29. Rzany B, DeLorenzi C (2015) Understanding, avoiding, and managing severe filler complications. Plast Reconstr Surg 136(5 Suppl):196S–203S.
30. Attila C, Ueda A, Wood TK (2009) 5-Fluorouracil reduces biofilm formation in Escherichia coli K-12 through global regulator AriR as an antivirulence compound. Appl Mi-

crobiol Biotechnol 82(3):525–533.
31. Tohidnezhad M et al (2012) Platelets display potent antimicrobial activity and release human beta-defensin 2. Platelets 23(3):217–223
32. Albeiroti S et al. (2015) Platelet hyaluronidase-2: an enzyme that translocates to the surface upon activation to function in extracellular matrix degradation. Blood 125(9):1460–1469.
33. Różalski MI et al. Antimicrobial/anti-biofilm activity of expired blood platelets and their released products. Postepy Hig Med Dosw (Online). 2013;67:321-325.
34. Lemperle G et al. Foreign body granulomas after all injectable dermal fillers: part 1. Possible causes. Plast Reconstr Surg. 2009;123(6):1842–1863.
35. Lemperle G, Gauthier-Hazan N. Foreign body granulomas after all injectable dermal fillers: part 2. Treatment options. Plast Reconstr Surg. 2009;123(6):1864–1873.
36. Alijotas-Reig J et al. Delayed immune-mediated adverse effects of polyalkylimide dermal fillers: clinical findings and long-term follow-up. Arch Dermatol. 2008;144(5):637–642.
37. Chrastil-LaTowsky B et al. Delayed inflammatory reaction to bioalcamid polyacrylamide gel used for soft-tissue augmentation. Arch Dermatol. 2009;145(11): 1309–1312.
38. Sachdev M et al. Facial granulomas secondary to injection of semi-permanent cosmetic dermal filler containing acrylic hydrogel particles. J Cutan Aesthet Surg. 2010; 3(3):162–166.
39. Dammak A et al. Granulomatous foreign-body reaction with facial dermal fillers after omalizumab treatment for severe persistent allergic asthma: a case report. Br J Dermatol. 2012;166(6):1375–1376.
40. Wiest LG et al. Electron microscopic documentation of late changes in permanent fillers and clinical management of granulomas in affected patients. Dermatol Surg. 2009;35 Suppl 2:1681–1688.
41. De Lorenzi C. Complications of Injectable Fillers, Part 2: Vascular Complications.Aesthet Surg J 2014;34:584–600.
42. Feinendegen DL et al. Autologous fat injection for soft tissue augmentation in the face: a safe procedure? Aesthetic Plast Surg. 1998;22(3):163–167.
43. Egido JA et al. Middle cerebral artery embolism and unilateral visual loss after autologous fat injection into the glabellar area. Stroke. 1993;24(4):615–616.
44. Lee DH et al. Sudden unilateral visual loss and brain infarction after autologous fat injection into nasolabial groove. Br J Ophthalmol. 1996;80(11):1026–1027.
45. Thaunat O et al. Cerebral fat embolism induced by facial fat injection. Plast Reconstr Surg. 2004;113(7): 2235–2236.
46. Yoon SS et al. Acute fatal stroke immediately following autologous fat injection into the face. Neurology. 2003;61(8): 1151–1152.
47. Sclafani AP, Fagien S (2009) Treatment of injectable soft tissue fill-

er complications. Dermatol Surg 35:1672–1680.
48. Kwon SG et al. Ischemic oculomotor nerve palsy and skin necrosis caused by vascular embolization after hyaluronic Acid filler injection: a case report. Ann Plast Surg. 2013;71(4):333–334.
49. Peter S, Mennel S. Retinal branch artery occlusion following injection of hyaluronic acid (Restylane). Clin Experiment Ophthalmol. 2006; 34(4):363–364.
50. Kim YJ et al. Ocular ischemia with hypotony after injection of hyaluronic acid gel. Ophthal Plast Reconstr Surg. 2011;27(6): e152–e155.
51. Grunebaum LD et al. The risk of alar necrosis associated with dermal filler injection. Dermatol Surg. 2009;35 Suppl 2:1635–1640.
52. Schanz S et al. Arterial embolization caused by injection of hyaluronic acid (Restylane). Br J Dermatol. 2002;146(5):928–929.
53. Coleman SR. Avoidance of arterial occlusion from injection of soft tissue fillers. Aesthet Surg J. 2002;22(6):555–557.
54. Cohen JL et al (2015) Treatment of hyaluronic acid filler induced impending necrosis with hyaluronidase: consensus recommendations. Aesthet Surg J 35(7):844–849.

NODULES AS A COMPLICATION IN AESTHETIC MEDICINE

Giuseppe Maria Izzo

Throughout our extensive experience as aesthetic practitioners, we have repeatedly noticed the formation of post-treatment nodules. Over these pages we will try to take stock of the possible causes and how we can intervene to address this complication. First of all, let us define what a nodule is: it is a cutaneous protuberance with solid content in a dermo-epidermal site of varying aetiology (table 1).

Filler nodules

Regardless of this classification, we are interested in nodules that may arise as a result of medical-aesthetic treatments, particularly those resulting from filler implantation.

An important distinction must be made between nodules from permanent fillers and those from resorbable fillers, as our corrective strategy will be completely different.

Nodules from permanent fillers (fig. 1) can occur either due to injection of an excessive amount of silicone or methacrylate or due to the excessive superficiality of the implant. Fortunately, this is happening less frequently nowadays due to the very rare use of these materials. There is, however, a very serious problem: permanent fillers can migrate and can also surface, giving rise to fistulous pathways with residual permanent scarring; they can also become the site of bacterial colonies, especially those once referred to as "water endoprostheses", a particular methacrylate preparation that quite often represented a veritable breeding ground for bacterial colonies.

Nodule removal techniques

But what can the aesthetic practitioner do to remedy this blemish? We have heard of all kinds of things in the past, from cortico-antibiotic infiltrations to high-energy radiofrequency to dissolve the granuloma capsule. We believe that two routes can be taken these days, both of which must be reserved for very experienced hands: surgical removal of the granuloma, while leaving as little aesthetic damage as possible, or the use of a 1,500 nm laser.

The laser light channelled into the nodule or granuloma through an microfibre optic acts on three levels. First, it warms the area, dissolving the filler. All permanent fillers, being sensitive to heat due to the thermal effect, go from a solid to a liquid state. The dissolved substance comes out of the micro-hole used to introduce the fibre optic. Secondly, the

TABLE 1 - NODULE AETIOLOGY

Nodule from infection	Pyoderma
Nodule from complication of dermatosis	Nodular acne (fig. 2)
Foreign body nodule	Filler or insect bite (fig. 3)
Neoplasm nodule	Epithelioma (fig. 4)

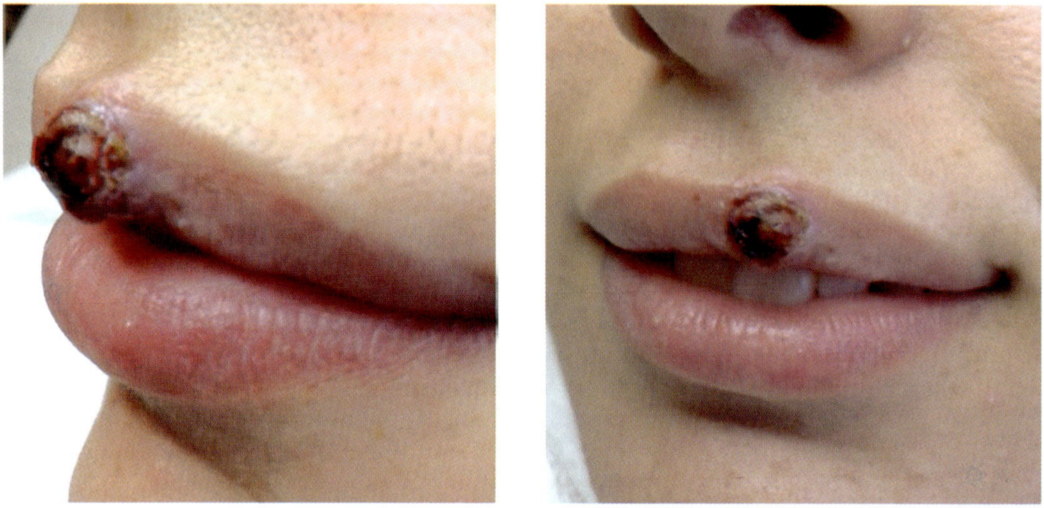

Figure 1 Nodule from permanent fillers

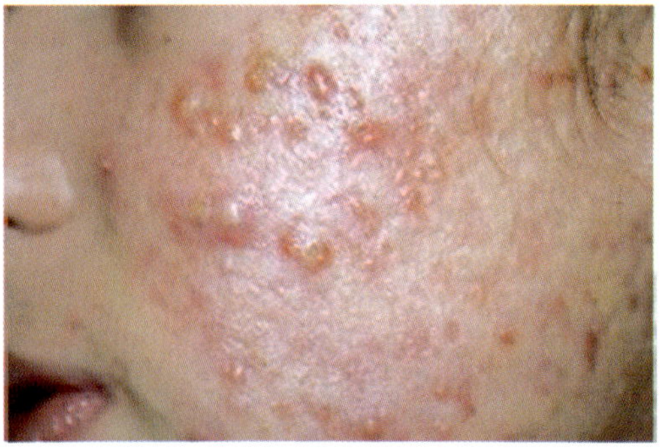

Figure 2 Nodulocystic acne

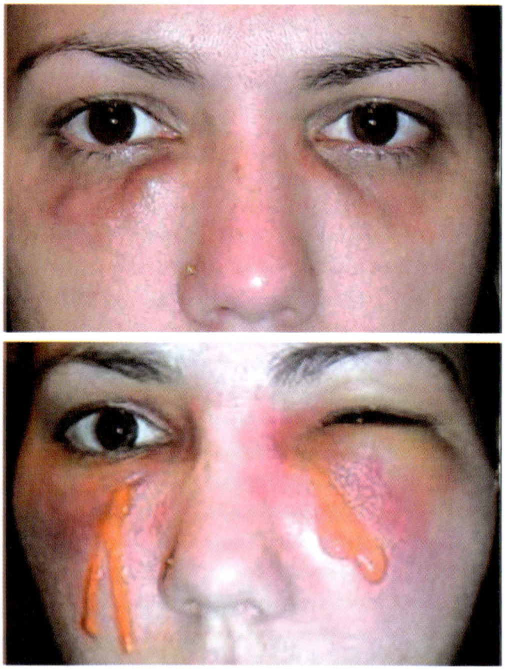

Figure 3 Filler

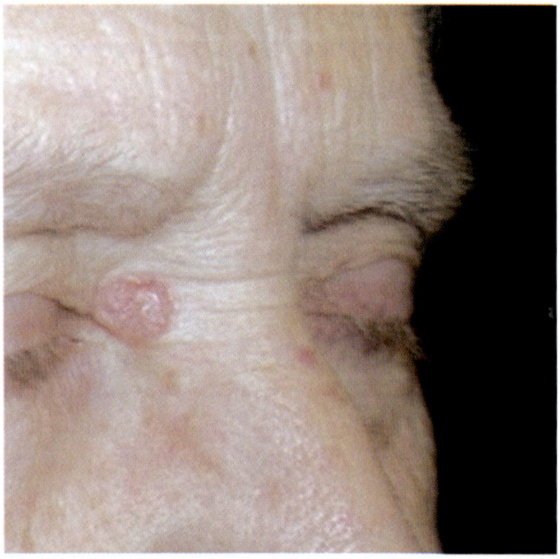

Figure 4 Basocellular epithelioma

increase in temperature caused by the laser coagulates the inflammatory tissue that always arises around the granuloma. Sterile pus is formed, and this too flows out of the small holes.
It is assumed that the laser acts on the so-called biofilm, a phenomenon that has yet to be proven but is increasingly accepted among experts in the field. The term biofilm refers to a mucopolysaccharide membrane created by bacteria, which surrounds and protects them: the immune system is ineffective against it and unable to destroy it. As a result, the inflammation no longer goes away and becomes chronic. This would explain why drugs are only temporarily successful: once their effect has worn off, the reaction flares up again. The presence of bacteria would explain the very high relapse rate after treatment with cortisone and other immunosuppressive agents.
There is another explanation for the lack of success in the case of surgery: the surgeon scatters the biofilm bacteria throughout the area when using the scalpel. Before long, they are reactivated, causing the inflammatory phenomenon to spread. The increase in temperature caused by the laser, on the other hand, kills the bacteria, permanently curing the inflammation.
For resorbable fillers, the matter is totally different. In this case, nodules can form due to:

- the implant being too close to the surface;
- an excessively large implant;
- sensitisation to the material

implanted.
In the first two cases, one or two treatments with hyaluronidase are sufficient, taking care not to damage the structure of the skin because the substance acts on any hyaluronic acid, including that of an endogenous nature.
This aside, it should be well emphasised that modern fillers should be injected into suitable areas of the skin and nowhere else, as in the case presented in figure 5.

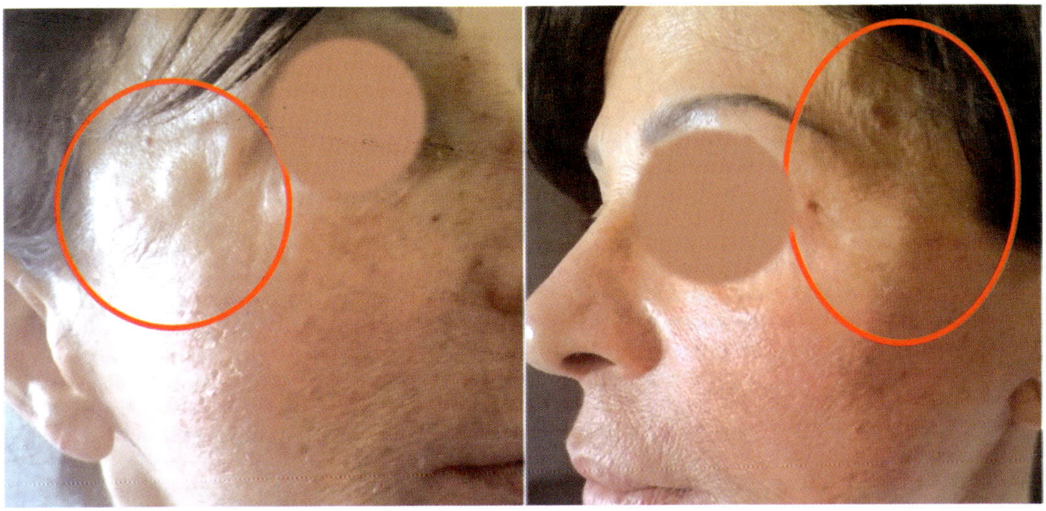

Figure 5 Macromolecular hyaluronic acid. Courtesy of Dr. Paola Tarantino

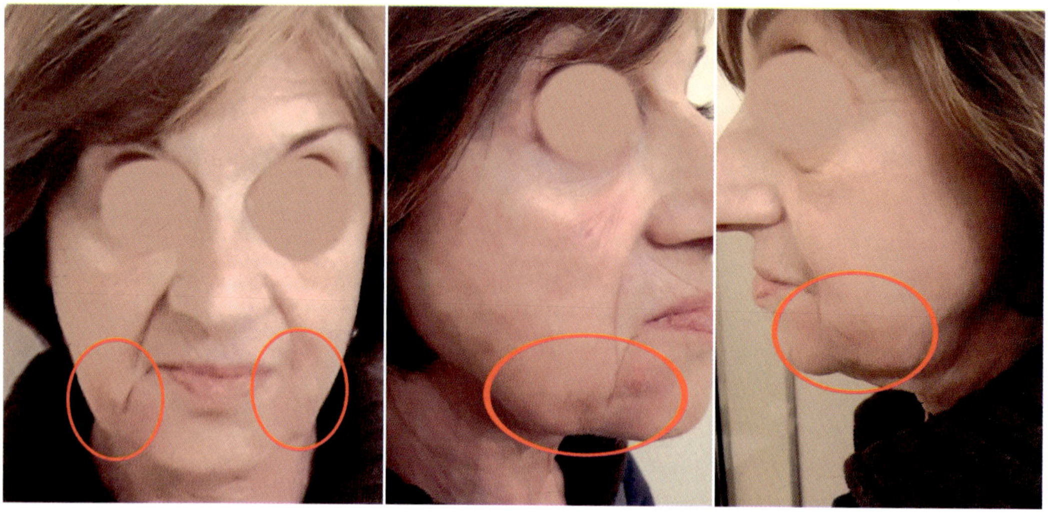

Figure 6 Hypersensitivity to hyaluronic acid filler. Courtesy of Dr. Paola Tarantino

As far as sensitisation to the molecule injected is concerned, the problem is more complex. Hyaluronidase may not be sufficient and general cortico-antibiotic therapy may be required, accompanied by infiltrations of the same substances, and even the possible mechanical extrusion of the material injected (fig. 6).

Conclusions

As we have seen, any filler can result in the occurrence of nodular lesions; obviously, the treatment of nodules from permanent fillers is very complex, whereas with modern fillers it is easier to achieve the complete elimination of the complication, except in the case of patient hypersensitivity to the molecule injected.

Bibliography

1. Correa-Selm LM, Rogachefsky A, Lee K. Management of Nodules Post-Filler Injection. Dermatology Learning Network, July 2017.
2. Bailey SH, Cohen JL, Kenkel JM. Etiology, prevention, and treatment of dermal filler complications. Aesthet Surg J. 2011;31(1):110-1121.
3. DeLorenzi C. Complications of injectable fillers, part I. Aesthet Surg J. 2013;33(4):561-575.

2

FORENSIC MEDICINE: THE PREVENTION AND MANAGEMENT OF LITIGATION

THE PREVENTION AND MANAGEMENT OF RISK IN AESTHETIC MEDICINE

Ruben Oddenino

Aesthetic medicine has taken on increasingly specific connotations within the medical and healthcare landscape over the last decade, so much so that it is now considered a specific discipline. As such, it is supported by qualified schools, capable of providing specialised training for professionals who intend to devote their medical practice to aesthetic treatment as well as to the well-being of their patients. At the same time, the expertise of forensic medicine has evolved, defining the damages that may result from such practice, leading to an increasingly clear definition of what we call "unfair" damage. Consequently, litigation management takes on fundamental importance with a view to a critical assessment of the claim for compensation.

The continuous desire on the part of patients to conform to the aesthetic canons [1] commonly accepted and shared by society today, supported by the availability of sometimes poorly trained professionals, has created the false illusion of being able to change our physical features at will and without any particular difficulty.

This, together with the impoverishment of relationships, an ever-increasing habit of self-isolation and the tendency to socialise almost exclusively through social networks, has led to the mystification of the human body image [2], which is falsely portrayed on the web as forever young and perfect. It therefore becomes extremely difficult and penalising to show ourselves as we really are, and the often disillusioned desire to look more and more like the fantasy we have built for ourselves leads to demands that are as pretentious as they are (sometimes) impossible to achieve.

Patient expectations and risk prevention

The correct prevention and management of risk in aesthetic medicine is a fine balancing act between the patient's expectations and failure to achieve the desired result.

Understanding the wishes of our patients without feeling obliged to comply with them is the first step towards maintaining a high professional profile. Refraining from performing a treatment when the likelihood of fulfilling expectations is low not only preserves the practitioner from medical-legal problems, but also often instils greater trust in them, precisely because they refute what could be an easy profit. Experience teaches us that this solid relationship of trust which is built up encourages patients to accept alternative treatments from the practitioner. If the patient understands that an unwillingness to operate is justified by the protection of their health and not by the insecurity or inability of the practitioner, the latter will always be their point of reference for a safe and suitable treatment.

Dysmorphias, which are much better

known and easier to diagnose when referred to eating disorders, are also frequent in aesthetic medicine, despite being less well known and less apparent. Individuals who ask for small, objectively insignificant retouches without paying attention to obvious imperfections are the order of the day [3]. These are patients who need to be understood and it can be counterproductive to divert their attention to imperfections that they themselves do not perceive as such. This could trigger a kind of "guided" dissatisfaction and subsequently create greater problems for them, which would inevitably affect the practitioner's work. The case of a perfectly stable person asking for advice on how to improve their appearance is different. They will be willing to accept advice, especially if the doctor is able to correctly assess the specific features of their face, highlighting their strengths and weaknesses without merely proposing generic therapies that are valid for most people.

The key to risk prevention is therefore represented by understanding the patient's desires and aligning them with their expectations. Paradoxically, to understand the importance of this concept, one only needs to imagine a patient wanting to rejuvenate their face and receiving anti-cellulite treatment instead. Even if the anti-cellulite treatment produces an excellent result, the patient will still be dissatisfied because her desire and expectations were of something completely different.

To quote M. Guillame: "*The subject looks, beyond the object, at what its image represents. But nothing exists behind the object and its image, so he steers his desire towards other images. The constantly renewed and entrapped desire is one of the springs of the growth in demand*". This must make us think about how desire does not know what it wants [4], especially in today's ever-changing society, where there is no lack of money but desire takes on a generalised dimension that refers not to real images but only to the images we desire.

Expectations must therefore be understood and discussed as part of the "aesthetic" therapy, which cannot be limited to the mere medical surgical act but must go further if it is to fully satisfy our patient. This concept is all the more important if we consider that the desire to achieve a youthful and pleasing appearance is often a necessity imposed by the standards that govern the society we live in. The older entrepreneur often loses out in comparison to a younger colleague who, despite being less experienced, inspires confidence due to his dynamism and desire to grow professionally. Similarly, female beauty offers better chances when it comes to romance, and more generally speaking, what we call good looks and beauty favour interpersonal relationships.

These apparently trivial concepts are present in our experience, often in a confused manner, and due specifically to the vague perception that we have of them, patients are often inclined to express their wishes in an imprecise manner. Hence the importance of a thorough discussion before embarking on medical aesthetic treatment aimed at satisfying the patient.

The right balance between body and soul leads to the recognition of beauty [5]. The Greeks, in their ancient wisdom, defined the nature of the true human being as follows: "*Kalòs kaì agathos*" meaning "*outer beauty can but coincide with inner beauty*" and vice versa.

Preventing litigation

A different and more purely legal issue is risk management in aesthetic medicine, as a measure to prevent litigation. Striving to understand the patient's reasons for dissatisfaction is the best way to maintain the relationship of trust between practitioner and patient. It is important not to underestimate the fact that the disappointment that ensues following an unsuccessful treatment often leads the patient to the conviction that they have been wronged. Many colleagues still believe that practitioners hold the privileged status that they held during the last century, when it was generally believed that the parish priest, doctor and notary were sacredly untouchable figures. As such, they are convinced that adopting a haughty and reticent attitude towards a disgruntled patient will somehow intimidate them to the point of avoiding any retaliatory action.

Nothing could be further from the truth. People today are perfectly aware of their rights and even if they aren't, lawyers step in to handle their claims.

The institute of mediation, which came into force fairly recently, represents the compulsory step before taking legal action against third parties and is aimed precisely at attempting an amicable settlement of a dispute by drawing up a conciliatory proposal.

Similar attempts can also be made out-of-court by means of a preventive technical assessment (pursuant to Article 696 bis of the Italian Code of Civil Procedure), in which the judge appoints a specialist in the field [6] and a forensic scientist, who, during the course of expert operations, attempt to settle the dispute by reaching an agreement between the parties. Only after the failure of the attempt at reconciliation does it become possible to take legal action. Once again, the problem of misunderstanding, unfulfilled expectations and poorly understood desires comes to the fore.

In this case, reconciliation does not mean admitting guilt, but rather clarifying positions with the intention of overcoming differences. A handshake may be sufficient but the agreement usually involves an economic transaction.

Health protection is rooted in various sources of law. Article 32 of the Italian Constitution protects health as a fundamental right of the individual; Article 4 of the Treaty of Oviedo (4 April 1997) regulates the professional obligations and rules of conduct of the health professional, while Article 5 governs consent to the medical act. In a more general manner, Article 2043 of the Italian Civil Code also provides for compensation following a tort [7]. This article states: "*Any wilful or unintentional act that causes unfair damage to others shall oblige the person committing the act to pay compensation for such damage*".

This last article, in fact, is of fundamental

importance in the management of the adverse event complained of by the patient, as it differentiates damage proper from so-called "unfair" damage, i.e. relating to medical liability. In practice, it separates complication from technical error. Complication is a more or less foreseeable but unavoidable event that occurs as a result of medical treatment despite the fact that the practitioner has taken all the necessary precautions to avoid it. However serious the damage may be, the practitioner will not be held liable for it, as long as the patient was properly informed of the risks before treatment. Things are different in the case of damage due to practitioner error, and it matters little whether this is due to malpractice, imprudence or negligence, because the practitioner will be required to pay compensation in all cases.

Insurance cover

As is easy to imagine, professional liability insurance cover, which became compulsory following the introduction of the Balduzzi law, is of paramount importance. It is worth clarifying some of the more complicated and controversial aspects of this matter. Given that concealing a claim from your insurance company in order to benefit from a reduced premium when taking out the policy risks invalidating all or part of the policy, just as not opening a claim in good time risks invalidating the insurance cover, the most important concepts to bear in mind when taking out insurance are the following.

All policies operate on a "Claims Made" basis. This means that the insurance clause triggers the claim by making the guarantees effective not from the moment the policyholder commits the tort, but from the first claim for damages received by the insurance company. This fact is not insignificant, so I shall try to explain the problems in more detail.

Let us suppose that a freelance practitioner carries out the activity of aesthetic practitioner for three years, covered by a policy that includes the risk arising from said activity, and that they then decide to abandon the activity of aesthetic practitioner in order to devote themselves solely to general medicine. They decide not to renew the previous policy, but to take out another, cheaper policy to cover the new activity. If, while working as a general practitioner, a claim for damages known to relate to the former activity should be received, there will be no cover either from the old policy, as it has expired, or from the new one, as it has been taken out only to cover damages arising from general practice. Don't forget that the law establishes a term of 10 years to file an action claiming compensation for damages.

Ascertaining, therefore, the existence of an extension of the policy's "retroactivity", i.e. covering professional errors committed in the past of which we are not yet aware, is very important to the validity of the insurance cover.

The second fundamental concept is that of "posthumousness", i.e. coverage for claims received after retirement, but referring to events that occurred during professional activity.

It seems clear, therefore, that the choice of the best insurance cannot and should not be limited solely to the amount of the annual premium but must take into account all the factors described above in order to benefit from full coverage in the professional field.

It is therefore easily to see how prevention and risk management are of no small importance when it comes to practising your profession with peace of mind, especially in a branch like aesthetic medicine, which often breeds misunderstanding between patient and practitioner.

Bibliography

1. Galimberti U. I miti del nostro tempo, Feltrinelli.
2. J. Hillman J. Il codice dell'anima, Adelphi.
3. Scafoglio D, Oddenino R. L'odore della bellezza: per una antropologia della corporeità nelle società tardo capitalistiche, Editoriale Delfino.
4. Galimberti U. Il Corpo, Feltrinelli.
5. Musitelli S, Oddenino R. Breve storia della chirurgia estetica, Edizioni Accademiche Italiane.
6. Oddenino R. La consulenza tecnica e la responsabilità civile e penale del chirurgo plastico e del medico estetico, SEE Firenze.
7. Trimarchi P. Istituzioni di diritto privato, Giuffrè Francis Lefebvre.

THE ASSESSMENT OF UNDESIRABLE EFFECTS IN FORENSIC MEDICINE. INFORMED CONSENT

Ruben Oddenino

On the subject of aesthetic medicine, the question that arises spontaneously is how and to what extent this activity is able to enhance individual beauty. Even before that, we must ask ourselves what the term "beauty" really means [1]. The answer is far from simple. Is beauty the acknowledgement of a universally accepted cultural standard? Or is it the objective acknowledgement of a well-known artist, to whom we can refer in terms of aesthetic sensitivity? Is it a matter of fashion? Probably all of the above and more, or none of the above at all [2].

An old Italian saying reminds us that "what we see as beautiful isn't that which is beautiful, what we see as beautiful is that which we like", and then there's the English saying "beauty is in the eye of the beholder", both of which imply that the standards of aesthetics depend on individual taste. Moreover, tastes change over time, to such an extent that there is a "macro-aesthetic" when the common orientation of aesthetics occupies a significant time span (see Renaissance aesthetics, Romanticism, Parisian Art Deco with the works of Paul Poiret, to name just a few currents separated by centuries, during which the artistic sense evolved), and a "micro-aesthetic", limited to our daily lives in which tastes can change radically from one day to the next.

Succeeding in navigating through such chaos becomes almost impossible when it comes to assessing the undesirable effects of aesthetic medicine. Here a different concept, to which forensic medicine refers when called upon to answer for the results of a procedure, prevails. It is no longer the sense of beauty that matters, but rather the improvement over the status quo ante. In other words, the result that one should expect, referring to the average of the results that can be achieved by a professional practising in that field, must be judged to be an improvement on the initial conditions.

To avoid totally subjective assessments by the medical examiner, criteria that can be traced back to what is called the "reduction of the aesthetic coefficient" have had to be adopted.

If we assume that we are all 100% beautiful, any change for the worse resulting from medical (aesthetic) error makes us 99%, 98%, 97%, 96% beautiful, and so on. Consequently, the reflection of the impairment of aesthetic efficiency is calculated on a percentage basis. It is clear, however, that such an impairment also has consequences at a psychological level depending on the sex, age and social status of the individual. The diversity of aesthetic damage can explain the difficulty in practically structuring its medical-legal assessment. Following various previous sentences, the Court of Cassation has confirmed that Italian Decree Law no. 158 of 2012 envisaged the application, also in the healthcare sector, of the criterion for the payment of com-

pensation for "biological" damage in compliance with the tabular system already adopted for road and boating accidents, as set out in articles 138 and 139 of the private insurance code, Legislative Decree no. 209 of 7 September 2005.
Under this directive, damage is classified as "slight", "slight to moderate", "moderate to severe" and "very severe". I am not going to dwell on the specifics of these categories of damage so as not to complicate things with further technicalities, but we need to understand how, following unfair damage, i.e. damage attributable to medical liability, the assessment of said damage is not left to chance or subjective opinion, but is structured in a precise manner according to the references shared also by the Italian Society of Legal Medicine (SIMLA).

Informed consent

What we call informed consent deserves a separate comment. The patient has a right to be properly informed about the medical act and the practitioner has a duty to provide the patient with clear and comprehensive information. Failure to provide such information constitutes a separate tort. This means that even if the treatment has the desired effect, the patient can present a claim for compensation justified by the fact that their right to be informed has been breached.
To better understand the importance of informed consent, which must not be considered as a mere, albeit dutiful, bureaucratic act, we must refer to the Italian Criminal Code [3].
As is well known, this is a collection of articles that specify the nature of offences and the punishments imposed upon them. Bearing in mind that Article 1 states that "*no one may be punished for an act that is not expressly envisaged by law as a criminal offence, nor with penalties that are not prescribed by law*", let us try to understand the relationship that exists between the consent given by the patient to the medical act and the medical treatment they intend to undergo.
As we all know, the Italian Criminal Code envisages a very severe penalty for anyone guilty of murder. This offence is regulated by Article 575 of the Criminal Code. Similarly, anyone who commits murder on a consenting person is punished, albeit with a less severe penalty (Article 579 of the Criminal Code). There is also an offence, set out in Article 583 of the Criminal Code, regarding the causing of bodily harm. However, there is no article that punishes those who cause injury to a consenting person. This is not an oversight that has resulted in a gap in the law, but it is due precisely to the absence of such an article that we doctors can practise our profession and use a scalpel [4].
Without the patient's explicit consent, surgery would be comparable to wilful bodily harm. The legislator has, however, also taken care to place "limits" on consent, but I am not going to dwell on them here as this would complicate the discussion. For purely illustrative purposes, I will mention the ban on carrying out experimental medical acts, even with the patient's consent, where these may endanger the life of either the patient or the unborn child.

The rule is quite complex, but we can summarise it by defining the medical act as lawful where the following three fundamental elements are all held at the same time: a university degree in medicine and surgery, successful completion of the state examination, and the patient's consent. Otherwise, the offences of abuse of profession, wilful bodily harm, violation of the obligation of informed consent and of the protection of the patient's self-determination and health, etc. could be committed.

From this perspective, consent becomes a determining element of healthcare practice. Other than in special cases [5], the law does not require such consent to be given in writing. However, a signature on a document is the simplest and most effective way of proving that all the necessary information has been provided.

Whichever form the information is given in, in order for it to be valid it must fulfil the following requirements: it must be personalised, clearly comprehensible taking into account the reader's intellectual level and thorough, stating not only the risks and complications but also any alternative therapeutic procedures. Consent must also be free, informed and can be withdrawn at any time.

Thanks to this last entitlement of the patient, the document can be signed shortly before the procedure. Please note, however, that this does not mean that the information must or can be given at the last moment. It simply means (and this must be stated on the written consent) that the patient is signing at that moment to state that they have received the above information during previous medical examinations. It often happens that, for fear of frightening and losing the patient, some practitioners issue a consent document containing scientific terms that only a medical graduate can understand, concealing risks and complications that might make the patient decide not to undergo the treatment. Nor can the closing phrase "*read, understood and accepted*" relieve the practitioner of responsibility for failure to provide complete information. A judge only needs to ask the patient with a limited educational background whether they actually understood the contents of the document they signed in order to invalidate the informed consent.

There are two important concepts to reflect on. The first concerns the relationship of trust that binds the practitioner to the patient. If the practitioner is proactive and calmly explains the critical points of a procedure without wanting to minimise adverse events at all costs, the bond between the patient and the practitioner will be strengthened, with the patient acknowledging the practitioner's trustworthiness and professionalism. There is nothing worse than being criticised for being careless.

The second point concerns informed consent once again, seen by a judge not as providing grounds for the practitioner's defence but rather as protection for the patient. It is therefore necessary to avoid including purely defensive phrases such as "*...I undertake not to take legal action...*" or "*...I am already satisfied...*", because in addition to violating the law and therefore being null and void, they would only serve to make the practitioner look bad in the eyes of the magistrate.

Forensic medicine in general is a very complex subject and it becomes much more so when the specialised branch concerns aesthetics, precisely because it lacks that functional justification that mitigates liability for the medical act.

Besides being compulsory, insurance cover must be carefully considered in all its contractual postulates to ensure that it does actually provide the necessary protection when required.

Bibliography

1. del Boca B. La dimensione umana, Bresci Editore.
2. Lipperini L. Non è un paese per vecchie, Feltrinelli.
3. Codice penale e leggi complementari, Hoepli.
4. Avecone P. La responsabilità penale del medico, Vallardi.
5. Presidential Decree no. 409 of 16/06/1977 on organ transplants; Law no. 135 of 05/06/1990 on AIDS; Ministerial Decree 15/01/1991 on treatment with plasma and blood by-products; Ministerial Decree 27/4/1992 on scientific experimentation; Law no. 201 of 12/08/1993 on cornea harvesting and grafting; Law no. 94 of 08/04/1998 on the use of medicines outside authorised indications; Law no. 40 of 19/02/2004 on assisted reproduction.

3

BOTULINUM TOXIN

COMPLICATIONS OF BOTULINUM TOXIN: PREVENTION AND TREATMENT

Patrizia Piersini, Giuseppe Sito

The use of botulinum toxin to correct blemishes related to the presence of dynamic wrinkles is increasingly established and widespread [1]. According to a survey carried out by the International Society of Aesthetic Plastic Surgery (Isaps), facial enhancement using botulinum toxin was the most popular cosmetic procedure in the world, with more than 6 million procedures worldwide in 2018 alone [2].

Its action is limited in time and completely reversible, and while this may be considered a limitation, it allows the resolution of most complications in a reasonably short period of time (usually 2 to 12 weeks).

Factors such as excessive dilution, diffusion of the substance, anatomical variability from patient to patient, inexperience of the injector or an error in the injection procedure may contribute to the occurrence of complications which are not very frequent in aesthetic medical procedures and, when they do occur, are mild and temporary. They can be divided into reactions to the injection and side effects of botulinum toxin [3].

Reactions to the injection

Mild bruising

The needles used for infiltration have a very fine diameter to minimise the pain of the implant and to make bruising less likely. Needles with a gauge of 32-33 G and very slow infiltration are recommended, firstly to prevent the substance from spreading, but also to prevent excessive pressure on the plunger from becoming the cause of bruising. In the case of bleeding, compression for a few minutes or the application of ice can prevent the occurrence of larger bruises, although it has been demonstrated that refrigeration delays the onset of the action of botulinum toxin. The application of creams containing vitamin K nano particles, escin or arnica 4-5 times a day, starting the day after inoculation, is recommended to speed up the reabsorption of bruising.

Mild rash or oedema

They may appear immediately after injection and recede spontaneously within a few hours.

Mild and temporary headache

A small number of patients complain of headaches after treatment. As this almost always occurs after the first inoculation, and rarely in subsequent injections, some suggest that this disorder can be blamed on the state of tension that often accompanies these treatments. It has also been suggested that headache may also occur as a result of contact between the tip of the needle and the periosteum.

Infection in the implant site

This is very rare and can be avoided by

thoroughly cleansing and disinfecting the skin before injection and by advising the patient not to apply make-up for two hours after inoculation.

Vasovagal syncope

They can occur in association with states of anxiety and tension in the patient and are characterised by a sudden drop in blood pressure and a slowing of the heart rate due to temporary inhibition of the sympathetic system and increased vagal tone. Prodromal symptoms may be cold sweating, blurred vision, pallor. Recovery usually occurs in about a minute. It is advisable to have an appropriate protocol to follow (e.g. lying the patient down with the legs raised) and, if necessary, medication to best manage this reaction.

Undesirable effects of botulinum toxin

These types of complication are definitely less frequent than reactions to injection. They can depend on the technique and their incidence tends to decrease as the injector becomes more experienced [1].

They are almost always due to a temporary effect on muscles adjacent to the predefined area of treatment due to unwanted spread of the toxin to surrounding areas.

Eyelid ptosis

Upper eyelid ptosis is generally observed one to two weeks after treatment (fig. 1). It is very rare, with an incidence of around 4% of all patients injected, temporary (average duration

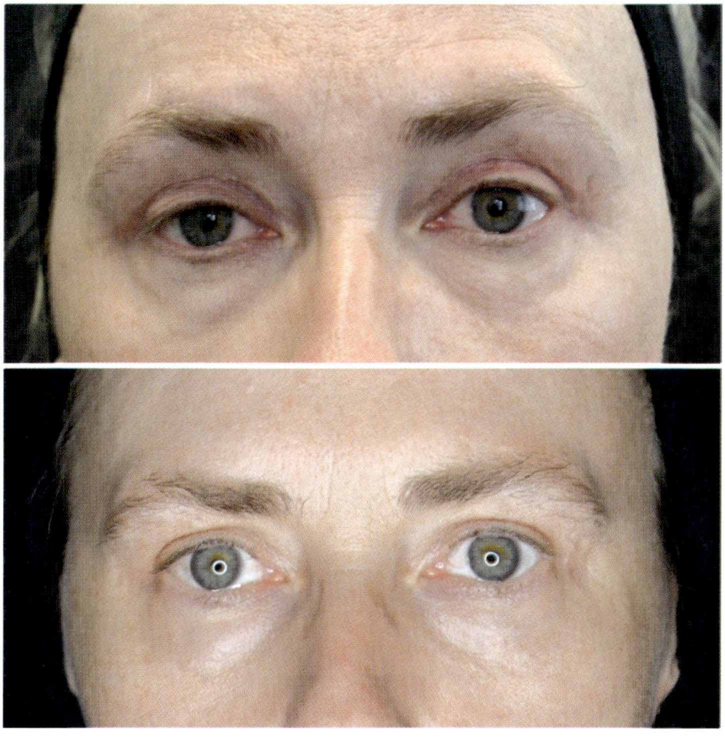

Figure 1
Right eyelid ptosis 15 days after infiltration and complete resolution 20 days after onset

of 2 to 4 weeks), but extremely stressful for the patient. It is almost always unilateral and the drooping of the eyelid can vary from 1 mm to total eyelid closure, becoming more evident towards the end of the day when muscle fatigue is greatest.

It is due to the deep diffusion of botulinum toxin through the orbital septum fascia to the elevator muscle of the upper eyelid due to overdose, excessive dilution or incorrect injection depth when treating glabellar lines. This complication often occurs when injections are performed too close to the supraorbital bone rim, particularly at the mid-pupillary line.

Its prevention consists in the careful inoculation of toxin into the established sites with the lowest possible dilution and dose. During the two hours following injection, it may be helpful not to massage the area, to avoid heat sources (hair dryer, hot shower, steam bath or sauna) and to refrain from wearing a motorbike helmet. Correction of slight eyelid ptosis, which can also occur spontaneously, can be speeded up using eye drops containing nafazolin nitrate + tonzilamine hydrochloride, in a dose of 1-2 drops per eye 4-5 times a day, with complete absence of side effects. In more severe cases, eye drops containing apraclonidine 5% (Iopidine 5 mg/ml), an alpha-adrenergic agonist that causes contraction of the Müller muscle and opens the eyelid, correcting the ptosis can be prescribed (dosage: one drop 3 times a day). These eye drops, which are routinely used in the treatment of glaucoma, must be used with great caution. Overdose can cause dry eyes, blurred vision and eyelid oedema. In this case, administration must be discontinued immediately [4]. Sethi et al. in 2021, in a cohort of 9,398 patients, reported an overall incidence of eyelid ptosis of 0.71% and eyebrow ptosis of 0.98% [1], but all figures are questionable due to the extreme variability of symptoms. An eye drop formulated with oxymetazoline hydrochloride, with excellent results and no side effects, has recently been approved. Oxymetazoline is a direct-acting agonist of the alpha-adrenergic receptor, which is believed to selectively act on the Müller muscle and lift the upper eyelid. Clinical studies show an improvement in 84% of cases.

Eyebrow ptosis

Eyebrow ptosis is a fairly common complication in treatment of the frontalis muscle with botulinum to smooth horizontal forehead lines. It occurs due to the excessive action of the botulinum protein on the lower and lateral portion of the frontalis muscle, with subsequent drooping of the eyebrow due to the pulling action of the orbicularis muscle and/or the corrugator muscle of the eyebrow. To avoid this complication, it is advisable to inject the frontalis muscle at least 2-3 cm above the supra-orbital border or 1.5-2 cm from the eyebrow, not to use too high a dilution and to use a superficial infiltration plane, possibly intradermal or subdermal [5].

If it does occur, it is a temporary complication and can be treated by blocking the eyebrow with 1 U Allergan or Speywood with natural conversion (2

Speywood) injected superficially in the caudal portion and 1 U below the medial margin.

Eyebrow asymmetry or Mephistophelian eyebrow

Eyebrow asymmetry is a relatively common complication that can result either from an asymmetry in the injection sites or different dosage between the two sides, or from anatomical variations in the individual patient. It can be easily corrected by injecting 1-2 U Allergan or Speywood with natural conversion above the wrinkles created by the lateral fibres of the frontalis muscle.

"Mephistophelian eyebrow" (fig. 2), which can be unilateral or bilateral, on the other hand, is the presence of an excessive upward curvature of the lateral portion of the eyebrow due to an imbalance between the treatment of the central portion of the frontalis muscle and the treatment of the lateral portion, leading to an excessive elevation of the tail of the eyebrow. This complication can be easily corrected by adding 1-3 U in the lateral portion of the frontalis muscle, along a line that starts vertically from the highest point of the eyebrow.

There is a simple semiotic manoeuvre to assess the possible occurrence of a Mephistophelian eyebrow: hold a thumb pressed over the procerus muscles, in the glabellar region, and ask the patient to look upwards and raise their forehead. If the patient has a predisposition towards this complication, an excessive elevation of the tail of the eyebrow will be noticed. Treatment of the lateral portion of the frontalis muscle is sufficient to prevent it.

Diplopia

This very rare complication can be caused, in the treatment of periocular wrinkles, by diffusion of the toxin into the orbit, with action on the lateral rectus muscle of the eye. Prevention involves superficial inoculation of botulinum into the orbicularis muscle of the eye and at a distance of about 1 cm from the outer canthus of the eye.

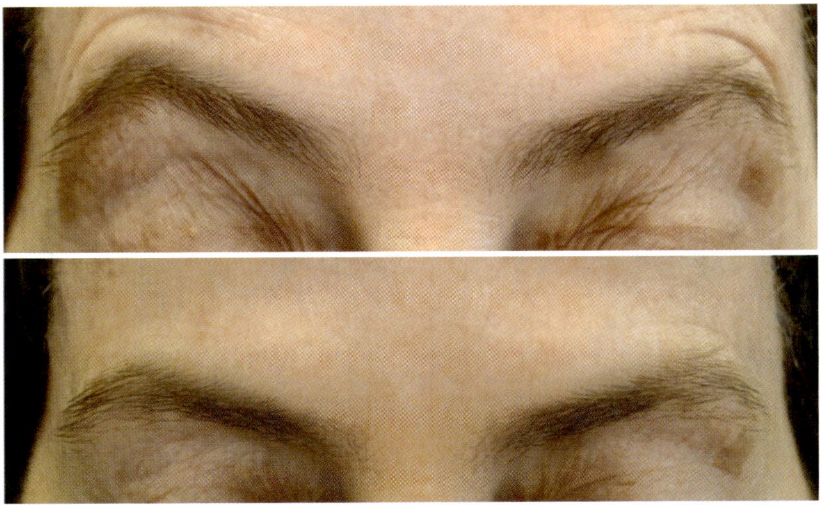

Figure 2
A case of Mephistophelian eyebrow before and after correction

Lower eyelid oedema

The lymphatic drainage of the sub-palpebral region can be made less efficient by the use of botulinum toxin in the treatment of periocular wrinkles potentially causing eyelid oedema, especially in patients with significant laxity of the orbicularis muscle and periocular wrinkles extending to the malar region.

It is advisable to massage with an anti-oedematous cream containing arnica, escin or vitamin K 6-7 times a day, performing Vodder lymphatic drainage and waiting for spontaneous remission.

Smile alterations

When treating periocular wrinkles, even if they extend downwards beyond the orbital rim, the most caudal injection must be assessed carefully so as not to interfere with the action of the zygomaticus major muscle, which lifts the corner of the mouth upwards and sideways and pushes up the malar fat pad.

Relaxing or blocking the zygomaticus major muscle with the action of botulinum can lead to a lack of cheek and lip lift in the smile, resulting in an unnatural expression.

Ectropion

Eyelid ectropion may become evident in patients with eyelid laxity if they are treated in the pretarsal region near the rim of the lower eyelid. Increased visibility of bags under the eyes can also occur when an overly lax orbicularis muscle is treated.

Prevention involves performing a "snap back test" on the lower eyelid before injection to carefully assess eyelid laxity. This is performed by pulling the lower eyelid down towards the lower orbital rim. If the eyelid does not return to its position immediately before blinking but takes at least one to three blinks to return to its position, this patient must be considered unfit for treatment.

Lagophthalmos and dry eye syndrome

Lagophthalmos, incomplete closure of the eyelid resulting in dry eye syndrome, can occur due to excessive paralysis of the orbital portion of the orbicularis muscle, resulting in weakening and difficulty maintaining proper muscle function. Early symptoms include irritation of the eye, foreign body sensation and slight intermittent watering especially in dry or windy environments. Botulinum injections should be slowed or stopped and the eye should be treated with eye drops and lubricating gels. [6].

Morphea-like lesions (localised scleroderma)

Several cases of morphea-like lesions (fig. 3), atrophic circular depressions, following botulinum toxin inoculation have been reported in literature. [7] The authors suggest that they may be due to a temporary loss of neural stimulation (focal neurogenic atrophy). This assumption is supported by the circular shape of the atrophic lesions, which would resemble the area of action of the neuroprotein. Another assumption suggested by the authors is related to the possible displacement of minute amounts of lubricant in the

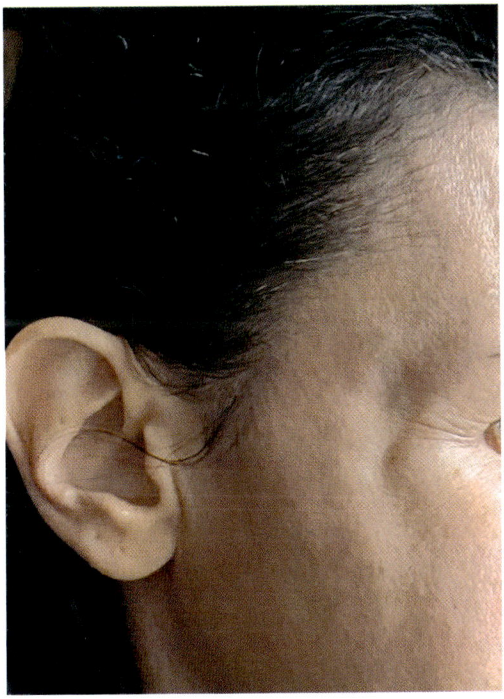

Figure 3
Morphea-like reaction to botulinum toxin

syringe, silicone oil, within the injected substance, which would subsequently be removed by tissue macrophages.

Reduction of strength and grip of the hand

Palms affected by hyperhidrosis are very debilitating psychologically and socially. The superficial injection of botulinum toxin can greatly help counteract hyperhidrosis, but injections should only be made into the superficial dermis. This maximises the paralysing effect on the eccrine units while minimising the total dose, approximately 50 U Botox per hand, required to achieve regression of the disorder. A certain degree of weakness in the hands is a common consequence of this therapy, but this complication can sometimes become clinically significant. Firm grip with the distal fingers and rotational movements of the entire hand may be impaired. This weakness is temporary and resolves spontaneously after a few weeks [8].

Dysphagia

Injections of large amounts of botulinum toxin (more than 200 U Botox per session) for the treatment of platysmal bands can lead to diffusion to the sternocleidomastoid muscle and the muscles of the larynx with the onset of dysphagia and weakness of the neck, especially when trying to raise the head in a supine position [9].

Lip asymmetry and lip ptosis

The treatment of peribuccal wrinkles with small amounts of botulinum may prove to be a very satisfactory treatment, but it can also easily give rise to complications. To avoid them, it is very important to use only a few units of botulinum (1-2 LU), injected very superficially into the orbicularis muscle, always keeping inoculation symmetrical to the medial line of the face. If these instructions are not followed, asymmetry can easily occur (fig. 4), the mouth may appear twisted when resting, and speaking or chewing may accentuate this effect. Functional deficits may include the inability to sip from a straw, to pronounce the letters "P" and "S" clearly, to whistle or to play a wind instrument. [10]

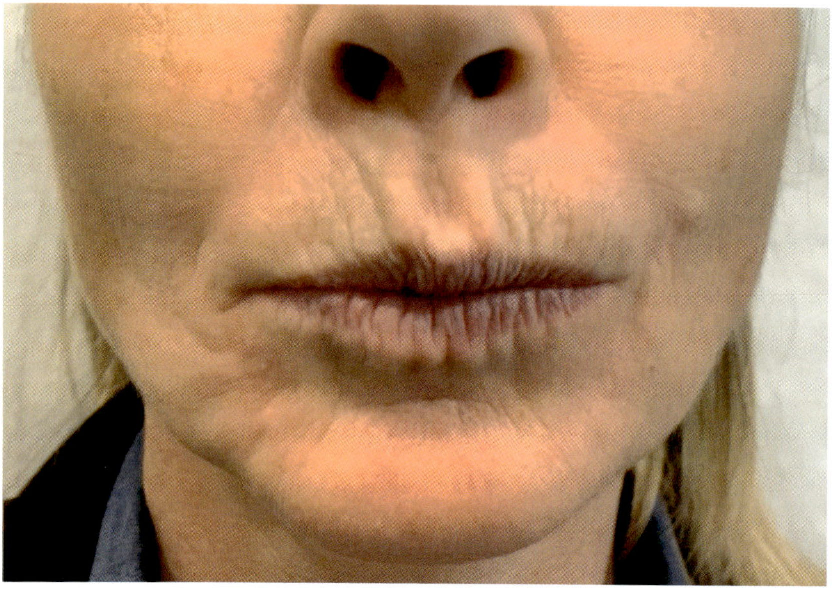

Figure 4
Asymmetry of the lips occurring 4 days after infiltration of botulinum toxin into suprabuccal lines

Allergic reactions and neutralising antibodies

The possible formation of antibodies resulting in immune resistance has always been a concern for doctors using botulinum toxin. Although hypersensitivity to the substance does not occur, the effectiveness of treatment may be reduced. However, the antigenicity of a material is almost uniformly proportional to the protein burden, and the greatly reduced amount of protein present in the various types of botulinum toxin currently used may allow the application of higher doses of product per treatment session, without fear of immunogenicity.
The prevalence of resistance to botulinum toxin is less than 5% and is associated with the dose and frequency of treatment sessions, but not with the duration of the overall treatment regimen. With regard to the frequency of injection, many practitioners carry out an additional touch-up, when appropriate, approximately two weeks after the initial treatment. As the doses used in aesthetic medicine are usually very small (<100 U), limiting the frequency of injection does not seem to be crucial [10].

Necrotising fasciitis

Necrotising fasciitis is considered to be a serious and very rare side effect of treatment with botulinum toxin, usually involving the subcutaneous fat and fascia. Certain debilitating diseases, such as diabetes, alcoholism and polymyositis, are predisposing factors for this condition.
In recent years, only one case has been described after inoculation with botulinum toxin for the treatment of blepharospasm, in which the infection, caused by bacterial inoculation of the patient's skin, spread through the fascial planes and led to muscle necrosis [11].
It has been suggested that this complication resulted from immobilisation due to the toxin, which was not for cosmetic use.

Certainly it must be considered as a rare but very severe risk in the inoculation of botulinum toxin in immunocompromised individuals, so more precautions, such as the use of a sterile field for performing the injections, should be taken.

Conclusions

It is clear from the discussion in this chapter that complications due to the use of botulinum toxin are not frequent, are always temporary, and are often resolved by the subsequent inoculation of a few units of botulinum toxin or the use of a drug.
Although the complication disappears very quickly, it is always extremely important for the injecting practitioner to be thoroughly familiar with the anatomy of the area treated, the characteristics and dilutions of the protein used, and the most up-to-date inoculation techniques.
It is necessary for the patient to be adequately informed about the possible side effects and complications of the treatment and to sign an informed consent form.

Bibliography

1. Sethi N, Singh S, De Boulle K, Rahman E. A Review of Complications Due to the Use of Botulinum Toxin A for Cosmetic Indications. Aesthetic Plast Surg. 2021 Jun;45(3):1210-1220. Erratum in: Aesthetic Plast Surg. 2022 Feb;46(1):595.
2. International Society of Aesthetic Plastic Surgery (ISAPS) International survey on aesthetic/cosmetic procedures performed in 2018. https://www.isaps.org/wp–content/uploads/2019/12/ISAPS–Global–Survey–Results–2018–new.pdf. Accessed May 29, 2020.
3. Small R. Botulinum toxin injection for facial wrinkles. Am Fam Physician. 2014 Aug 1;90(3):168-75.
4. Chen S, Long J. Zhong Nan Da Xue Xue Bao Yi Xue Ban. Adverse events of botulinum toxin A in facial injection: mechanism, prevention, and treatment. 2019 Jul 28;44(7):837-844.
5. Borba A, Matayoshi S, Rodrigues M. Avoiding Complications on the Upper Face Treatment with Botulinum Toxin: A Practical Guide. Aesthetic Plast Surg. 2022 Feb;46(1):385-394.
6. Ozgur OK et al. Dry eye syndrome due to botulinum toxin type-A injection: guideline for prevention. Hawaii J Med Public Health. 2012 May;71(5):120-3.
7. Landau M, Emelyanova E, Hirsch R. Morphea-like lesions after botulinum toxin A injection. JAAD care Rep. 2020Nov; 6(11): 1185-1187.
8. Kontis TC, Lacombe VG. Iniezioni di Tossina Botulinica e Filler in Medicina Estetica. Edizioni Piccin.
9. Brandt FS, Bellman B. Cosmetic use of botulinum A exotoxin for the aging neck. Dermatol Surg 1998;24: 1232-4.
10. Klein AW. Complications with the use of botulinum toxin. Dermatol Clin. 2004 Apr;22(2):197-205, vii.
11. Latimer PR et al. Necrotizing fasciitis as a complication of botulinum toxin injection. Eye (Lond). 1998;12 (Pt 1): 51-3.

4

REVITALISATION AND TRACTION THREADS

THE COMPLICATIONS OF REVITALISATION THREADS AND TRACTION THREADS: PREVENTION AND TREATMENT

Alberto Diaspro, George Sulamanidze

The facial ageing process is the result of a combination of alterations in bone structure and the superficial and deep adipose structures of the soft facial tissues and the skin that covers them.

As the collagen network deteriorates and the elastic fibres become depleted, the tissues of anatomical areas with greater projection and definition, which are consequently more susceptible to the action of gravity, such as the mid-facial area and the jaw line, weaken considerably [1].

The efficiency of suspension threads is related to the focal nature of soft tissue ptosis, as some areas manifest the effect of gravity more than others.

Partial knowledge of the basics of the topographical anatomy of facial ageing and of the vectors along which gravitational ptosis occurs prevents optimal results from being achieved with this method, as it is not a question of "pulling tissue over an inert volume", but rather of defining contours and projections by restoring the physiological position of the superficial facial tissues [2].

Volume depletion plays an important role in the central part of the face, due to the gravitational ptosis of the deep and superficial fat compartments. Its restoration is consequently the main aim of any mid-facial rejuvenation technique.

The jawline, on the other hand, loses definition due to gravitational ptosis and the action of the platysma major depressor muscle in this area, the hypertrophy of cheek fat and loosening of the masseter skin ligaments, resulting in loss of definition between the face and the neck. The use of these techniques in the lower part of the face allows the suspension of the superficial tissues, exploiting the residual volume of subcutaneous fat in the area of the mandibular angle and allowing the repositioning of the skin of the jaw line along a posterior-superiorly oriented vector, reversing the gravitational effect [3,4].

The use of suspension threads has progressively aroused considerable interest, because it allows the treatment of initial dermatochalasis and signs of moderate gravitational ptosis by means of a minimally invasive procedure [5]: in areas where the dermal adipose layers can be mobilised without surgical dissection and in the desired direction, their use allows the return of the tissues to their original position.

However, the details and basic principles of the techniques have often been neglected during their application, resulting in modest, if not questionable, and short-lived results due to early loss of suspension stability, as well as adverse events, side effects and complications.

The aforementioned problems are also often attributed to technical details, such as the morphology of the thread and barbs, and generally to the presumed ineffectiveness of the method rather than to partial knowledge of the gravitational ageing process of the face and its vectors, to a lack of respect for patient selection criteria, and to the inappropriate application of the technique due to a lack of knowledge or insufficient familiarity with it.

Anatomy

The treatment of the normal facial anatomy is not covered in this chapter, so reference should be made to dedicated texts.
With respect to suspension thread or biostimulation implantation procedures, anatomical structures such as foramen with their nerve trunks, major arteries and veins of the face are located at a greater depth than the correct plane of insertion and implantation of the threads. As a result, they do not constitute areas of danger, other than in the case of technical error.
To ensure the reliability of the result, the points of insertion and stabilisation of the threads are located in areas where the ligamentous structures of the face flare into a terminal arborization where they are inserted into the skin: stabilising a thread by anchoring it to a ligament is anatomically incorrect and poses the risk of complications due to implantation in the wrong anatomical plane, being too deep and close to the neuro-vascular structures mentioned above.
The subcutaneous adipose tissue, the correct plane for the implantation of the threads, is a lax structure with connective tissue septa: these septa and the terminal subcutaneous portions of the facial ligaments are the insertion and attachment points which allow a safe and reliable implantation procedure and predictable results.

Indications

The correct selection of the ideal candidate is crucial in order to obtain a predictable result: initial or moderate facial soft-tissue ptosis, usually in patients between the ages of 35 and 50, is the optimal selection criteria for reliable results.
Compliance with the rules of asepsis proper for outpatient surgery must be guaranteed during the thread implantation procedure, as this is the most effective way of preventing inflammatory and infectious complications: a sterile table must be set up with the materials needed to perform the procedure and hands must be washed with iodine or chlorhexidine-based antiseptic solutions. Cleanse the patient's face and neck with the same antiseptic solution and set up the working area with sterile sheets, using sterile gloves.
The use of local anaesthetic with adrenalin injected through a blunt cannula ensures the comfort of the patient during the procedure, facilitates the implantation of the thread for minimal hydro-dissection and avoids bruising due to vasoconstriction of the superficial blood vessels.
The prescription of broad-spectrum antibiotic therapy, which is usually unnecessary, can be assessed depending on the number of thread insertion points, particularly in the case of use in multiple areas of the face, and the patient's ability to cleanse and disinfect at home.

Complications

Any procedure using suspension threads can result in post-op discomfort, slight bleeding with linear bruising, oedema, asymmetry, dimples and uneven contours.

Side effects are common but temporary and may include:

- asymmetry (fig. 1);
- localised pain;
- bruising due to slight bleeding;
- oedema;
- formation of skin folds or dimples (fig. 2);
- localised depressions or irregularities of the skin.

They are expected to resolve spontaneously within a few days (7 to 10) after thread implantation.

Any situation which does not resolve spontaneously within 2 weeks of thread implantation must be considered a complication. Such situations include:

- persistent asymmetry;
- haematoma;
- persistent inflammation (fig. 3);
- suppuration of the insertion points;
- infection (fig. 4);
- migration or exposure of the thread (fig. 5);
- persistent skin folds or dimples;
- persistent skin depressions or irregularities;
- visibility of the thread (figs. 6-7-8);
- persistent focal overcorrection;
- (early) insufficient result due to weakening or loss of attachment (fig. 9).

Any injury to nerves, blood vessels or tissues of the salivary glands or ducts is to be considered secondary to errors in technique and therefore not a complication related to the method.

Lastly, it should be noted that overcorrection of the area treated represents a decision made by the operator, sometimes because it is necessary, or an error in technique when it is not required by the technique chosen or for the area treated: it usually corrects itself spontaneously in the days following the implant, but, if particularly pronounced, it may take a few weeks (2 or 3), or may persist beyond that, causing embarrassment in social situations for the patient who complains of it.

In general terms, the approach to the above-mentioned sequelae and complications must be considered with respect to the time of onset: within the first 7-10 days after thread implanta-

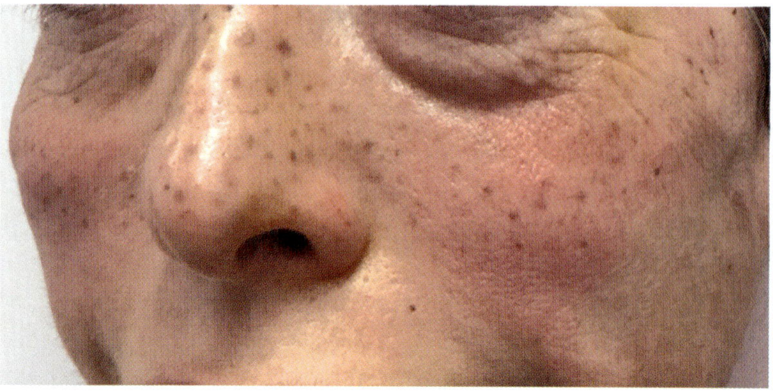

Figure 1
Asymmetry after thread implantation in the right mid-facial region

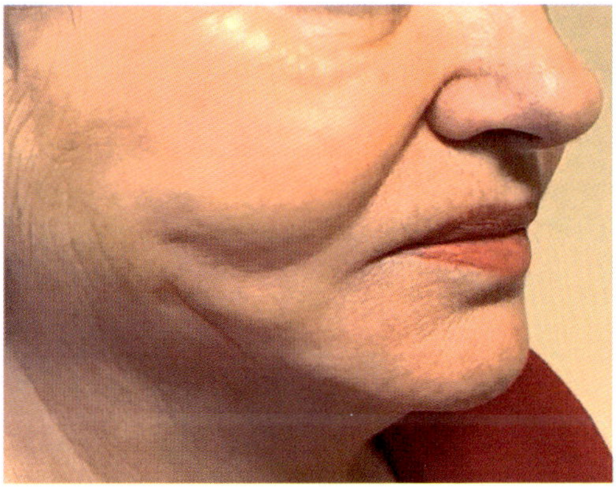

Figure 2 Presence of skin folds and umbilications due to placement of the thread too close to the surface. Courtesy of Dr. G. Sulamanidze

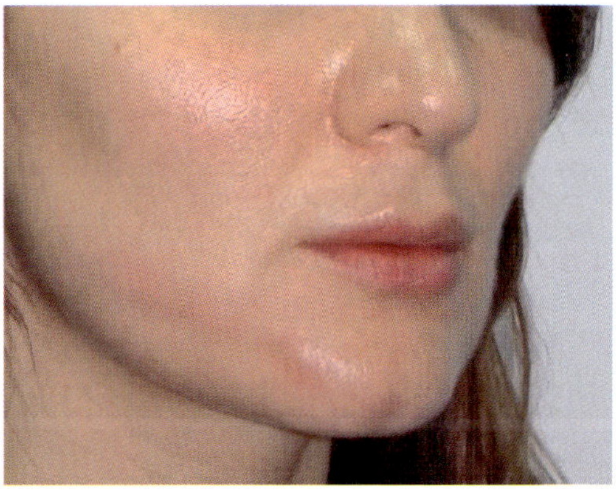

Figure 3 Chronic inflammation of the implanted thread from the pretragal region to the marionette line. Courtesy of Dr. G. Sulamanidze

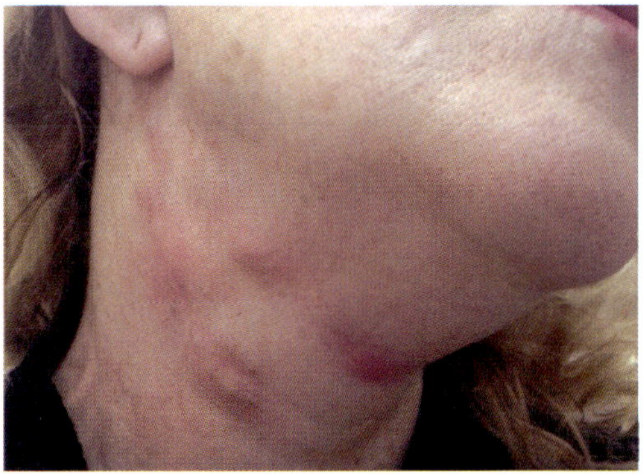

Figure 4 Abscess along the thread implanted in the submandibular region. Courtesy of Dr. G. Sulamanidze

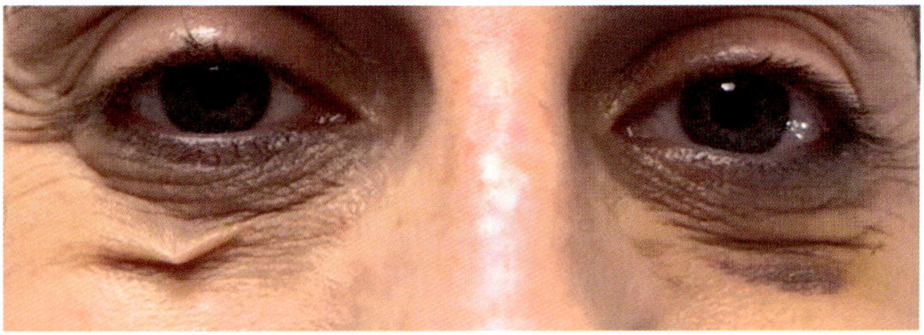

Figure 5 Visibility of non-barbed thread implanted in eyelid area and subsequently migrated: visible due to thin skin and absence of subcutaneous fatty tissue. Courtesy of Dr. G. Sulamanidze

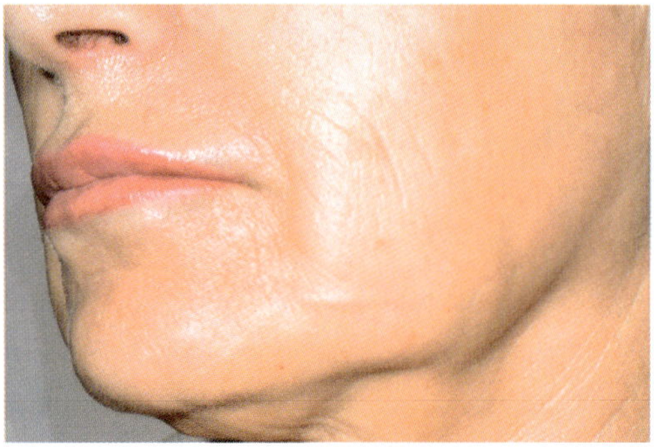

Figure 6 Visibility due to placement of the thread too close to the surface, in static mimicry

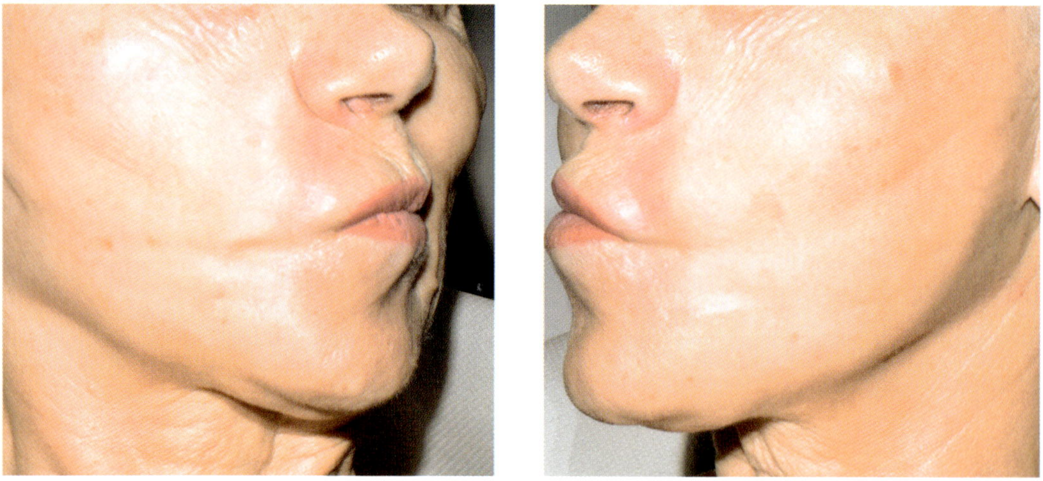

Figure 7 Visibility due to placement of the thread too close to the surface, in active mimicry

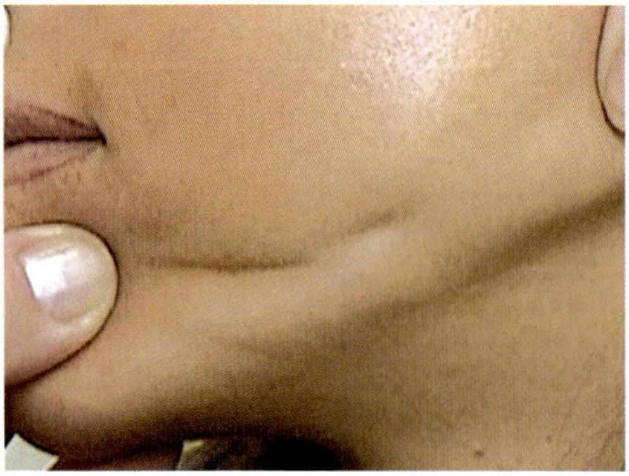

Figure 8 Visibility due to placement of the thread too close to the surface, in static mimicry. Courtesy of Dr. G. Sulamanidze

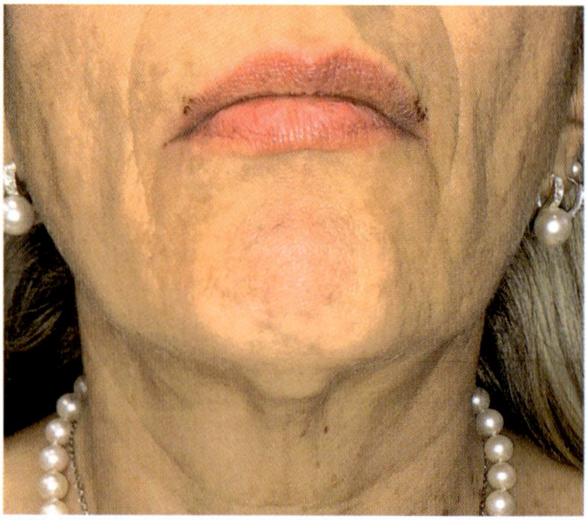

Figure 9 Loss of median attachment of the thread implanted in the submandibular region

VIDEO 4.1

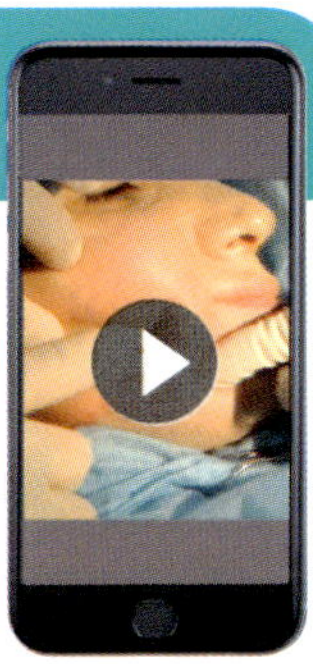

Removal of resorbable thread from the cheek (fig. 3)
Courtesy of Dr. G. Sulamanidze

VIDEO 4.2

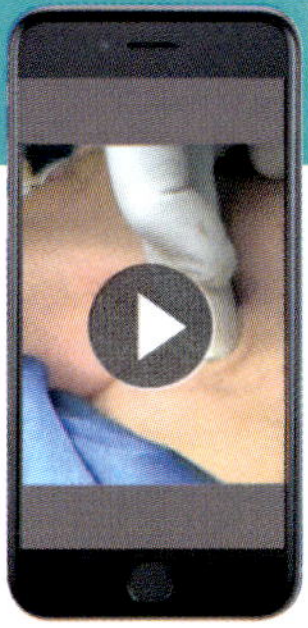

Removal of non-resorbable thread from the cervical region
Courtesy of Dr. G. Sulamanidze

tion, watchful waiting is always the first choice, because any interaction in this early period potentially leads to a poorer outcome.

Any symptoms that do not present clinically suspect acuity and which resolve spontaneously with ordinary painkillers should not be a cause for concern. Any remaining oedema can be treated with appropriate medication.

During this initial period, attention must be paid to the insertion points, checking that the thread is not extruded or there is no local inflammation which, if left untreated, would result in infection and contamination of at least the terminal portion of the thread.

At the post-implant check-up, the presence of asymmetries or alterations in the tissue profile should be treated exclusively with gentle massage in the critical areas, practised by the doctor and never by the patient.

The first 15 days are particularly critical: problems that persist beyond that require intervention by the doctor so that they do not become more severe. Any persistent asymmetries or

VIDEO 4.3

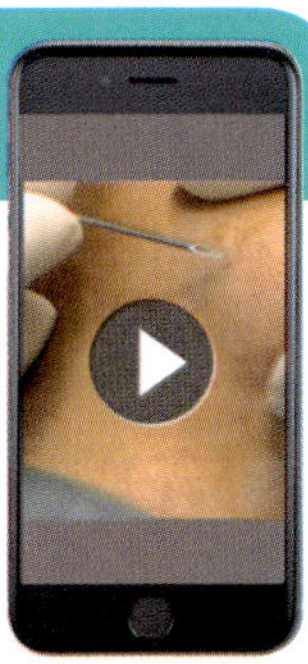

Removal of non-resorbable thread from the submandibular region
Courtesy of Dr. G. Sulamanidze

irregularities in tissue contours must be massaged by pinching the skin in order to favour the loss of grip by the barbs on the cutaneous plane. This usually results in complete resolution. If this does not occur, it can be helpful to use a blunt cannula and, under local anaesthetic, to locally determine the detachment of the barbed portion of the thread from the cutaneous plane.

Every inflammatory sign and symptom of the insertion points or localised along the path of the thread, with the appearance of redness, localised skin tenderness or possible serohaematic formations, must be treated with drugs and reassessed in the short term. If it does not resolve or if it recurs, it is advisable to schedule removal of the thread to prevent infection, which often represents the evolution of the inflammatory situation but above all the most worrying complication, both in terms of acute problems and possible outcomes.

The presence of extensive bruising or haematomas which do not resolve spontaneously in the first 15 days requires reassessment with a view to possible antibiotic therapy (if not already prescribed after implantation) to avoid overinfection, given the presence of the implanted thread.

If it becomes necessary to remove the thread, usually due to recurrent infection or malpositioning, it is possible to proceed through a small skin incision, hooking up the thread with a vascular hook after locating it precisely on the cutaneous plane and administering a small dose of local anaesthetic: despite the stability of the suspension of the tissues affected by ptosis, the thread has no further resistance and, once hooked up and extracted from the skin using surgical tweezers, can be removed gently without discomfort for the patient, with the possible addition of anaesthetic at a greater distance (videos 4.1, 4.2 and 4.3).

Conclusions

As a general rule in medicine and surgery, most complications related to the use of suspension threads can be prevented when the practitioner has acquired adequate preparation with regard to facial anatomy and the ageing process, patient selection criteria have been met, basic principles and techniques have been followed and mastered, and the right thread the defect to be treated has been selected [6,7].

Sterile conditions during all procedures are essential as the implants inserted are characterised by slow resorption.

It is necessary to observe that the results that can be obtained concern a static correction of ptosis: this procedure is frequently performed in the mid-facial and zygomatic area (45.5%), along the jawline (17%) and in the submental region (16.2%), all areas in which the superficial soft tissue planes can be easily repositioned [8].

When the use of threads in areas with significant mimicry is envisaged, proper selection of a thread with adequate elasticity must be considered.

Lastly, it must be pointed out that effective subcutaneous repositioning is only feasible at local level and that soft tissue suspension techniques along the jawline using long threads anchored mostly in the temporal or parietal area are to be discouraged, because physiological facial mimicry and chewing would lead to detachment of the barbs or to lesion of the subcutaneous tissues with loss of suspension. These areas are also crossed by important superficial blood vessels that expose the patient and the practitioner to major complications, due more to imprudence than to inexperience and negligence [9].

Knowledge of the possible complications must always be combined with an understanding of how to handle them, whether they be mild and temporary or severe: the thread to be used must be chosen not only on the basis of mechanical and morphological characteristics, but also considering the possibility of acquiring the aforementioned skills with respect to the results to be proposed to patients, always guaranteeing safety as well as reliability.

Bibliography

1. Flament F, Bazin R, Piot B. Influence of gravity upon some facial signs. Int J Cosmet Sci. 2015 Jun;37(3):291-7.
2. Abbate V, Dell'Aversana Orabona G, Seidita F et al. Facial Soft Tissue Ptosis: A Quantitative Analysis using 3d Facial Scan App For iPhone. J. Maxillofac Oral Surg 2022.
3. Diaspro A, Luni M, Rossini G. Thread Lifting of the Jawline: A Pilot Study for Quantitative Evaluation. J Cutan Aesthet Surg. 2021 Jan-Mar;14(1):47-54.
4. Diaspro A, Rossini G. Thread lifting of the midface: A Pilot Study for Quantitative Evaluation. Dermatol Ther. 2021;34(4):e14958.
5. Gülbitti HA et al. Thread-Lift Sutures: Still in the Lift? A Systematic Review of the Literature. Plast Reconstr Surg. 2018 Mar;141(3):341e-347e.
6. Rachel JD, Lack EB, Larson B. Incidence of complications and early recurrence in 29 patients after facial rejuvenation with barbed suture lifting.Dermatol Surg. 2010 Mar;36(3):348-54.
7. Sarigul Guduk S, Karaca N. Safety and complications of absorbable threads made of poly-L-lactic acid and poly lactide/glycolide: Experience with 148 consecutive patients. J Cosmet Dermatol. 2018 Dec;17(6):1189-1193.
8. Sulamanidze M et al. Avoiding Complications with Aptos Sutures. Aesthet Surg J. 2011 Nov;31(8):863-73.
9. Sulamanidze M, Vozdvizhenskiy I, Sulamanidze G, Sulamanidze K, Azizyan E. Experience in Preventive Measures and Treatment of Complications at Face and Neck Thread Rejuvenation. In: Serdev N, editor. Miniinvasive Face and Body Lifts - Closed Suture Lifts or Barbed Thread Lifts [Internet]. London: IntechOpen; 2013 [cited 2022 Jun 26]. Available from: https://www.intechopen.com/chapters/45724 doi: 10.5772/56250.

5

FILLER

FILLER COMPLICATIONS IN THE UPPER THIRD OF THE FACE: GLABELLA AND TEMPLES

Giuseppe Sito, Silvia Silenzi

Hyaluronic acid (HA) injections are among the most popular treatments for the correction of facial imperfections, erasing the signs of ageing, such as wrinkles, and restoring skin volume and firmness [1]. Fillers have become so popular because they are medical devices with a high safety profile that guarantee immediate and long-lasting results with a shorter recovery time than plastic surgery.

Nevertheless, aesthetic treatments with hyaluronic acid gel are not without side effects. Mild, moderate or severe adverse events (AEs) may occur following filler treatments. Clinical manifestations include pain, swelling, redness, oedema, nodules, granulomas, skin discolouration, necrosis, infection and biofilm formation. Depending on the moment at which they occur, adverse events are classified into acute, delayed and late.

While the use of fillers is relatively simple, to ensure safe treatment, the injector must have a thorough anatomical knowledge and must also take precaution to avoid areas of risk and the occurrence of severe adverse events.

Anatomy

The anatomy of the face is complex and intricate. We, as doctors, aim to guarantee our patients the highest level of care and safety. A thorough anatomical knowledge of the face is essential to avoid complications following aesthetic treatments. The ability to predict the position of deep anatomical structures such as blood vessels and nerves, based on signs on the surface, is of fundamental importance to the injector.

The aim of this chapter is to examine the upper third of the face, particularly the glabella and temples, providing an overview of the anatomy and highlighting aspects relevant to the safe treatment of this area of the face.

Anatomy of the glabella

The glabella represents the glabrous (hairless) area between the two eyebrow arches and it is the craniometric point corresponding to the maximum prominence, on the median sagittal plane of the skull, of the lower part of the frontal bone. The glabella is closely related to the frontal sinuses, the nasion, and provides attachment to the fibres of the orbital part of the orbicularis oculi and the procerus muscle. The transverse ends of the more superficial corrugator muscle merge with the fibres of the orbicularis oculi [2,3].

The central part of the forehead plays an important role in facial expression. The combination of the frontal fibres, the procerus muscle, the eyebrow corrugator and depressor muscles and the pars medialis of the orbicularis oculi form the glabellar complex [3,4]. Over time, the continuous and repeated contraction of these hyperdynamic muscles causes the formation of distinctive horizontal and vertical lines (fig. 1).

The glabellar rhytids are important

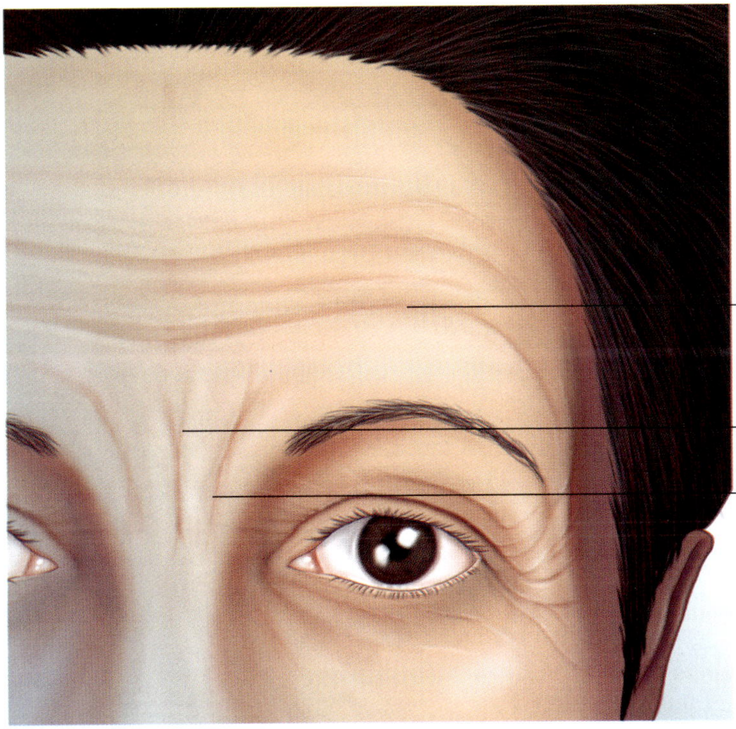

Figure 1 Vertical and horizontal folds of the glabella and forehead

as they are dynamic and functional in determining the position of the underlying anatomical structures. The glabella, along with the forehead lines, is often treated in aesthetic medicine with injections of fillers and botulinum toxin; as a result, topographical analysis of this area is important to avoid complications.

The vertical crease, also known as the corrugator, is considered as a point of reference for locating the course of the supratrochlear artery, which supplies the soft tissue of the central forehead, as well as the position of the fat compartments, nerves and muscles (fig. 2) [5].

The central frontal fat compartment is distinguished by the vertical crease of the corrugator and the midline of the forehead. This compartment has been clearly highlighted by anatomical studies on cadavers using coloured gels that can identify the edges of the various fat compartments of the face (fig. 3).

The corrugator wrinkle also seems to form parallel to the path of the supratrochlear artery (fig. 4) [5]. This peculiar feature makes it possible to use the topography of the superficial folds as indicators to predict the position and direction of the underlying blood vessels. Knowledge of the vascularisation of the glabella is particularly important as the injection of gel directly into a fold in this area risks damaging the regional blood supply. This is one of the possible causes of prolonged haematoma or ischaemia as well as other severe adverse events

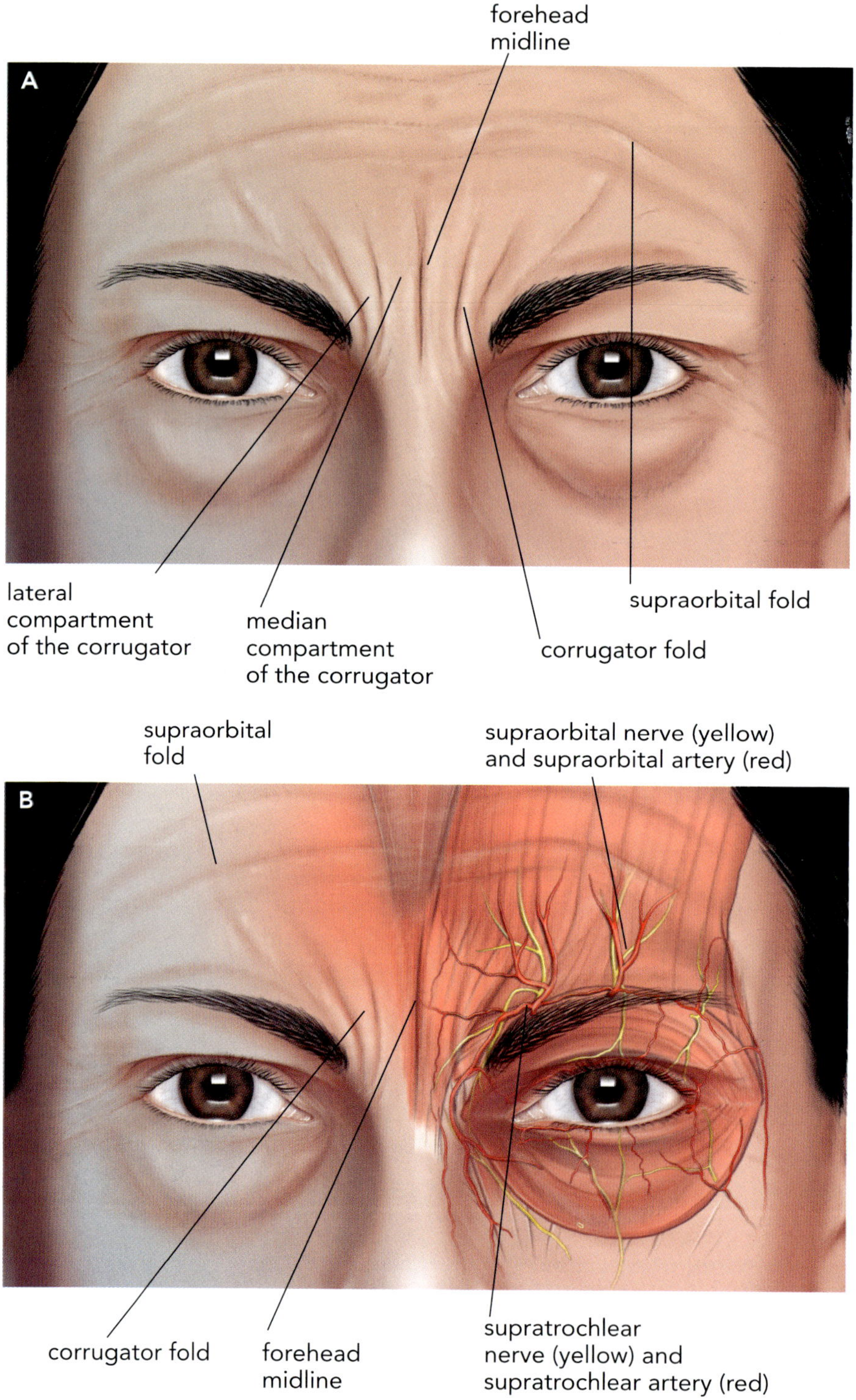

Figure 2 Glabellar lines and underlying structures. Topographical analysis of the superficial folds helps to identify the relative position of the underlying anatomical structures

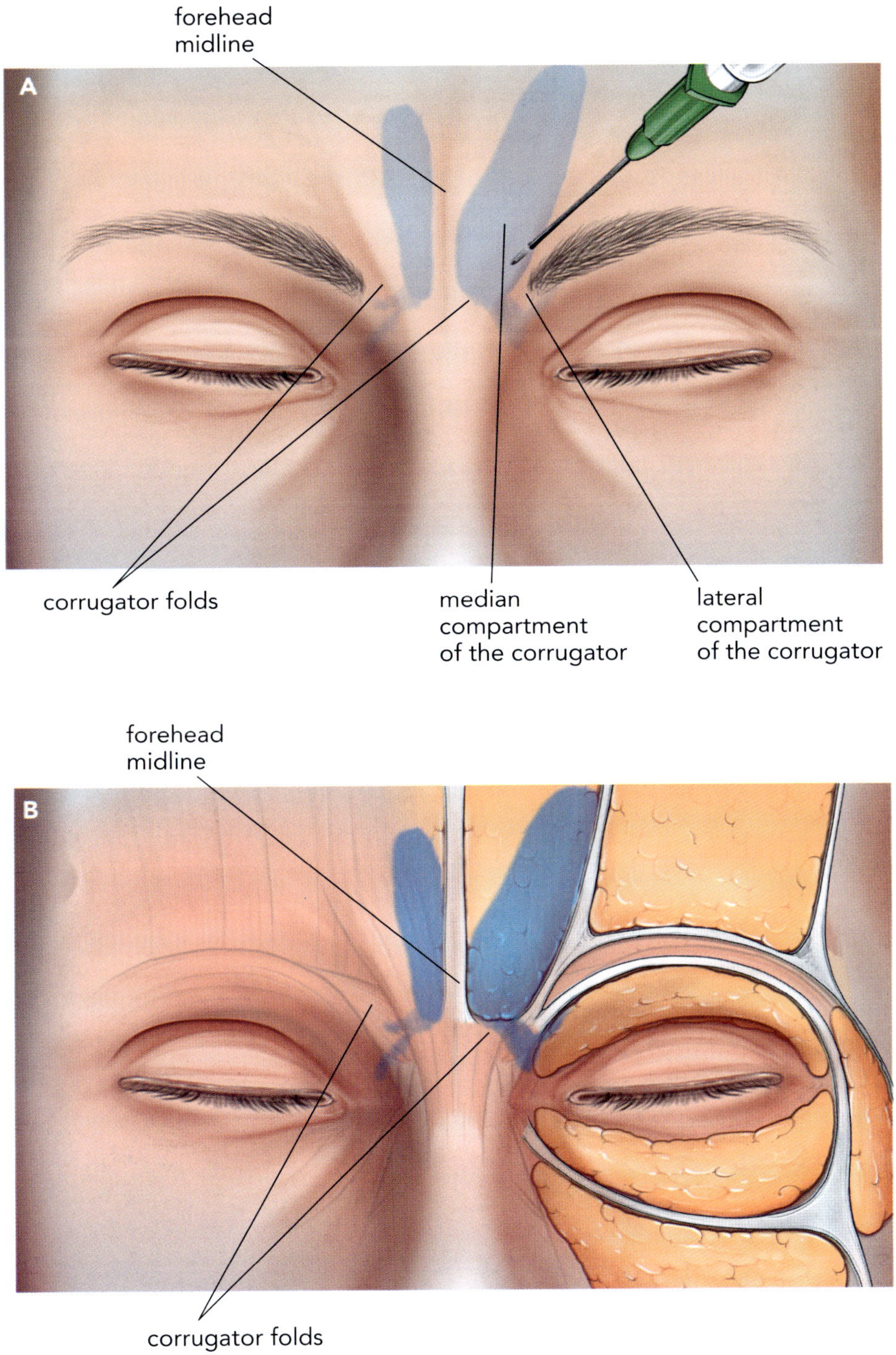

Figure 3 Glabellar lines and underlying structures. The vertical lines of the corrugator and the midline of the glabella demarcate the fat compartments of the face. Anatomical studies performed on cadavers using coloured injectables. The fat compartments of the face are distinct and separate: the dye injected into one compartment does not spread to the adjacent compartment

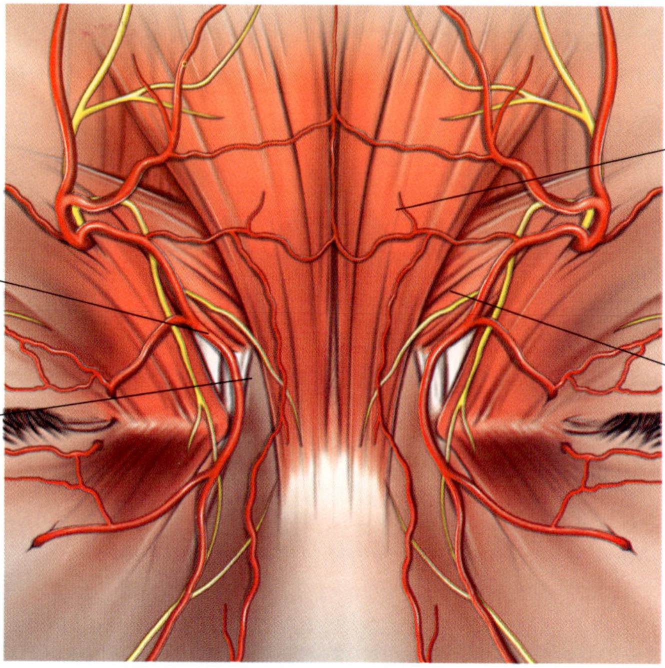

Figure 4 Glabellar lines and underlying structures. The vertical line of the corrugator marks the relative position of the supratrochlear artery

described in literature. Complications can be avoided by adopting the right medical practices based on in-depth anatomical knowledge. In a 2020 paper by Cotofana S. et al. [6], ultrasound examination was performed on healthy volunteers to identify the path of the superficial branch of the supratrochlear artery and the deep branch of the supraorbital artery with respect to the ipsilateral vertical glabellar line. The mean distance between the superficial branch of the supratrochlear artery and the ipsilateral vertical glabellar line was 10.59 mm in males and 8.21 mm in females; while for the supraorbital artery, this distance was 22.4 mm and 20.7 mm in males and females, respectively.

When frowning, a medial displacement in the position of the supratrochlear artery of 1.6 mm in males and 1.8 mm in females and of 3.9 mm in the supraorbital artery position for both sexes were observed. Lastly, the average depth of the supratrochlear artery at rest and of the supraorbital artery with respect to the skin surface was 3.3 mm and 3.5 mm, respectively [6].

The vertical fold of the corrugator and the glabellar midline help to identify the relative position of other important structures in this area such as the supraorbital and supratrochlear nerves. Anatomical studies of the path of the supraorbital and supratrochlear nerves indicate that they follow well-defined routes [7,8]. The supraorbital nerve originates approximately 21 to 35 mm from the glabellar midline

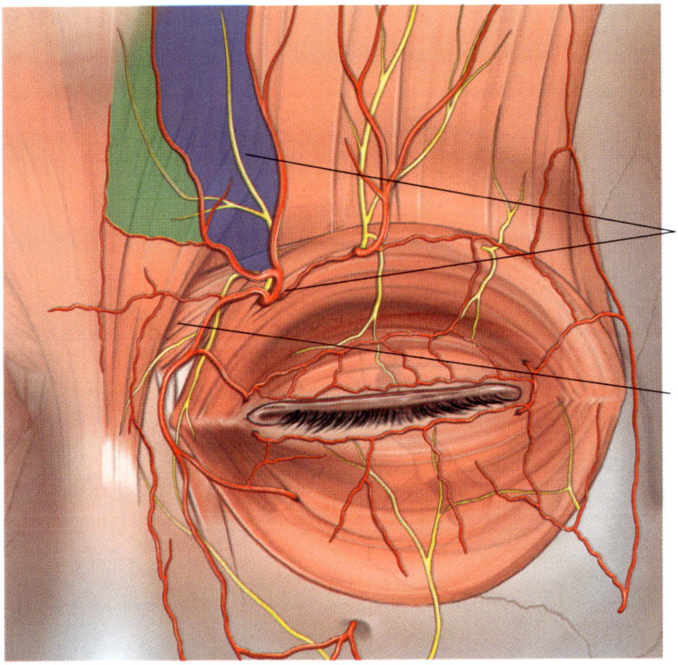

Figure 5 Glabellar lines and underlying structures. The vertical line of the corrugator marks the relative position of the supratrochlear artery and nerve

and divides into superficial and deep branches. The superficial branch penetrates the frontalis muscle and runs superiorly in the subcutaneous plane to the vertex of the scalp. The deep branch runs deeply towards the frontalis muscle and the eyebrow corrugator muscle, travelling superiorly and laterally between the periosteum and the galea towards the temporal fusion line [9,10]. The supratrochlear nerve, on the other hand, exits the orbit between the pulley of the superior oblique muscle and the supraorbital foramen. Passing underneath the corrugator muscles, it runs upwards together with the supratrochlear artery to innervate the skin of the glabella, medial forehead, upper eyelid and medial conjunctiva (fig. 5) [11].

Complications of the glabella: description and critical analysis

While HA-based fillers have a high safety profile, adverse events (AEs) have been reported at glabella level. Minimal and self-limited complications, such as bruising, redness and swelling, are relatively common and resolve spontaneously without any consequences for the patient. However, more serious adverse events, such as visual impairment, necrosis and anaphylaxis, have also been reported.

In the case of ischaemic events, therapeutic recommendations include prompt administration of high-dose hyaluronidase (HYAL) and warm compresses. The half-life of hyaluronidase is short, so it should be reconstituted shortly before use, with repetition of injections every two hours

until the capillary refill time improves.
Skin necrosis is a rare complication, a consequence of untreated vascular impairment, which can be detrimental to a patient's health if not treated properly. Possible causes are direct trauma to the vessel wall, accidental intravascular injection of a filler or direct pressure of the filler on the vessel, causing obstruction of the lumen. Injection-related oedema is another possible mechanism of impaired blood flow, as it contributes with external force to the compression of the vessel wall [13]. All this can lead to tissue anoxia, ischaemia with possible progression to necrosis [12,14].
Initial (though not pathognomonic) signs and symptoms of altered blood flow include: pain during administration of the product with blanching of the skin (immediate); *livedo reticularis* (marbling) with or without numbness of the area (minutes-hours); blue or grey-blue skin discolouration (1-2 days); presence of blisters (2-4 days) followed by demarcation of a distinct margin of hyperaemia surrounding frank necrosis with flaking and ulceration (days-weeks) if the occlusion persists [12,14].
In patients with "impending necrosis", the symptoms and related ischaemic signs resolve with prompt intervention without causing permanent damage. However, there are cases of delayed compression of vessels by the product that do not trigger immediate signs. Occlusion of an artery causes immediate pain and whitening of the area, while venous obstruction usually manifests with a delayed, purplish reticulated appearance [13,15].
Numerous methods are used to resolve vascular compression and the choice of treatment varies depending on when the patient is seen by the injecting practitioner. In the case of immediate manifestation of signs of an ischaemic event, it is advisable to stop injecting and gently massage the area [12,16,17]. Hyaluronidase should be administered promptly at a high dosage, with the application of hot compresses and cream or nitro-glycerine patches [12,16,17]. Injections of hyaluronidase, at decreasing concentrations, should be administered at predetermined short intervals until vascular flow is restored [12,16-18]. In the event of blistering, antibiotics (by mouth and/or cream) should be prescribed [16,19]. Anticoagulant therapy (7-day course of low-dose ASA6) should also be considered [12,19,18], with hyperbaric oxygen in severe cases [19]. It is advisable to assist the patient, without sending them home, at least until the symptoms begin to disappear.

Anatomy of the temporal fossa

The temporal fossa has a very complex anatomy due to the multiple layers that make it up and the vessels that run through them. Anatomical knowledge of this area can be helpful in critically analysing the reasons for the hollowing of the temples due to ageing and the most successful aesthetic correction techniques (fig. 6).
The layers of the temporal region, from the outside to the inside, are: the skin, the subcutaneous tissue, the temporoparietal fascia (TPF), the deep temporal fascia, the superficial fat pad and the temporalis muscle [20,21]. The temporal fossa has well-defined boundaries and a reproducible method for understanding the anatomy of this area is to divide it into the superior and inferior temporal compartments [22].

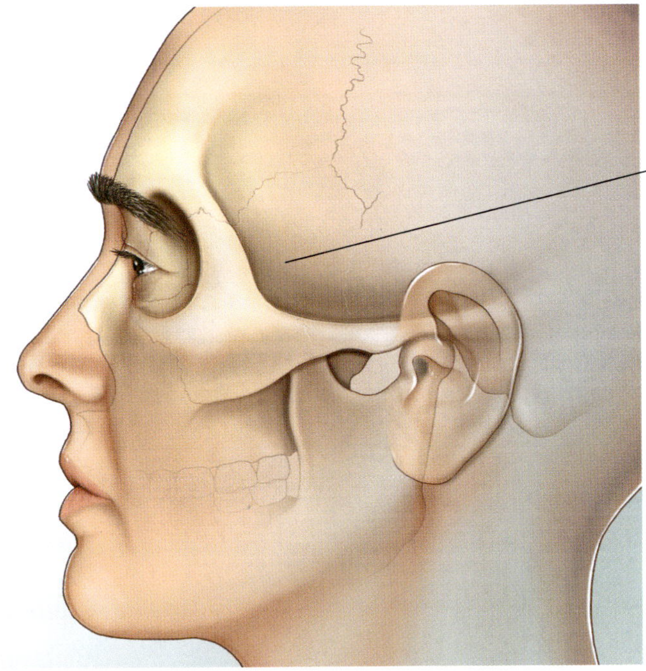

Figure 6 Temporal fossa

The superior temporal compartment is delimited superiorly by the superior temporal septum. This septum represents the deep boundary between the central forehead and the temporal fossa where the periosteum fits into the line joining the superficial temporal fascia and the galea (fig. 7) [23]. This joining line lies anteriorly between the superficial temporal fascia and the galea that covers the deep surface of the lateral edge of the frontalis muscle; while posteriorly it forms a large area of adhesion located 30 mm from the supraorbital rim known as the temporal triangular ligamentous adhesion (TLA) [20]. The TLA represents the convergence of the superior and inferior temporal septa.

There are no vital structures in the superior temporal septum and it is within the limits of this space that it is possible to see the transzonal passage of the temporal fat compartment by the two laminae of the deep temporal fascia.

The inferior temporal compartment is delimited by the cephalic border, which represents the inferior septum. This septum is located on average 27 mm above the zygoma at the level of the temporal border of the frontal process. The inferior septum is oblique and forms a line extending from the lateral angle of the temporal ligament to the external acoustic meatus. This septum forms the upper edge of a triangular fibro-adipose compartment between the underlying superficial and deep temporal fascia. This fascia condenses as it travels caudally towards the lower cheekbone, merging with the zygomatic-cutaneous ligaments and forming the lower border of the compartment (fig. 8) [20,23].

A thorough knowledge of the vascular anatomy of the temporal region is impor-

Figure 7
Temporal fossa. Schematisation of the superior and inferior temporal layers and septa

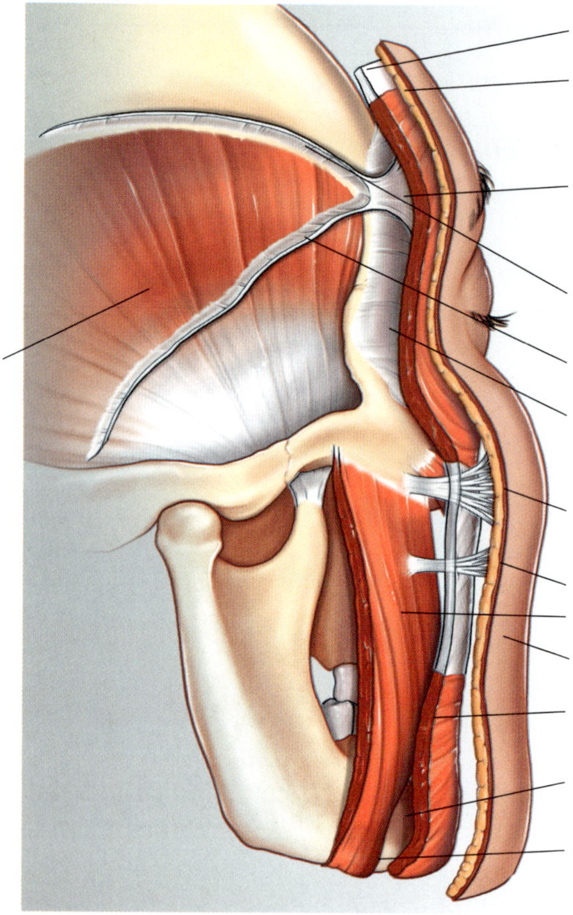

tant to avoid possible complications. The proximity of the dense fascia zone and tight muscular and vascular network in this region may involve the risk of performing a perivascular injection with its associated undesirable effects. The temporal region receives its vascular supply from three separate branches of the external carotid artery. The superficial temporal artery (STA) runs within the temporoparietal fascia (TPF) and its anterior branch runs with the temporal branches of the facial nerve and often communicates with the supraorbital artery (fig. 9). The mid and deep temporal arteries are located within the deep temporal fascia. The deep temporal artery originates from the internal maxillary artery. Unintentional injection into one of these arteries can cause retrograde vascular occlusion resulting in significant complications including retrograde thrombosis of the ophthalmic system with occlusion of the central retinal artery, and cause blindness [23].

Injections with a needle in the lower medial quadrant of the temporal fossa only are recommended to avoid these undesirable effects. The use of cannulas is recommended for the rest of the temple, in both the superior temporal compartment, which is a vessel-free plane, and in the superficial temporal fat compartments.

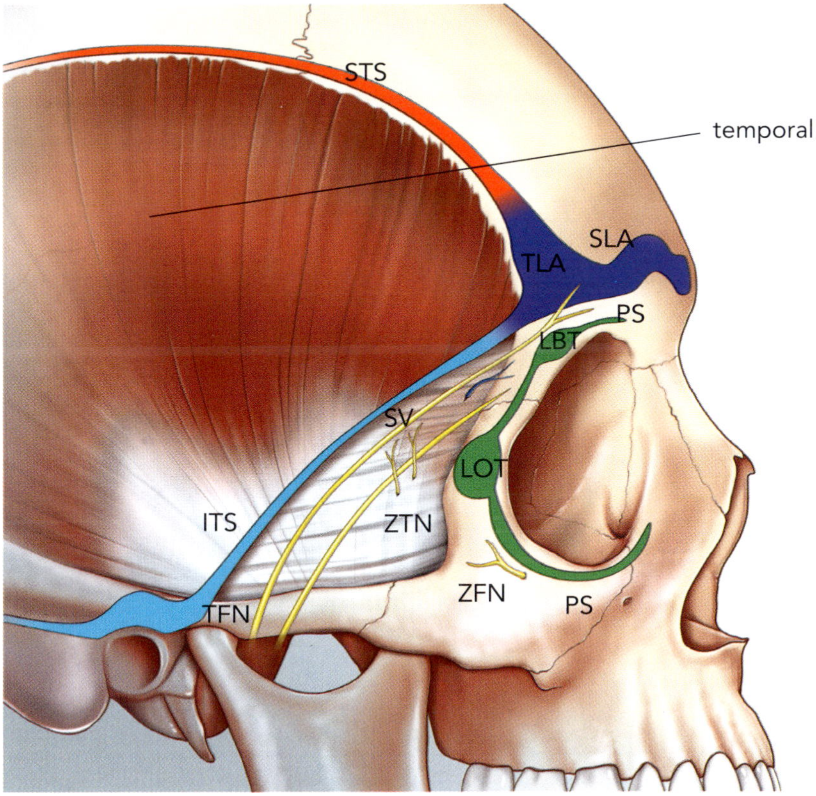

Figure 8 Periorbital and temporal ligamentous attachments with the main neurovascular relationships: lateral view. Temporal ligamentous attachment (TLA), supraorbital ligamentous attachment (SLA), superior temporal septum (STS), inferior temporal septum (ITS), periorbital septum (PS), lateral thickening of the front of the periorbital septum (LBT) lateral orbital thickening of periorbital septum (LOT), sentinel vessel (SV), temporal branches of the facial nerve (TFN), zygomatic-temporal nerve (ZTN), zygomatic-facial nerve (ZFN)

Complications of the temples

Most of the complications affecting the temples as a result of the use of HA fillers are severe. However, the adverse events recorded in this area are extremely rare and, where present, they are hard to illustrate with mere pictures. The authors of this book have not had any cases of complications related to treatment of the temples during their experience. This is why reference is made to the cases described in literature.

Bibliography

1. Wollina U, Goldman A. Facial vascular danger zones for filler injections. Dermatol Ther. 2020;33(6).
2. Knize DM. Muscles that act on glabellar skin: A closer look. Plast Reconstr Surg. 2000;105(1).
3. Pessino K, Patel J, Patel BC. Anatomy, Head and Neck, Frontalis Muscle; 2020.
4. Brown TM, Krishnamurthy K. Anatomy, Head and Neck, Procerus Muscle; 2019.

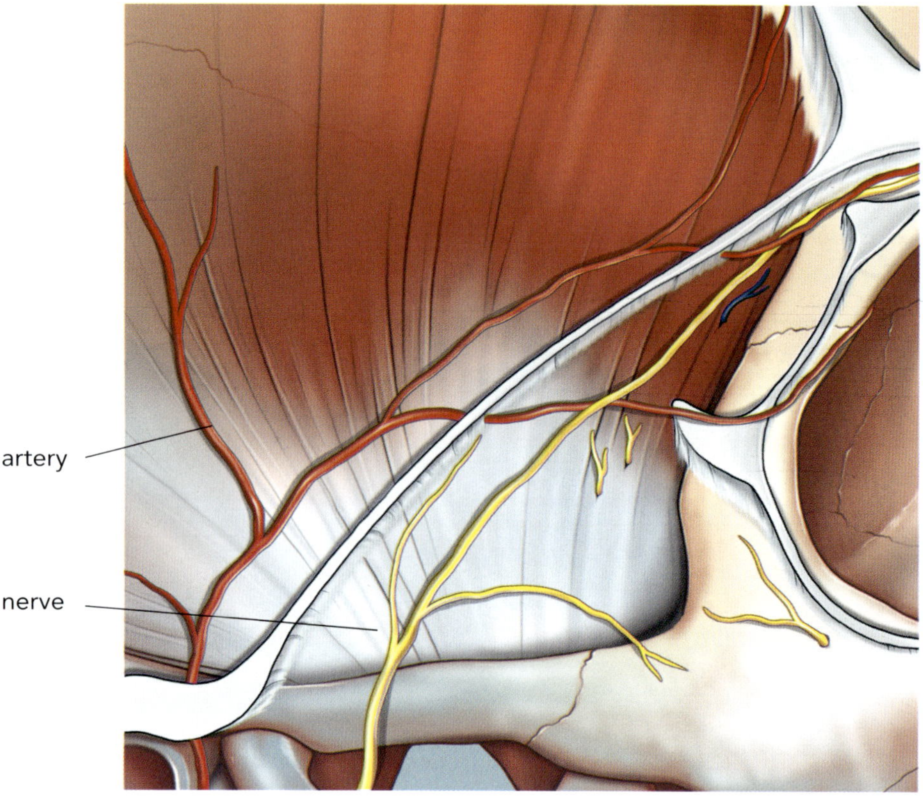

Figure 9 Intersection of the frontal branch of the facial nerve and the anterior branch of the superficial temporal artery

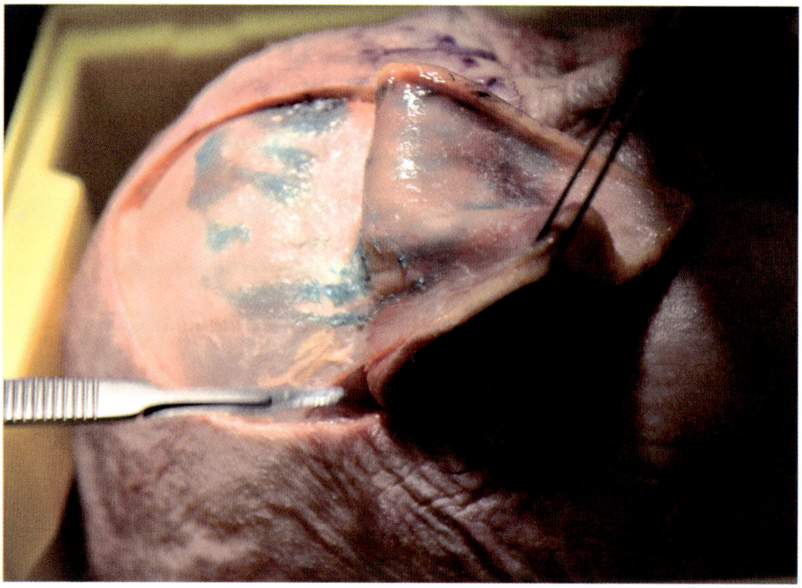

Figure 10 Dissection of the temporal fossa

5. Pessa Joel E., MD, Joel E. Pessa and MD RJR. Facial Topography : Clinical Anatomy of the Face. In: CRC Press LLC; 2012:14-46.
6. Cotofana S, Alfertshofer M, Frank K, et al. Relationship between Vertical Glabellar Lines and the Supratrochlear and Supraorbital Arteries. Aesthetic Surg J. 2020;40(12).
7. Knize DM. A study of the supraorbital nerve. Plast Reconstr Surg. 1995;96:564-569.
8. Beer GM, Putz R, Mager K, Schumacher M KW. Variations of the frontal exit of the supraorbital nerve: an anatomic study. Plast Reconstr Surg. 1998;102:334-341.
9. Malet T, Braun M, Fyad JP, George JL. Anatomic study of the distal supraorbital nerve. Surg Radiol Anat. 1998;19(6).
10. Christensen KN, Lachman N, Pawlina W, Baum CL. Cutaneous depth of the supraorbital nerve: A cadaveric anatomic study with clinical applications to dermatology. Dermatologic Surg. 2014;40(12).
11. Huff T, Daly DT. Neuroanatomy, Cranial Nerve 5 (Trigeminal); 2019.
12. Snozzi P, Van Loghem JAJ. Complication management following rejuvenation procedures with hyaluronic acid fillers-an algorithm-based approach. Plast Reconstr Surg - Glob Open. 2018;6(12).
13. Daines SM, Williams EF. Complications associated with injectable soft-tissue fillers: A 5-year retrospective review. JAMA Facial Plast Surg. 2013;15(3).
14. Funt D, Pavicic T. Dermal Fillers in Aesthetics: An Overview of Adverse Events and Treatment Approaches. Plast Surg Nurs. 2015;35(1):13-32.
15. Vidič M, Bartenjev I. An adverse reaction after hyaluronic acid filler application: A case report. Acta Dermatovenerologica Alpina, Pannonica Adriat. 2018;27(3).
16. Sito G, Manzoni V, Sommariva R. Vascular complications after facial filler injection: A Literature Review and Meta-analysis. J Clin Aesthet Dermatol. 2019;12(6).
17. DeLorenzi C. New high dose pulsed hyaluronidase protocol for hyaluronic acid filler vascular adverse events. Aesthetic Surg J. 2017;37(7).
18. Cohen JL, Biesman BS, Dayan SH, et al. Treatment of hyaluronic acid filler-induced impending necrosis with hyaluronidase: Consensus recommendations. Aesthetic Surg J. 2015;35(7).
19. De Boulle K, Heydenrych I. Patient factors influencing dermal filler complications: Prevention, assessment, and treatment. Clin Cosmet Investig Dermatol. 2015;8:205-214.
20. Moss CJ, Mendelson BC, Taylor GI. Surgical anatomy of the ligamentous attachments in the temple and periorbital regions. Plast Reconstr Surg. 2000;105(4).
21. Cotofana S, Lachman N. Anatomie der Fettkompartimente des Gesichts und ihre Bedeutung für die ästhetische Chirurgie. JDDG - J Ger Soc Dermatology. 2019;17(4).
22. Mendelson B, Wong CH. Anatomy of the aging face. In: Neligan PC, ed. Plastic Surgery. 3rd Philad. Philadelphia; 2013:78-92.
23. Lamb JP, Surek CC. Facial Volumization: An Anatomic Approach. In: Thieme Medical Publisher Inc, ed. Facial Volumization: An Anatomic Approach; 2017:61-66.

FILLER COMPLICATIONS IN THE MIDDLE THIRD OF THE FACE: RHINOFILLER

Alberto Diaspro, Cristina Sartorio

The nose is in the middle of the face and is key to its aesthetic balance. Any alteration in its length, width or position of the tip, or a deformity such as hump or deviation, affects all the facial features. It changes during the ageing process, the most important changes being the altered projection of the tip, often due to hypertonia of the nasal septum depressor muscle as well as gravitational ptosis.
Surgical rhinoplasty is the therapy of choice but many patients prefer to consider so-called "non-surgical rhinoplasty" or "liquid rhinoplasty" thanks to its minimal invasiveness. While allowing only the correction of "minor" defects and with a temporary result, this technique is interesting for patients who prefer to avoid or are unsuitable for surgery under general anaesthetic. It also allows the correction of residual imperfections without having to undergo a new surgical procedure.
As with surgical rhinoplasty, three-dimensional reshaping is performed by means of grafts [1-3], the treatment plane must be addressed and the injections must be performed according to the same rules [4]. Consequently, the practitioner who intends to perform this technique is required to have a sound knowledge of the surgical anatomy, as well as the structural and vascular anatomy of the nose.
The most common complications of non-surgical reshaping are of significant severity and are hard to manage for both patient and physician. [5-6]
The nasal region is highly vascularised and this chapter presents the safest reshaping techniques using injectables to avoid injury to these structures, which are the most effective way to avoid complications, even severe ones.

Anatomy

The correct knowledge of the anatomical planes is necessary to allow a safe procedure and predictable results, as with any surgical or non-surgical intervention on the face (fig. 1) [5,8,9,10].
The superficial intradermal plane is avascular, but the subcutaneous layer of superficial fat contains major blood vessels, so inoculation of the product in this area must be carefully avoided. The superficial musculoaponeurotic system (SMAS) of the nose still has blood vessels on the inside, while the underlying layer is the safest for injection, as it is relatively avascular. Lastly, the perichondrium and periosteum adhere closely to the cartilage and bone respectively (figs. 2-3).

Injectable materials

Non-surgical nose reshaping techniques using hyaluronic acid were first mentioned in 2006 [11], while those using collagen were mentioned in 2007 [12], with the first comprehensive article on the use of hyaluronic acid and botulinum toxin published by an Italian author in 2008 [13].
Injectable polylactic acid, polyacryla-

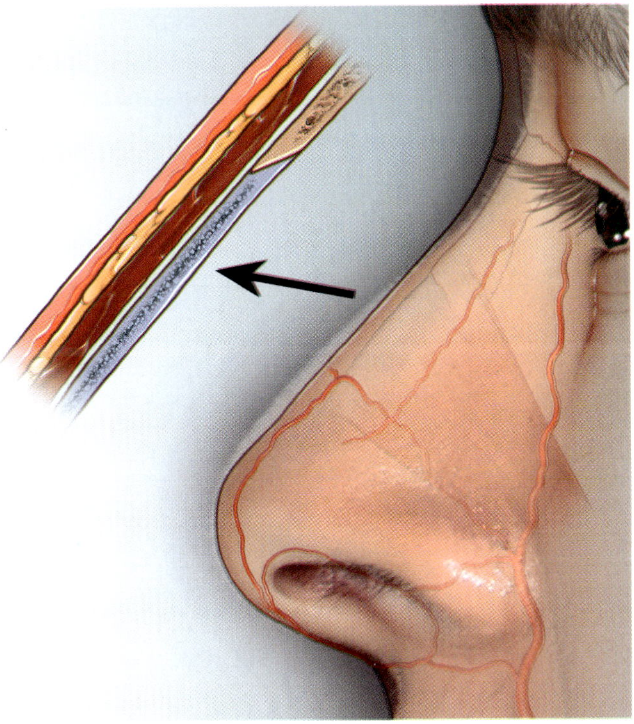

Figure 1 Anatomical layers of the nasal region: detail. Epidermis and dermis; subcutaneous fatty tissue (of varying thickness); nasal muscles (nasal SMAS); areolar lax connective tissue; perichondrium/ periosteum

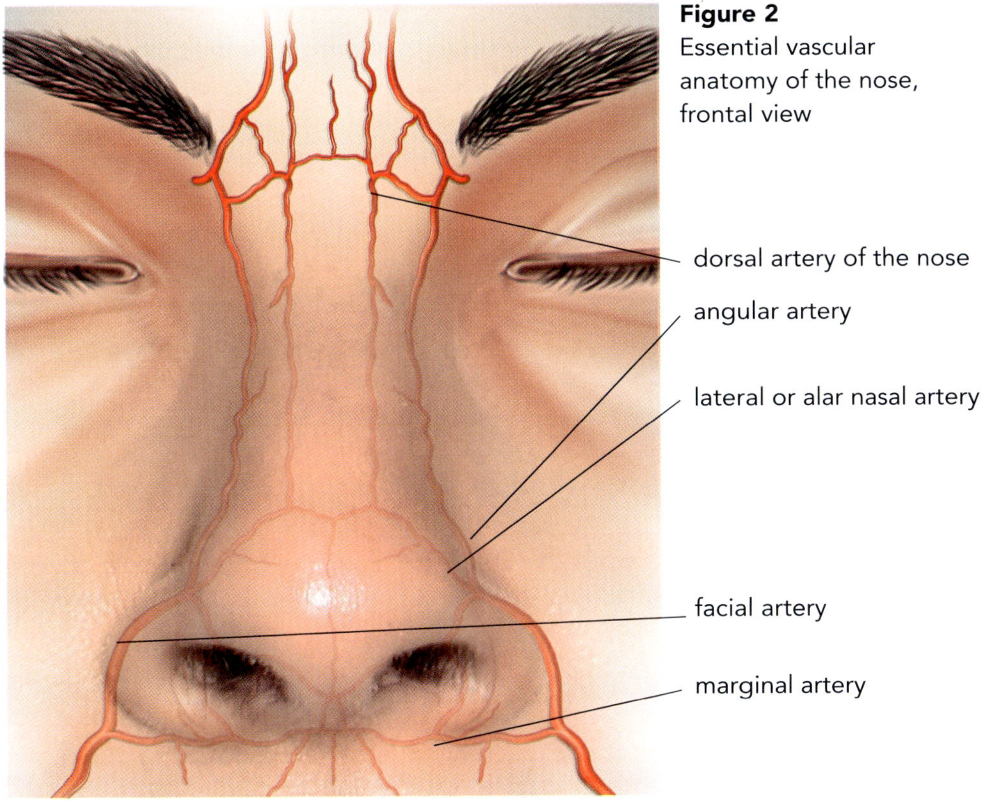

Figure 2 Essential vascular anatomy of the nose, frontal view

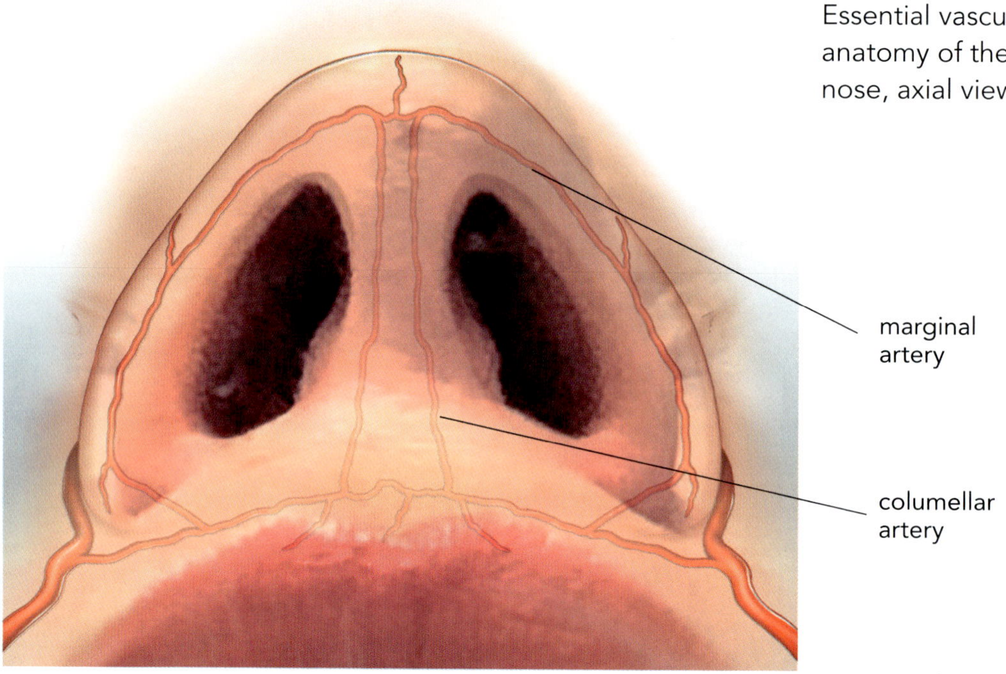

Figure 3
Essential vascular anatomy of the nose, axial view

mide and tricalcium phosphate [14][15] were subsequently used and, in 2019, the use of carboxymethylcellulose [16] was reported for the first time, with submucosa injection for functional purposes, to improve upper airway aerodynamics in a patient with "empty nose syndrome". This use of hyaluronic acid to functionally improve the external nasal valve had already been published in 2012 [17].

Key points to maximise the safety of infiltration

Hyaluronic acid filling agent can always be dissolved by hyaluronidase, which makes it the product of choice. The injection must always be performed in a deep plane, either supraperiosteal or supraperichondral, and the pressure applied to the syringe plunger must be very measured, with slow infiltration so that the tissues can adapt to the product injected, always in small quantities to avoid sometimes delayed oedema.
Gentle massage after injection allows the best possible shaping of the implant.
The strictly intradermal plane allows the injection of small amounts of product when minor corrections are required [7].
Never inject into any layer of the alar groove area, the tip or the edge of the nostril, as the lateral nasal arteries, which are terminal, run through these areas (figs. 4-6).
Patients who have undergone previous septorhinoplasty surgery have an altered anatomy and the anatomical planes are no longer identifiable: this puts them at significantly increased risk and they may be considered unsuitable for the procedure [18].

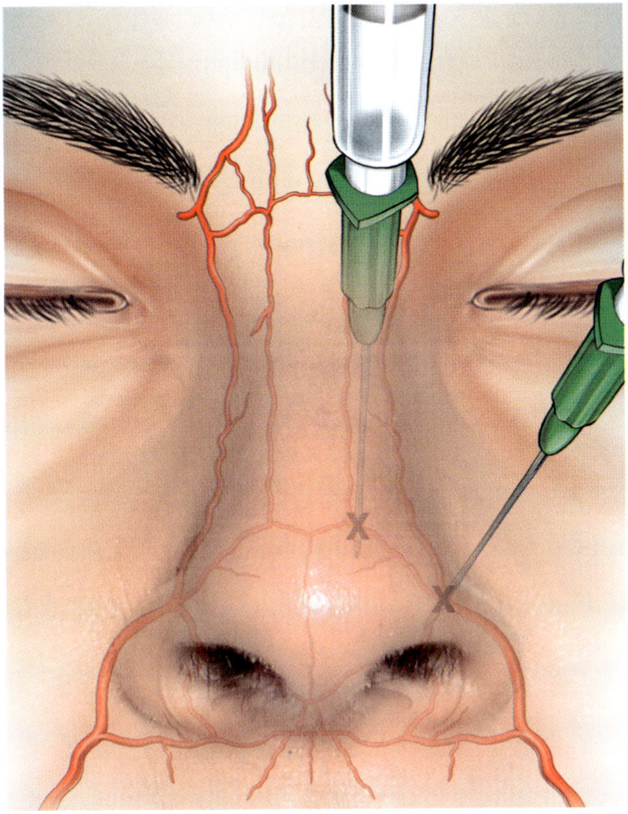

Figure 4
Incorrect technique with needle on upper and middle third of the nose, in the superficial plane: frontal view. Lesion of dorsal artery, angular artery and/or lateral (or alar) nasal artery

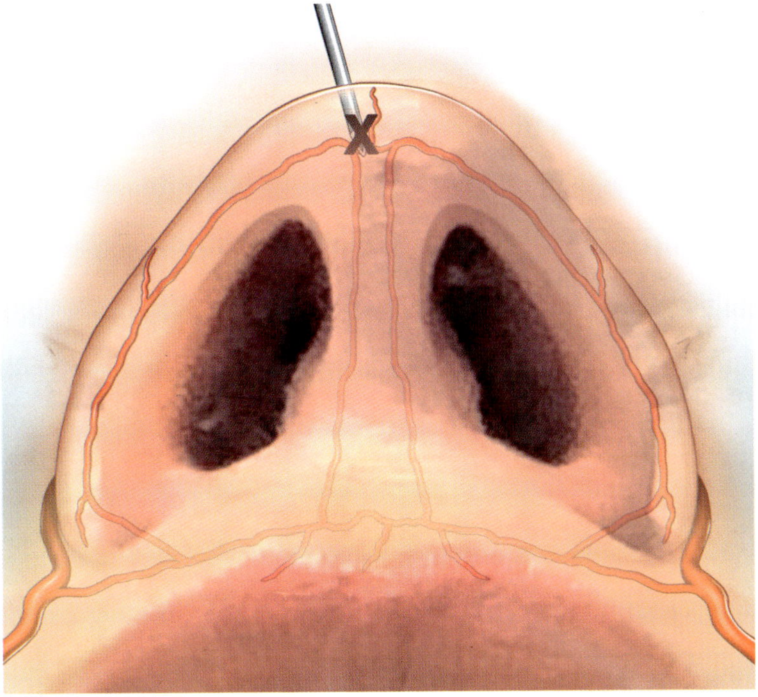

Figure 5
Incorrect technique with needle in the tip, in the superficial plane: axial view. Marginal artery lesion

Treatment phases:

- collection of informed consent and written post-treatment instructions;
- removal of make-up and disinfection;
- possible topical anaesthetic;
- injection: vertical with a 13 mm 30 G needle or with a 40/50 mm 25 G cannula and bolus technique. Strictly intradermal with a 4 mm long 30/32 G or less needle when minor corrections are required;
- massage (ensure adequate distribution of the gel);
- have the patient wait for about 15/30 minutes after implantation and then make a follow-up appointment;
- telephone availability to receive call regarding any suspicious signs or symptoms.

A number of injection techniques have been developed to enable a specific clinical result [4,7,19]. From an operational point of view, we recommend being comfortable and assuming a correct posture when performing the implant: holding the syringe with the dominant hand and using the other to place pressure on the injection site when necessary. With frontal vision we are able to appreciate and therefore correct deviations of the nasal pyramid and the aesthetic lines of the nose. Correction of deviations of the nasal pyramid is achieved by selectively filling the lateral wall of the nose on the opposite side to the deviation, with a vertical deposit technique that allows us to achieve the maximum projection effect using the smallest amount of product,

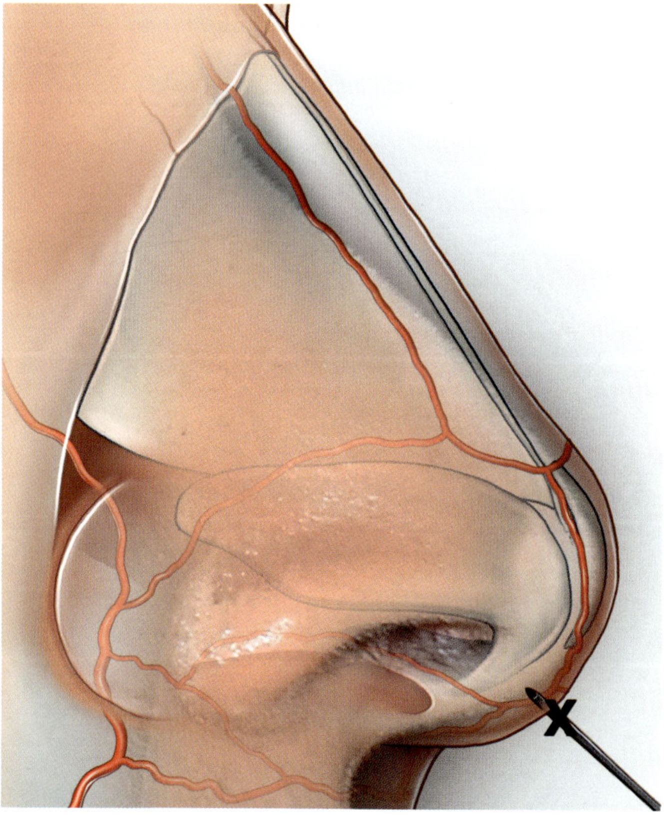

Figure 6
Incorrect technique with needle in the tip, in the superficial plane: oblique view. Marginal artery lesion

with visual improvement of even significant soft tissue deficits. The use of high G′ gels which tend not to spread to the adjacent tissues is advisable.
When preparing for the correction of the aesthetic lines of the nose, we use a retrograde linear technique instead: with both techniques it is best to inject the product into a median or lateral site (figs. 7-8) avoiding the para-median and basal areas (fig. 9).
With lateral vision, on the other hand, we focus on the correction of the hump and the projection and rotation of the nasal tip. When we undertake the correction of the hump, we address the filling of the cephalically depressed area at the angle of curvature, using a bolus technique with implantation in the periosteal plane. When we wish to harmonise the tip of the nose, we do so with the selective filling of the cephalic portion of the tip, using a fanning technique, finally projecting it with a bolus into the nasal spine [10].

Planning the technique in view of the desired results

It is absolutely essential to be aware of the main angles in order to achieve a harmonious profile:

- naso-frontal angle at the centre of which we identify a point called the Nasion at the root of the nose, on the nasofrontal suture, 12-14° wide;
- naso-facial angle, between the nasal spine and the facial plane (forehead-chin line), usually about 30°;

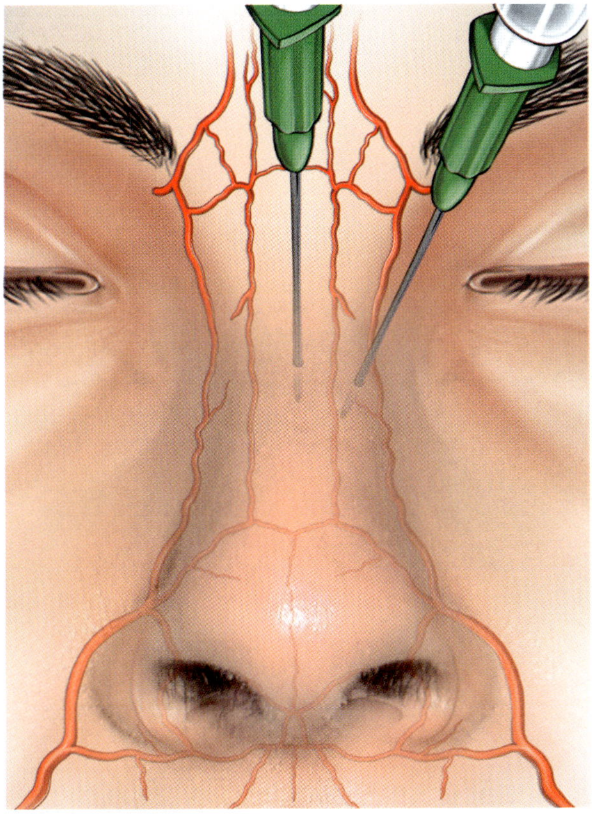

Figure 7
Injection technique with needle on upper and middle third of the nose, in the deep pre-periosteal plane: safe areas, frontal view

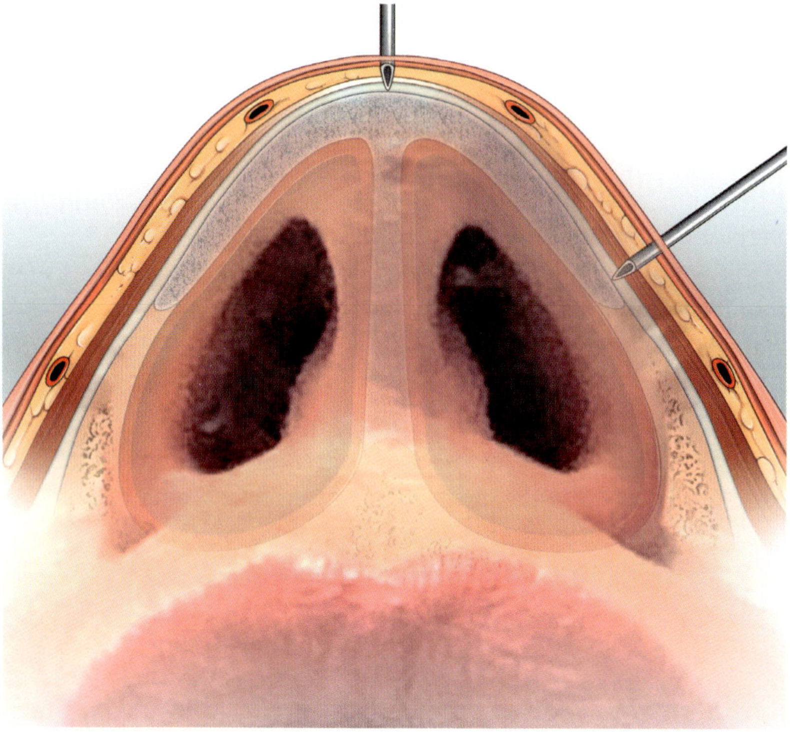

Figure 8
Injection technique with needle on upper and middle third of the nose, in the deep pre-periosteal/ perichondral plane: safe areas, frontal view

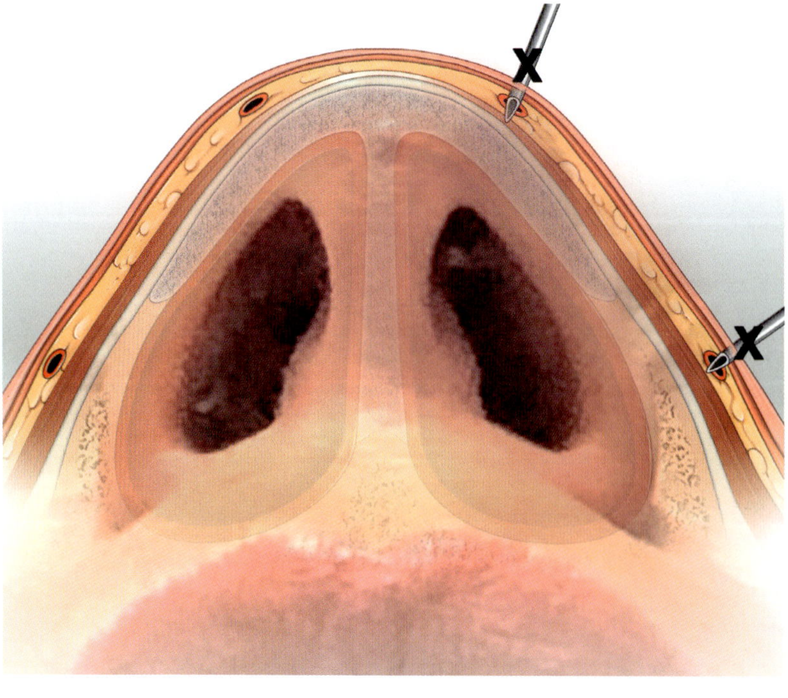

Figure 9
Incorrect technique with needle on upper and middle third of the nose, in the superficial plane: axial view. Lesion of the dorsal artery and angular artery

- naso-labial angle;
- naso-mental angle between the aesthetic line of Ricketts and the vertical line passing through the tip of the nose, usually 115°-130° wide because it is their variation that gives the nose a pleasing shape after injection therapy.

To open up the naso-frontal angle, correcting the retruded nasal root, the following points must be considered.

- Technique: bolus injection.
- Depth: periosteum.
- Injection site: periosteal root of the nose.
- Volume: 0.2-0.5 ml total.
- Instrument: 30 G needle (0.3 x 13 mm).

To straighten the nasal spine in the case of a twisted nose, i.e. concave on the right and convex on the left, or a crooked nose with unilateral concavity when viewed from the front, it is necessary to proceed as follows.

- Technique: bolus/linear retrograde injection, depending on the anatomy with micro-bumps until symmetry is restored.
- Depth: periosteal.
- Injection site: lateral, to prevent unintentional injury of the dorsal nasal artery and angular artery.
- Volume: 0.3-0.8 ml total.
- Instrument: 30 G needle (0.3 x 13 mm).

Infiltration into a superficial or perichondral plane along the cephalic margin of the alar cartilages should be avoided, as it can lead to vascular impairment of the lateral nasal artery.

To raise the tip of the nose by projecting it anti-clockwise, upwards, it is necessary to inject using the following methods.

- Technique: vertical.
- Depth: periosteal directly under the nasal septum.
- Injection site: proximal part of the nasal septum.
- Volume: 0.1-0.3 ml total.
- Instrument: 30 G needle (0.3 x 13 mm).

Never perform superficial infiltrations into the midline of the tip, as this can damage the columellar artery.

The practitioner uses two fingers of the non-injecting hand to gently compress the tissue, asking the patient to breathe through the mouth.

The injection is administered above the bone directly below the nasal septum. The injection depth and volumetric increase are controlled by palpation.

Complications

The complications involved in non-surgical nasal reshaping mainly concern vascular impairment from intravascular injection (fig. 10) like vascular-ophthalmic [20,21], neuro-ophthalmic [22,23], cutaneous-ophthalmic [24] and cutaneous [25] adverse events (video 5.1 and figs. 11-12) while migration of the injected material has been reported [26].

Most cases occurred with the use of hyaluronic acid [27] or calcium hydroxypapatite [28,29], which are the two most commonly used agents.

This is followed by the use of fatty tissue, also in association with the aforementioned products [30].

Non-vascular complications include migration [26] and skin dysesthesia [31], while adverse events reported with other materials such as acrylamide and silicone are related to inflammatory and infectious reactions: granulomatosis [32], intranasal

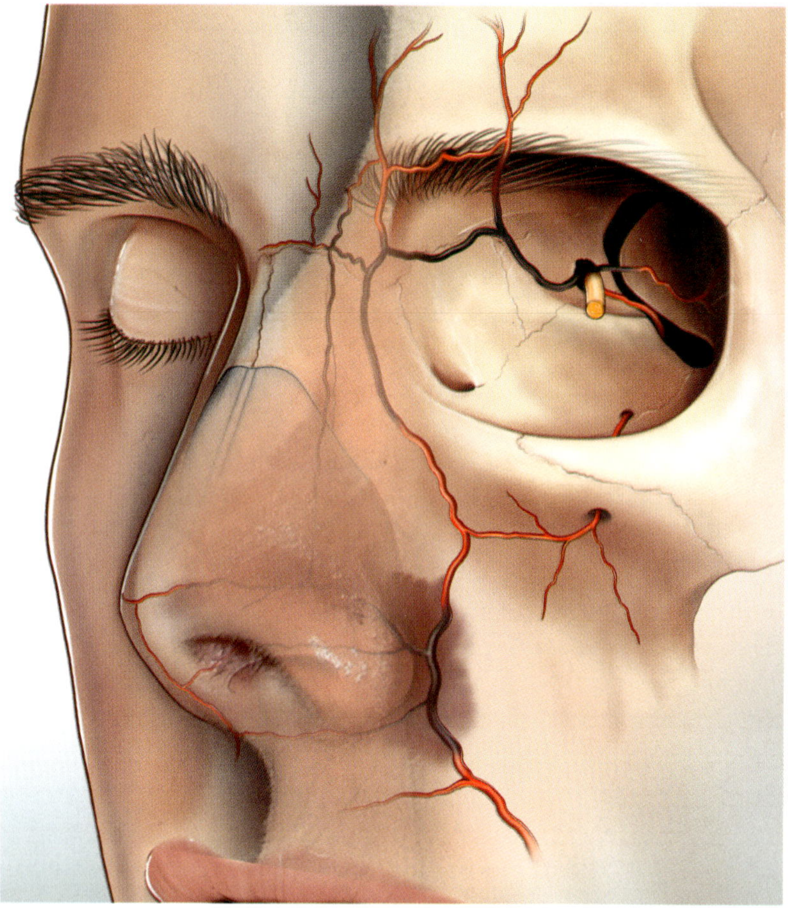

Figure 10
Neuro-ophthalmic impairment caused by retrograde embolisation to the ophthalmic vessels is more likely with injection into: the angular nasal artery; dorsal artery.
Vascular impairment of the cutaneous tissues of the tip, nasal ala and dorsal portion is more likely with superficial plane injections into: cephalic and caudal margin of the alar cartilages; tip; columella.

VIDEO 5.1

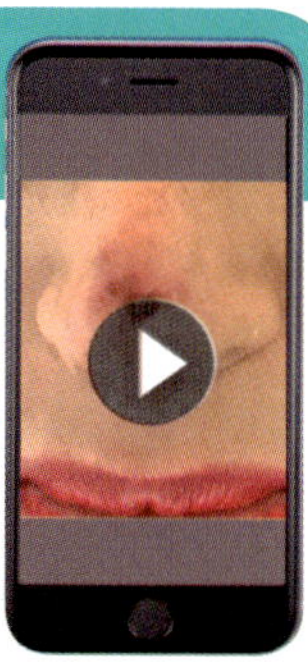

Cutaneous necrosis of the nasal tip: evolution and healing

abscess [33] and dermatomyositis [34].
Articles related to complications have been published since 2008. During the following six years, their presence in international literature was constant, becoming relative in subsequent years until there was a peak of interest culminating in 2018-2019. This is a sign of a consolidated awareness of the problem and its severity.
The papers cited include only one systematic review [35], the others being case series or case reports.

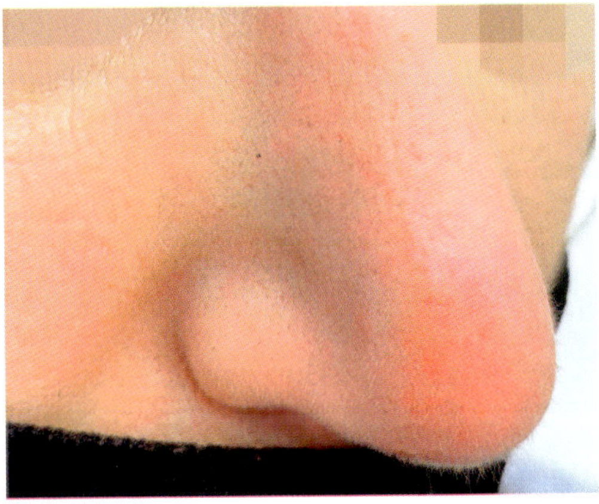

Figure 11 Vascular impairment without necrosis in the tip and nasal spine area

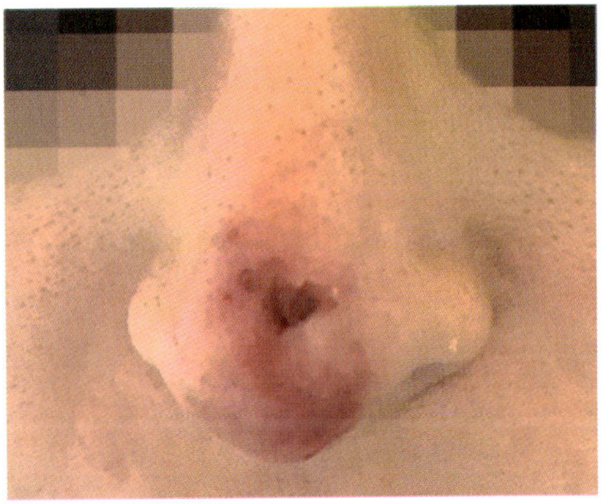

Figure 12 Cutaneous necrosis of the nasal tip

Conclusions

Nasal reshaping using injectables can be a reliable and effective camouflage technique with a high rate of patient satisfaction [36].

The correction of post-surgical deformities requires further attention, given the alterations in the vascular anatomy and the internal characteristic of the residual scar tissue: it is advisable to inject a minimal amount of product and wait an adequate length of time after inoculation.

Unfortunately, despite a conscious choice of material, sound anatomical knowledge and the use of a reliable technique, complications are more likely to occur in the treatment of the nose than in other facial regions.

Bibliography

1. Giacomini PG, Rubino S, Mocella S, Pascali M, Di Girolamo S. Approach to the correction of drooping tip: common problems and solutions. Acta Otorhinolaryngol Ital. 2017 Aug;37(4):295-302.
2. Boccieri A, Macro C, Pascali M. The use of spreader grafts in primary rhinoplasty. Ann Plast Surg. 2005 Aug;55(2):127-31.
3. Boccieri A, Pascali M. Septal crossbar graft for the correction of the crooked nose. Plast Reconstr Surg. 2003 Feb;111(2):629-38.
4. Segreto F, Marangi GF et al. Nonsurgical rhinoplasty: a graft-based technique. Plast Reconstr Surg Glob Open 2019;7:e2241
5. De Lorenzi C. Complication of injectable fillers, part 1. Aesthet Surg J 2013; 33:561-75
6. Li KT, Huang YH, Chen CH et al. Delayed onset of cerebral infarction after cosmetic facial injection using hyaluronic acid. J Formosan Medical Association 2016; 115:587-588
7. Romeo F. Profiloplasty in One Session Versus Single Treatment Areas. Dermatol Surg. 2021 Jul 1;47(7):953-958.
8. Y, Andretto Amodeo C, Bouaziz D, Polselli R. Nasal arterial vasculature: medical and surgical applica-

tions. JAMA Facial Plast Surg. 2012 Nov;14(6):429-36.
9. Saban Y, Amodeo CA, Hammou JC, Polselli R. An Anatomical Study of the Nasal Superficial Musculoaponeurotic System: Surgical Applications in Rhinoplasty. JAMA Facial Plast Surg. 2008;10(2):109–115.
10. Saban Y, Polselli R, Bertossi D, East C, Gerbault O. Facial Layers and Facial Fat Compartments: Focus on Midcheek Area. Facial Plast Surg. 2017;33(5):470–482.
11. Beer KR. Nasal reconstruction using 20 mg/ml cross-linked hyaluronic acid. J Cosmet Dermatol. 2006;5(5):465–466.
12. de Lacerda DA, Zancanaro P. Filler rhinoplasty. Dermatol Surg. 2007;33 Suppl 2:S207–S212.
13. Redaelli A. Medical rhinoplasty with hyaluronic acid and botulinum toxin A: a very simple and quite effective technique. J Cosmet Dermatol. 2008 Sep;7(3):210-20
14. Rokhsar C, Ciocon DH. Nonsurgical rhinoplasty: an evaluation of injectable calcium hydroxylapatite filler for nasal contouring. Dermatol Surg. 2008;34(7):944–946.
15. Braccini F, Dohan Ehrenfest DM. La rhinoplastie médicale : de l'usage de la toxine botulique et des produits de comblement pour un remodelage atraumatique du nez [Medical rhinoplasty: rationale for atraumatic nasal modelling using botulinum toxin and fillers]. Rev Laryngol Otol Rhinol (Bord). 2008;129(4- 5):233–238.
16. Borchard NA, Dholakia SS, Yan CH, Zarabanda D, Thamboo A, Nayak JV. Use of intranasal submucosal fillers as a transient implant to alter upper airway aerodynamics: implications for the assessment of empty nose syndrome. Int Forum Allergy Rhinol. 2019;9(6):681–687.
17. Redaelli A, Limardo P. Minimally invasive procedures for nasal aesthetics. J Cutan Aesthet Surg. 2012;5(2):115-20
18. Robati RM, Moeineddin F, Almasi-Nasrabadi M. The Risk of Skin Necrosis Following Hyaluronic Acid Filler Injection in Patients With a History of Cosmetic Rhinoplasty. Aesthet Surg J. 2018;38(8):883–888.
19. Bertossi D, Lanaro L, Dorelan S, Johanssen K, Nocini P. Nonsurgical Rhinoplasty: Nasal Grid Analysis and Nasal Injecting Protocol. Plast Reconstr Surg. 2019 Feb;143(2):428-439. doi: 10.1097/PRS.0000000000005224. Erratum in: Plast Reconstr Surg. 2019 Aug;144(2):538. PMID: 30531619.
20. Chen W, Wu L, Jian XL, et al. Retinal Branch Artery Embolization Following Hyaluronic Acid Injection: A Case Report. Aesthet Surg J. 2016;36(7):NP219–NP224.
21. Bae IH, Kim MS, Choi H, Na CH, Shin BS. Ischemic oculomotor nerve palsy due to hyaluronic acid filler injection. J Cosmet Dermatol. 2018;17(6):1016–1018.
22. Kim SN, Byun DS, Park JH, et al. Panophthalmoplegia and vision loss after cosmetic nasal dorsum injection. J Clin Neurosci. 2014;21(4):678–680.
23. Kim YJ, Kim SS, Song WK, Lee SY, Yoon JS. Ocular ischemia with hypotony after injection of hyaluronic acid gel. Ophthalmic Plast Reconstr Surg.

2011;27(6):e152–e155.
24. Wibowo A, Kapoor KM, Philipp-Dormston WG. Reversal of Post-filler Vision Loss and Skin Ischaemia with High-Dose Pulsed Hyaluronidase Injections. Aesthetic Plast Surg. 2019;43(5):1337–1344.
25. Robati RM, Moeineddin F, Almasi-Nasrabadi M. The Risk of Skin Necrosis Following Hyaluronic Acid Filler Injection in Patients With a History of Cosmetic Rhinoplasty. Aesthet Surg J. 2018;38(8):883–888.
26. Chae SY, Lee KC, Jang YH, Lee SJ, Kim DW, Lee WJ. A Case of the Migration of Hyaluronic Acid Filler from Nose to Forehead Occurring as Two Sequential Soft Lumps. Ann Dermatol. 2016;28(5):645–647.
27. Kim EG, Eom TK, Kang SJ. Severe visual loss and cerebral infarction after injection of hyaluronic acid gel. J Craniofac Surg 2014;25(2):684-6
28. Tracy L, Ridgway J, Nelson JS, Lowe N, Wong B. Calcium hydroxylapatite associated soft tissue necrosis: a case report and treatment guideline. J Plast Reconstr Aesthet Surg. 2014;67(4):564–568.
29. Marumo Y, Hiraoka M, Hashimoto M, Ohguro H. Visual impairment by multiple vascular embolization with hydroxyapatite particles. Orbit. 2018;37(3):165–170.
30. Yoon SS, Chang D, Chung KC. Acute fatal stroke immediately following autologous fat injection into the face. Neurology 2003;61(8):1151-2
31. Alharethy S. Alterations in Nasal Sensibility Following Calcium Hydroxyapatite Dorsal Augmentation. J Craniofac Surg. 2018;29(2):e104–e106.
32. Colombo G, Caregnato P, Stifanese R, Ferrando G. A vast intranasal filler-induced granulomatous reaction: a case report. Aesthetic Plast Surg. 2010 Oct;34(5):660-3
33. Chang C, Lee SB. Unusual long-term complication of polyalkylimide hydrogel manifesting as nasal septal abscess. J Craniofac Surg. 2015 May;26(3):e197-9
34. Hu HC, Cho HY, Chiu YH. Dermatomyositis Induced by Filler Rhinoplasty Using Liquid Silicone. JAMA Otolaryngol Head Neck Surg. 2019 Nov 21
35. Chatrath V, Banerjee PS, Goodman GJ, Rahman E. Soft-tissue Filler-associated Blindness: A Systematic Review of Case Reports and Case Series. Plast Reconstr Surg Glob Open. 2019;7(4):e2173.
36. Harb A, Brewster CT. The Nonsurgical Rhinoplasty: A Retrospective Review of 5000 Treatments. Plast Reconstr Surg. 2020 Mar;145(3):661-667.

FILLER COMPLICATIONS IN THE LOWER THIRD OF THE FACE

Raffaella Sommariva, Lucia Calvisi

As with all aesthetic procedures, the treatment of the mandibular region and chin requires a preliminary assessment of the patient before a filler is injected. Particular attention should be paid to the mandibular angle, mandibular profile, chin, prejowl and marionette lines (fig. 1). The patient should be examined statically and dynamically and photographed from the anterior, oblique and posterior positions.

The chin is a key element in profile aesthetics as it contributes to the definition of the mandibular border and the harmony of the region, curves and contours of the face. A receding chin can give the profile an austere, stern or sometimes unassertive appearance, with the chin's features seeming to reflect the individual's personality (fig. 2). However, the patient is often unaware that their chin is flawed.

In women, symmetry, roundness and harmony are synonymous with beauty, the lips are elements of primary attraction, the chin is generally small and round, the jaw slender and with rounded angles, while in men the facial features are more pronounced, the jaw and chin are wide and square and should exude energy, vitality and masculinity (fig. 3).

As time goes by and with the sagging of the soft tissues of the cheek, in addition to bone resorption, the mandibular

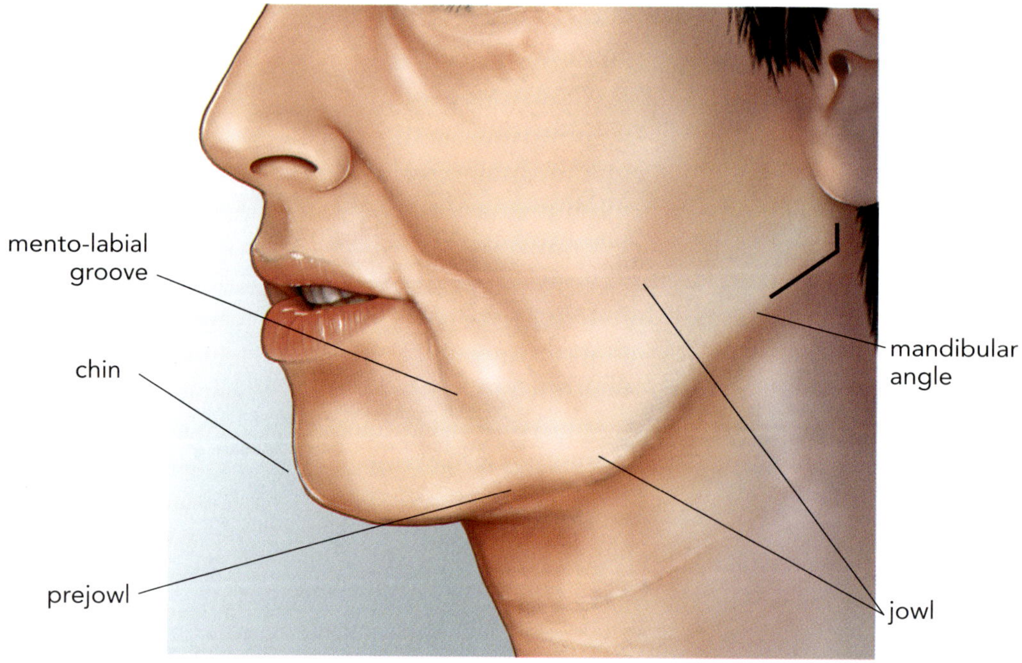

Figure 1 The gravitational drooping of the soft tissues of the cheek alters the mandibular profile and contributes to the appearance of the mento-labial grooves

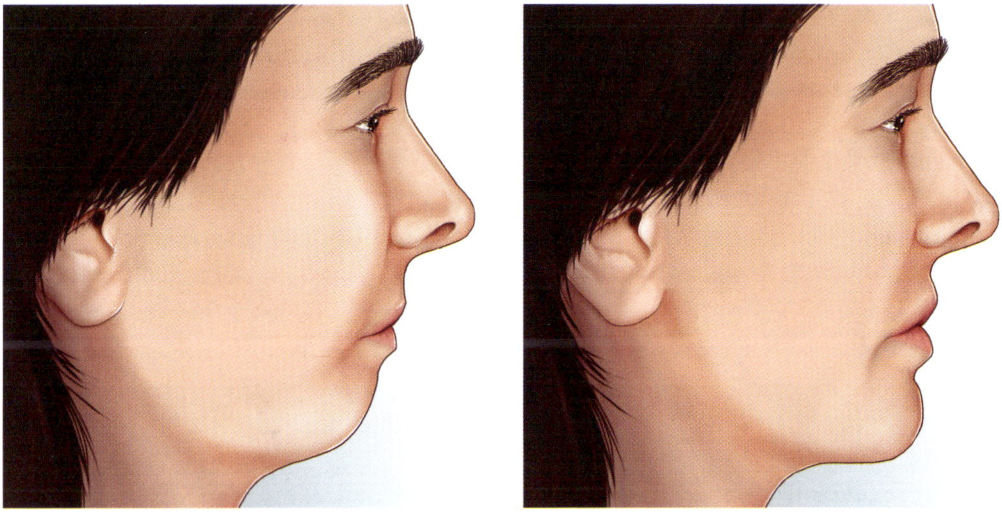

Figure 2 Chin and personality. A receding chin changes the physiognomy and makes the profile austere, sad or unassertive as the case may be

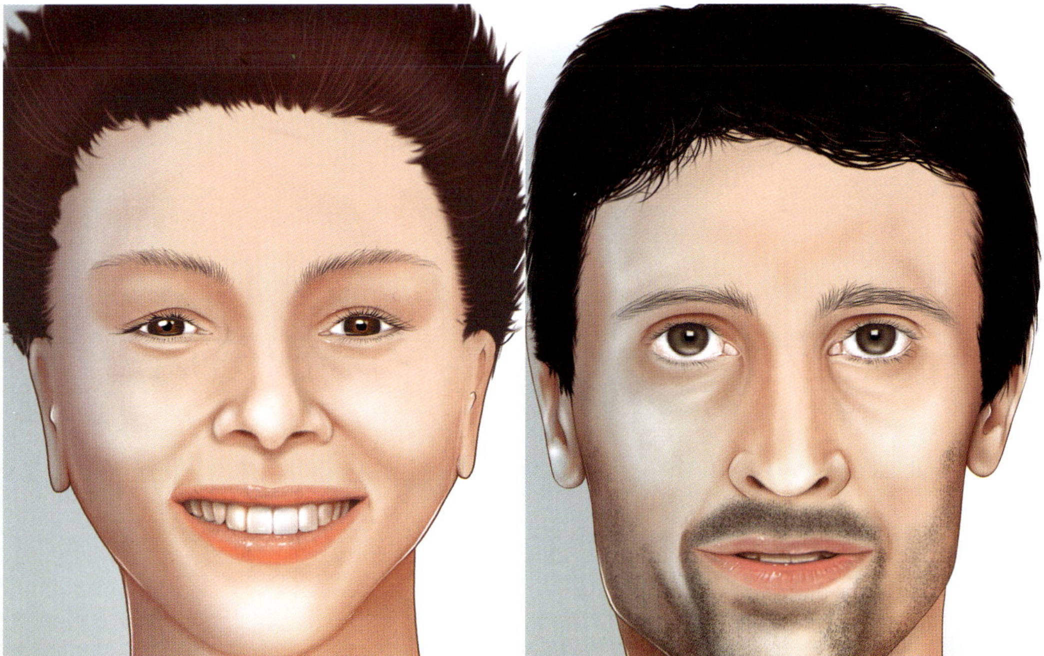

Figure 3 Gender differences in the appearance of the chin and jaw, reflecting the different male and female skeletal structure

contour becomes less well-defined and requests for non-surgical correction are becoming increasingly common. Soft tissue ptosis can also occur in the chin, but this can be made less obvious with a minimally invasive mentoplasty.

When assessing the profile, the mento-labial cleft and angle, the convexity of the chin and the position of the chin in relation to the lips and nose must be evaluated (fig. 4A).

The chin should be positioned between two vertical lines that descend at right angles to the Frankfurt plane: the anterior line descends from the forehead and the posterior line from the orbital. If the chin and lower lip are recessed in relation to the anterior plane, we speak of mandibular micrognathia, whereas if the chin and lower lip protrude beyond the anterior plane, we are dealing with mandibular prognathia (fig. 4B). Mandibular micrognathia and prognathia are the speciality of the maxillofacial surgeon.

With regard to the proportions of the lips in relation to the nose and chin, reference is made to their position in relation to Ricketts' aesthetic plane (fig. 4C): the lips remain within the plane which is traced tangentially from the tip of the nose to the chin. The upper lip is slightly further back (about 4 mm) than the low-

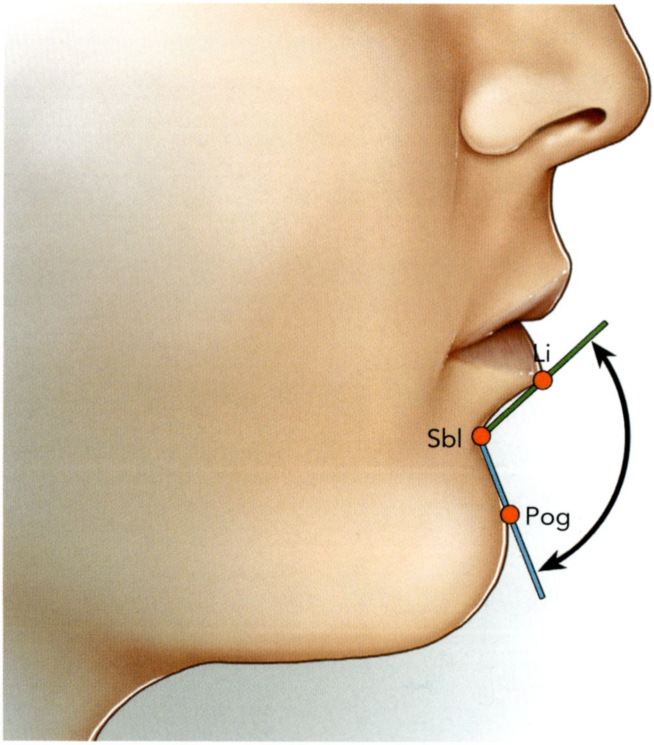

Figure 4A Chin: gender differences. The mento-labial cleft is usually more pronounced in men, with apparent greater prominence of the chin. The mento-labial angle, an important factor in the perception of the beauty of the profile, is considered attractive when it is between 107° and 118° (acceptable up to 140°) and is more acute in men than in women

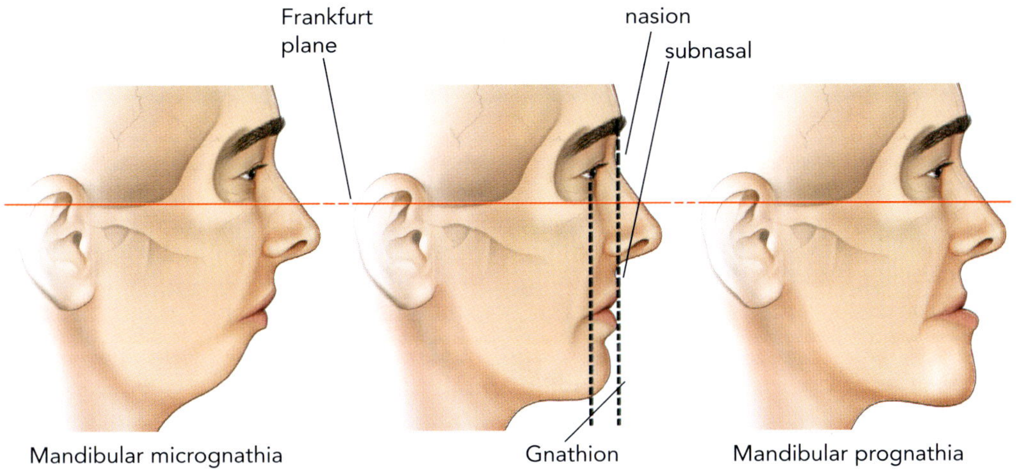

Figure 4B The chin and lower lip. The central figure shows the correct anteroposterior position of the chin, the left figure shows micrognathia and the right figure shows mandibular prognathia

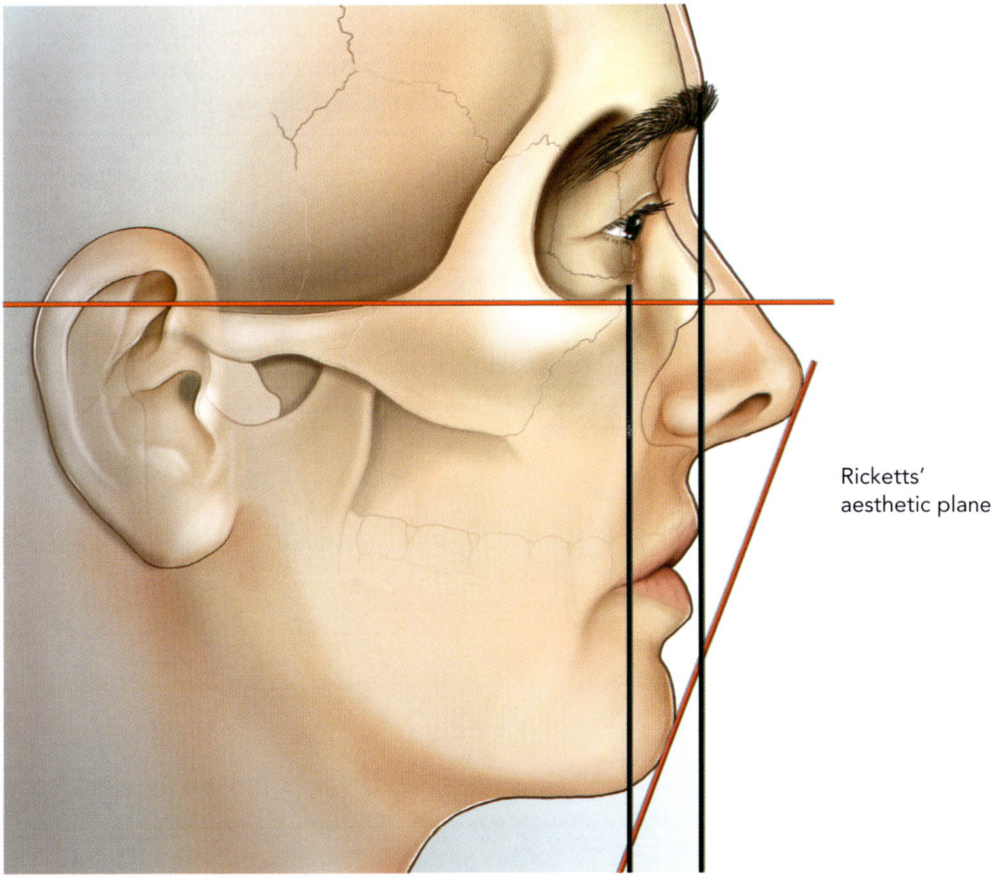

Figure 4C Ricketts' aesthetic plane: position of lips in relation to chin and nose

er lip (about 2 mm).
When observed frontally, it is necessary to assess symmetry, the mento-labial cleft and the possible presence of hyperactivity wrinkles of the chin muscle ("cobblestone" chin). The goal of the treatment is to make the jaw line straighter, to soften the transition between the chin and jowl and to lengthen the jowl anteriorly.
The aesthetic endpoint in men differs from that of women because men should have a squarer and more prominent jaw, compared to women, and a broader chin.
In the ideal male profile, the chin should reach the vertical line, descending from the nasion to the pogonion, whereas in the female profile, it is usually slightly behind (0.5-1 cm) this line. If it is further back, then correction is advisable (fig. 5). Minimally invasive mentoplasty can be performed with injectables or, in more severe cases, with the insertion of chin implants. Of course the most severe cases should be handled by the maxillofacial surgeon.

Injection technique

The materials used in minimally invasive mentoplasty are calcium hydroxyapatite, autologous fat and preferably high G' hyaluronic acid.
As always, knowledge of the structural and vascular anatomy of the anatomical region is essential for good results, placing the filler in the least risky plane and so reducing the risk of complications.
Five overlapping layers of tissue can be distinguished in the chin: the skin, su-

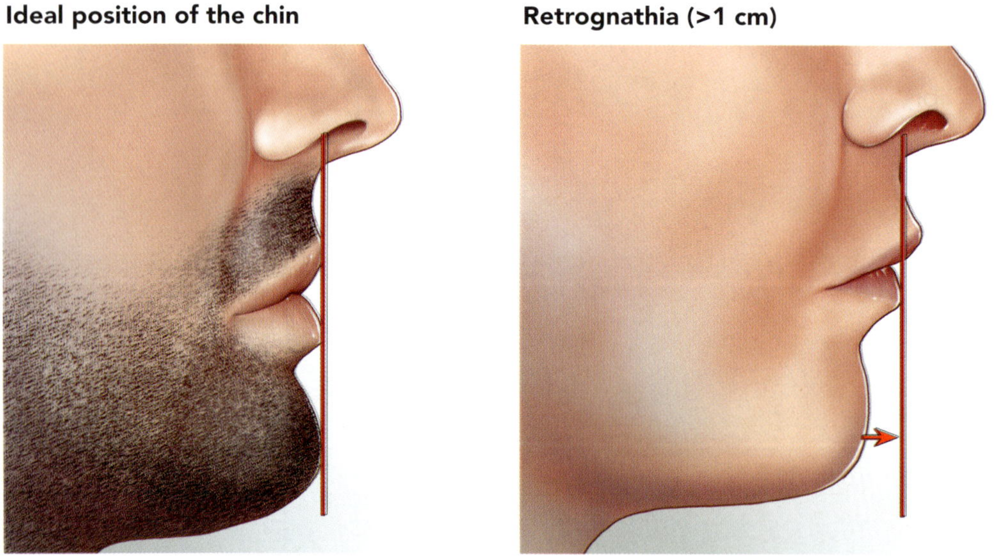

Figure 5 The chin should reach the vertical line that descends from the border of the vermilion to the pogonion (male gender), or be slightly (0.5-1 cm) behind it (female gender): if it is set back by more than 1 cm, we have first-degree retrognathia; up to 2 cm, second-degree retrognathia; more than 2 cm, third-degree retrognathia, which requires surgery

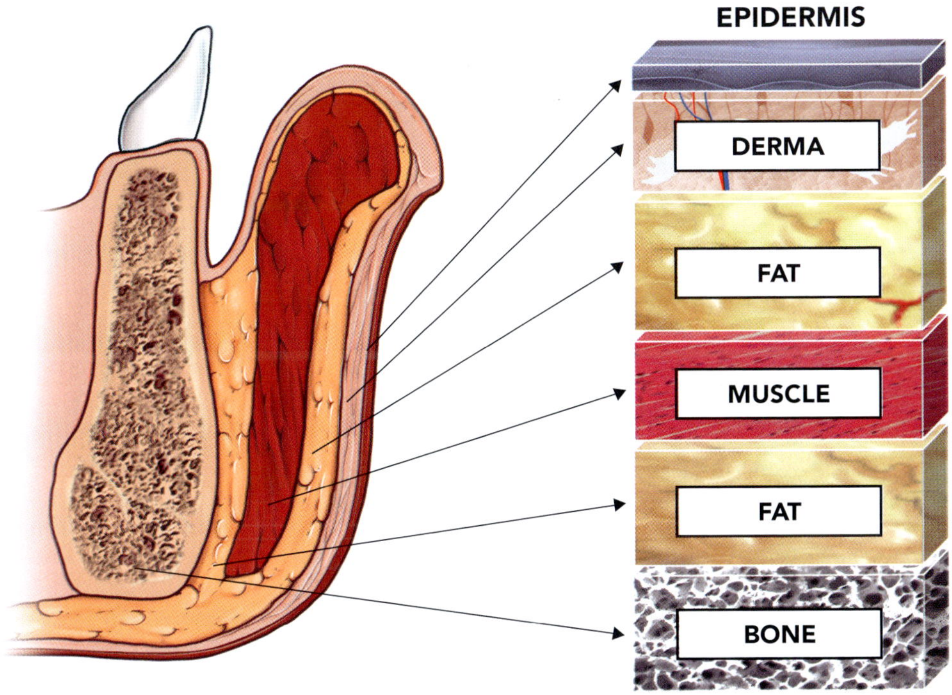

Figure 6 Five overlapping layers of tissue can be distinguished in the chin: the skin, superficial fat, muscle, deep fat and the jawbone

perficial fat, muscle, deep fat and the jawbone (fig. 6). Vascularisation is the responsibility of the submental artery, the inferior labial artery and the mental artery, which are often largely anastomosed to each other.

To increase the projection of the skeletal structure, it is necessary to inject into the parasinaphyseal region, particularly with a needle on the midline in the supraperiosteal site (fig. 7), while to increase the projection of the soft tissues it is appropriate to use a 25 G microcannula for implantation in the subcutaneous layer, where the vascular system is prevalent, performing a real "multilayer" technique. If hyaluronic acid is used, it should be high G′ if injected in the supraperiosteal site, softer and more dynamic if implanted subcutaneously.

It is essential to disinfect the area with an antiseptic preparation, followed the deposit of small boluses of 0.5 cc of the product at the angle of the mandible, with the intention of making the jaw profile straighter. Alternatively, a 25 G cannula can be used to draw the mandibular angle.

With regard to the anterior part, injection is into the jowl with a 25 G cannula, shaping the chin and then proceeding along the remaining part of the jawline. In the lateral regions of the chin, on either side of the parasymphyseal region (and between a vertical line passing through the canines and a vertical line descending 1 cm from the labial commissures), the filler implant must be subcutaneous, with a microcannula, and never on the periosteum to avoid the

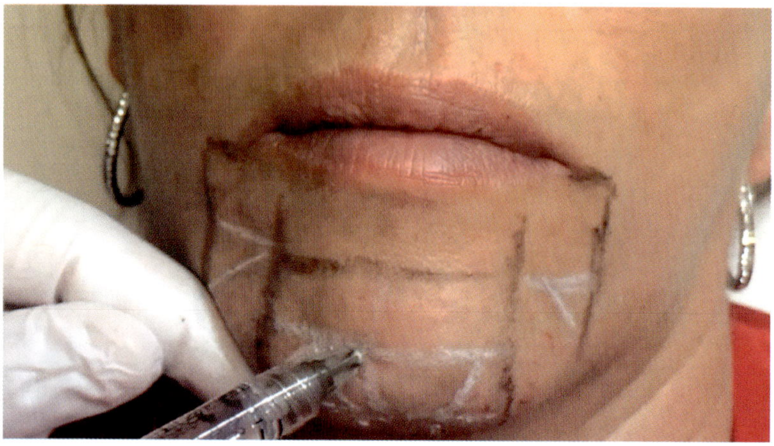

Figure 7 Implant with multilayer technique in the chin: high G′ hyaluronic acid in supraperiosteal site, softer hyaluronic acid in subcutaneous site

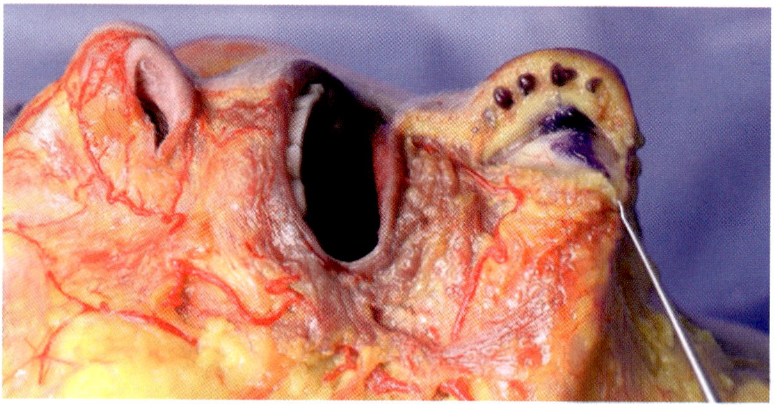

Figure 8 Precise sites of hyaluronic acid implantation in the chin using the multilayer technique: high-G′ "static" hyaluronic acid directly on the supraperiosteal plane and more "dynamic" hyaluronic acid near the surface, in the subcutaneous plane. Courtesy of E2e

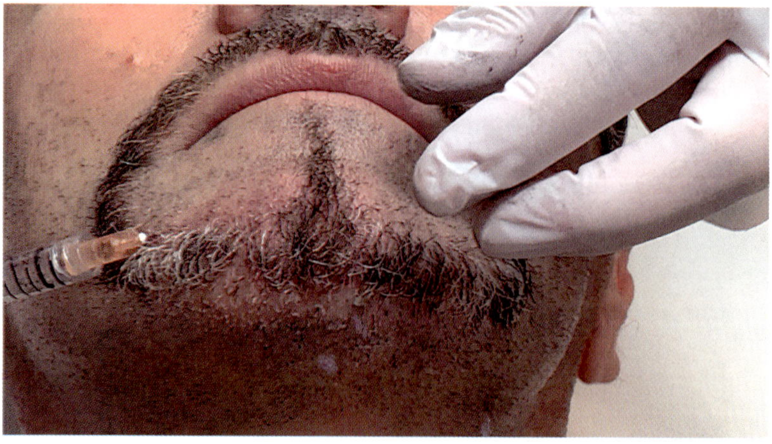

Figure 9 Implantation in the lateral regions of the chin: subcutaneously and with a microcannula

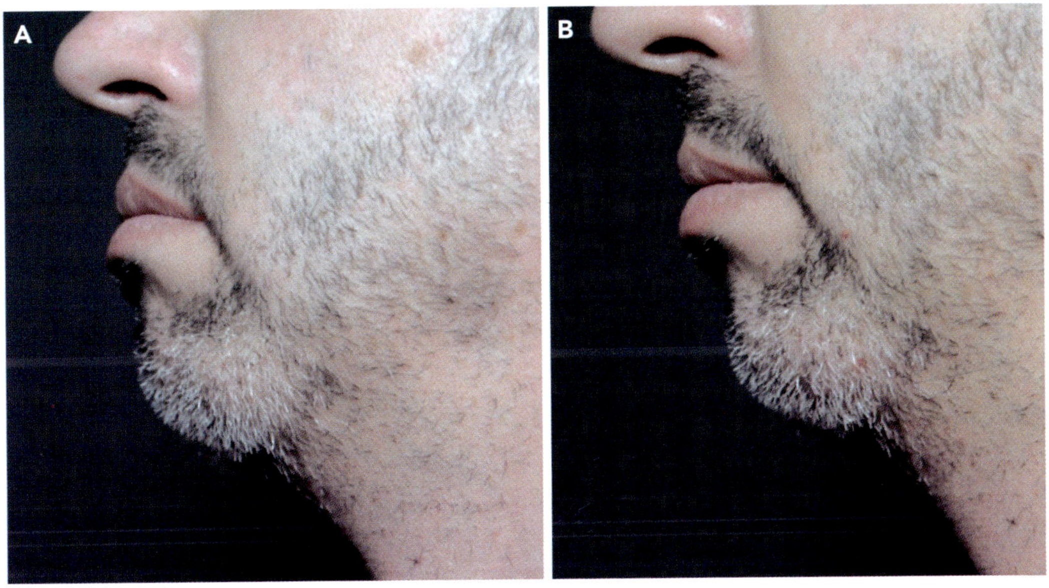

Figure 10 Multilayer technique. In men, the implant must adapt to the anatomy of the squarer and broader chin and generally higher doses of filler are required. Courtesy of Prof. Giuseppe Sito

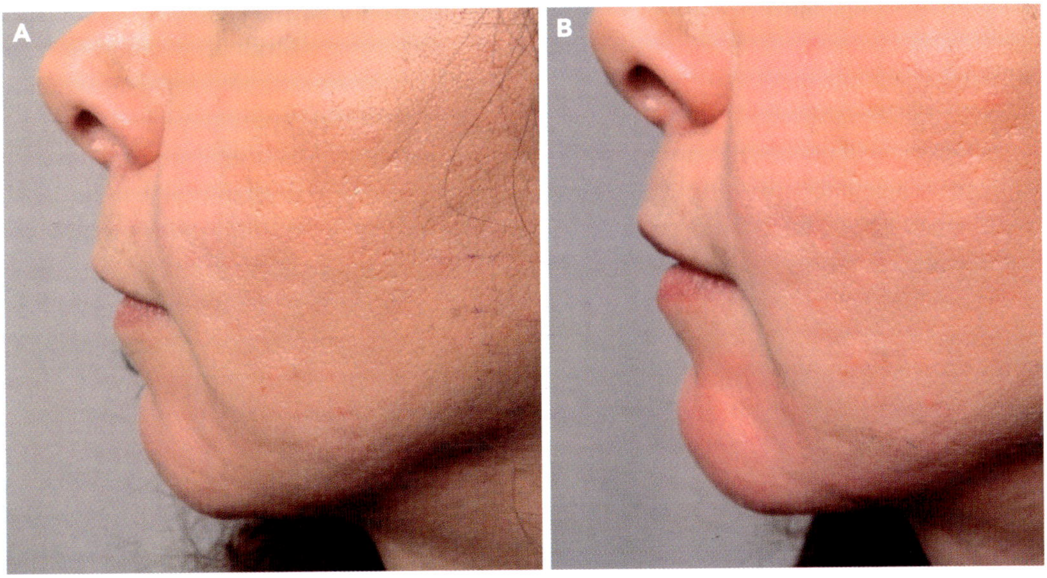

Figure 11 Multilayer technique: there are no age limits for correction of chin prominence. Courtesy of Prof. Giuseppe Sito

VIDEO 5.2

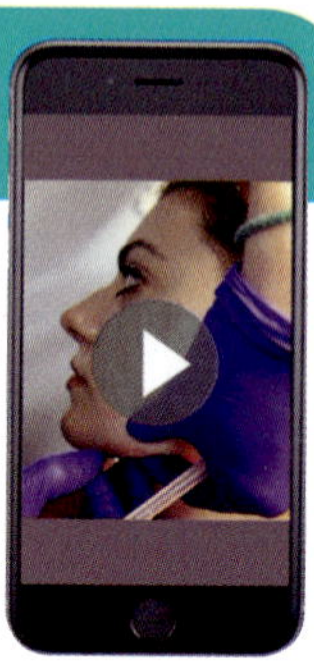

Jawline correction with filler

mental artery emerging from the mental foramen.

In the lateral regions, the mento-labial cleft and the right paramedian region, injection with a needle should only be intradermal to avoid the superficial mental artery.

Complications

In this site too, complications from injectables are very rare if the right implantation plans and techniques are observed. In the past, before the advent of microcannulas, bruising was common and sometimes severe, while vascular complications are described in literature focusing on the chin.

The most common complications of jawline fillers are redness, bruising and oedema.

Other less frequent complications are infection and the formation of foreign body granuloma.

Accidental intravascular injection of the filler causes pain and blanching along the arterial distribution area, which, if not recognised and treated, then leads to tissue ischaemia and consequent necrosis. At the first signs of the onset of vascular occlusion, it is essential to intervene promptly with infiltrations of hyaluronidase (the use of hyaluronidase in Italy is off-label).

Literature reports that, in addition to vascular damage, improper injections in the mandibular region can cause damage to the parotid gland and duct. Trauma to the parotid gland can lead to its infection, duct occlusion, mucocele or salivary fistulae.

The use of a cannula, as opposed to a needle, usually protects us more from vascular complications.

In a study reported in literature, however, where the lipofilling technique was used instead of hyaluronic acid, a vascular complication in the chin was reported.

Although the correction of wrinkles and skin laxity in the lower third is performed almost exclusively using hyaluronic acid fillers, more experienced injectors now have the option of combining hyaluronic acid treatment with botulinum toxin treatment. Obviously, this type of injection is more delicate and requires more experience on the part of the operator, but the result that can be obtained is highly satisfactory.

The treatment of what we call marionette lines, acting on the depressor muscle of the corner of the mouth, allows us to lighten that unattractive "downturned mouth" look; the treatment of the chin, on the other hand, relaxing the mental muscle, acts on the "orange peel" effect.

Clearly, these methods are not free of complications, but in general, as is always the case with the use of botulinum, the side effects are moderate and, above all, temporary: bruising at the injection site, asymmetry of a half-lip, drooling, and the appearance of dimples in the chin.

Bibliography

1. Vazirnia A, Braz A, Fabi SG. Nonsurgical jawline rejuvenation using injectable fillers. J Cosmet Dermatol. 2020;19(8):1940-1947.
2. Bertossi D, Robiony M, Lazzarotto A, Giampaoli G, Nocini R, Nocini PF. Nonsurgical Redefinition of the Chin and Jawline of Younger Adults With a Hyaluronic Acid Filler: Results Evaluated With a Grid System Approach. Aesthet Surg J. 2021;41(9):1068-1076.
3. Müller D, Prinz V, Sulovsky M, et al. Longevity and subject-reported satisfaction after minimally invasive jawline contouring. J Cosmet Dermatol. 2022;21(1):199-206.
4. Yeh LC, Fabi SG, Welsh K. Arterial Penetration With Blunt-Tipped Cannulas Using Injectables: A False Sense of Safety?. Dermatol Surg. 2017;43(3):464-467.
5. Galadari H, Galadari I, Smit R, Prygova I, Redaelli A. Use of AbobotulinumtoxinA for Cosmetic Treatments in the Neck, and Middle and Lower Areas of the Face: A Systematic Review. Toxins (Basel). 2021;13(2):169.
6. Jabbour SF, Kechichian EG, Awaida CJ, Tomb RR, Nasr MW. Botulinum Toxin for Neck Rejuvenation: Assessing Efficacy and Redefining Patient Selection. Plast Reconstr Surg. 2017 Jul;140(1):9e-17e.
7. Gassia V, Beylot C, Béchaux S, Michaud T. Les techniques d'injection de la toxine botulique dans le tiers inférieur et moyen du visage, le cou et le décolleté. Le "Néfertiti lift" [Botulinum toxin injection techniques in the lower third and middle of the face, the neck and the décolleté: the "Nefertiti lift"]. Ann Dermatol Venereol. 2009 May;136 Suppl 4:S111-8. French.
8. D'Emilio R, Rosati G. Full-face treatment with onabotulinumtoxinA: Results from a single-center study. J Cosmet Dermatol. 2020 Apr;19(4):809-816.
9. Bae GY, Na JI, Park KC, Cho SB. Nonsurgical correction of drooping mouth corners using monophasic hyaluronic acid and incobotulinumtoxinA. J Cosmet Dermatol. 2020 Feb;19(2):338-345.

6

LASER

LASER INDUCED SIDE EFFECTS AND COMPLICATIONS IN AESTHETIC MEDICINE

Leonardo Longo

The possible side effects and complications of laser therapy have been described by various authors and are caused mainly by two factors: malfunctioning of the instrumentation and/or errors in the method of application [1-3].

Knowledge of the possible side effects and complications in the use of lasers in aesthetic medicine and surgery, along with the analysis of their causes, could help in their prevention and possible treatment.

The side effects and complications that have occurred over approximately 40 years of practice were analysed and compared with what has been described in literature. Their specific treatment was then proposed.

Most patients who presented side effects and complications, but continued with the practitioner who performed the procedure, recovered successfully, with exceptional cases of sequelae. By contrast, patients who turned to someone other than their practitioner presented irreversible lesions in the majority of cases.

Laser therapy and surgery solve numerous aesthetic problems, which is why they are being used more and more often. In-depth knowledge of the methods of application must, however, be acquired by attending specific and objective training courses and regular refresher courses, and by choosing instruments that are as unsophisticated and reliable as possible.

Medical examination and patient selection

When a patient requests an aesthetic medical consultation, it is important to remember that we are doctors and that the patient must always be examined thoroughly, because first a diagnosis has to be made and only then can a treatment be proposed.

Unfortunately, social networks, the mass media and uncontrolled advertising by public and private companies and organisations often lead the patient to make a self-diagnosis, including treatment, depending on current trends. Superficial knowledge of the facts is mistaken for science and patients often come to the cosmetic doctor with their diagnosis already prepared and having decided on their treatment, asking for it directly.

This type of patient should never be treated in any way because they will invariably have and create problems.

When, on the other hand, the patient agrees to be examined, then it is possible to propose a diagnosis and the corresponding treatment, according to science and conscience, greatly reducing the risk of side effects.

Selection of the patient is very important, based on their medical history, the type of lesion and their expectations and those of the people around them.

Table 1 summarises the main points to be considered at all times. Based on this, the type of laser to be used is decided, along with when and how. There

TABLE 1 - PATIENT SELECTION

Skin type (skin examination)
Location
Medical history (acne, sunburn, scars)
Previous therapies (Vit, Roaccutane, other)
Diagnosis (general and specialist)
Type of lesion
Patient and family expectations

TABLE 2 - CONTRAINDICATIONS

Specific contraindications for each type of laser
Cancer, excluding laser surgery

are relatively few absolute contraindications (table 2), some general and some specific depending on the type of laser used.

It is always necessary to remember that:

- any laser induced effect, be it therapeutic or surgical, is strictly dose-dependent;
- laser and light are absorbed selectively by their complementary colour;
- the laser is always perfectly dose-dependent on the tissue, because it is coherent, i.e. composed of photons arranged neatly in time and space and all equal in terms of the quality (same wavelength) and quantity of light transported;
- a change in radiation dosage can result in the same type of laser having opposite effects on the same tissue;
- at the same dose, each laser is selectively absorbed by a substance, cell or tissue of complementary colour, known as a chromophore. The "colour" of the laser corresponds to the wavelength of the photons emitted;
- the laser is a light beam, subject to the laws of optics. Consequently, the irradiation of surfaces is maximum when the beam is perpendicular to the target surface, otherwise a part is lost due to the laws of reflection and refraction;
- the skin must be free of clothing or substances that alter its colour;
- lasers, pulsed light and LEDs are also subject to the laws of optics, but their radiation is never coherent, i.e. it can never be measured on the tissue but only at source, and is usually not even monochromatic, with several wavelengths being emitted at the same time;
- the choice between laser, pulsed light and LED, or their combination, depends on the specific case;
- the effects of lasers and light are never only photothermal but are, above all, photochemical and also photomechanical.

When all these factors are taken into account, the chances of side effects occurring decreases considerably.

Side effects and complications

The side effects and complications of laser treatment can be divided into three groups according to their severity: mild, moderate and severe [4-6].

Mild reactions often only require "watchful waiting" or topical medical intervention and are reversible.

Moderate reactions always require external therapeutic intervention, to varying degrees, and unfortunately do not always resolve completely.

TABLE 3 - SIDE EFFECTS AND COMPLICATIONS FROM EXTERNAL SURGICAL SKIN IRRADIATION

Mild	Moderate	Severe
Persistent rash	Reactive hyperpigmentation	Systemic infection
Persistent oedema	Reactive hypopigmentation	Hypertrophic scarring
Matting	Herpes	Ectropion
Haematoma	Mycosis	Introflected scarring
Itching, stinging		
Dermatitis		

TABLE 4 - SIDE EFFECTS AND COMPLICATIONS FROM ENDOLUMINAL IRRADIATION

Mild	Moderate	Severe
Persistent rash	Paresis	Systemic infection
Persistent oedema	Breakage of fibre	Hypertrophic scarring
Bruising	Puncture of the wall	Necrosis
Haematoma	Mycosis	Thrombosis
Endotheliitis	Embolism	
Contracture		

TABLE 5 - SIDE EFFECTS AND COMPLICATIONS FROM EXTERNAL NON-SURGICAL SKIN IRRADIATION

Mild	Moderate	Severe
Persistent rash	Second-degree burns	Systemic infection
Persistent oedema	Reactive hyperpigmentation	Third-degree burns
Blisters	Reactive hypopigmentation	Hypertrophic scarring
Dermatitis	Herpes	
	Opposite effects	

Severe reactions require more in-depth and specific treatment and almost never resolve completely.
Depending on how the lasers are used, the complications can be different, based on whether they result from external surgical irradiation (tab. 3), endoluminal laser therapy and/or surgery (tab. 4) or photobiomodulation with external irradiation (tab. 5).

Treatment of complications following laser surgery with external irradiation

When surgical lasers are used, postoperative erythema and oedema are normal and last from two days to about a month, depending on the type of procedure. Several specific medications are available, containing anti-inflammatory, disinfectant, regenerative and emollient substances, to be applied immediately after surgery to minimise recovery time. The same protocol applies to the possible onset of itching, stinging, matting and superficial dermatitis.
There are specific treatments for moderate complications such as herpes and mycosis. Discolouration, on the other hand, must be treated if it lasts longer than a month. Treatment can be medical, physical or both. Persistent reactive hyperchromia can be treated with 5% hydroquinone creams and, if particularly intense and persistent, with lasers with a wavelength complementary to the colour of the hyperchromia (532, 585, 755, 1064 nm). The prognosis is 1-3 months.
Hypopigmentation should be treated with intense pulsed ultraviolet light or with excimer lasers if available. Topical creams alone have little effect in these cases, although Vitamin E, for example, offers valuable help. The prognosis is 3-6 months.
In the case of severe complications, systemic infections require specific therapy, following blood tests and instrumental examinations. Hypertrophic scars and keloids can be treated with photobiomodulation laser and IPL, not surgery, to avoid recurrence and possible aggravation. The same goes for hypotrophic scars, possibly in combination with local restructuring therapies. Here the prognosis is an average six months. Ectropion requires surgical correction.

Treatment of the complications of endoluminal laser treatment

This procedure enables the resolution and simplification of many otherwise complex and/or impossible surgical operations. Its fortunately exceptional side effects always require a surgical approach to their resolution and almost always result in sequelae.
Mild complications often require only topical medical therapy. Infections and mycoses require specific systemic medical therapy. Rupture of the optic fibre or embolism require surgery. If paresis does not resolve spontaneously, it can be treated with a short one- or two-week course of anti-inflammatory/regenerative laser therapy of the nerve tissue, with successful recovery. Haematoma and bruising with topical and/or systemic draining substances. If irradiation is possible, photobiomodulation lasers can also be used. Vascular necrosis and thrombosis must be treated surgically, in a sterile surgical room.

Treatment of complications of non-surgical external laser treatment - photobiomodulation

Mild and moderate complications should be treated in the same way as above. First- and second-degree burns require treatment with appropriate topical medication. Third-degree burns also require photobiomodulation with lasers at different doses, although patients rarely agree to this. The other complications are similar to those described above and require the same treatment. In photobiomodulation, the dose is of considerable importance: if it is wrong, the opposite effects to those desired are achieved. To reverse them, all you have to do is reverse the dose.

Most frequent complications

Telangiectasias

Side effects and complications are often seen following the treatment of telangiectasias on the face and lower limbs with laser (tab. 6). We proposed a reasoned approach to this type of lesion many years ago, after treating thousands of them at the University of Siena's Phlebology Centre and our outpatient clinic in Florence.

In short, it can be said that the treatment of choice for facial telangiectasias is always laser, while those of the limbs require in-depth diagnosis first. Only primitive, high-flux teleangiectasias of less than a millimetre in diameter can be treated successfully and at low risk with lasers, otherwise sclerotherapy in all its variants continues to be the method of choice. Enormous advantages are obtained with combined laser sclerotherapy, in which lasers are used only to close the ends of the vessels and thereby reduce the flow, and sclerosants to close the perforating vessels at the same time. Given the reduced flow, the sclerosant remains on the lesion for longer and in a greater concentration, so less toxic doses can be used and larger areas can be treated at the same time. The side effects of this approach are almost nil. Otherwise, when faced with discolouration, matting, hypo- and hypertrophic scars, the therapeutic approach is always as indicated above (figs. 1-2-3). It must be remembered that the mechanism

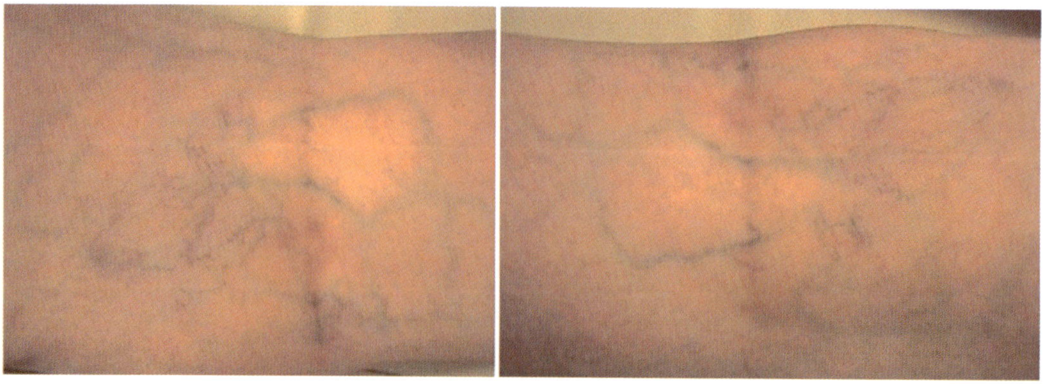

Figure 1 Reticular veins: laser treatment is not suitable. Red telangiectasias: laser treatment is indicated

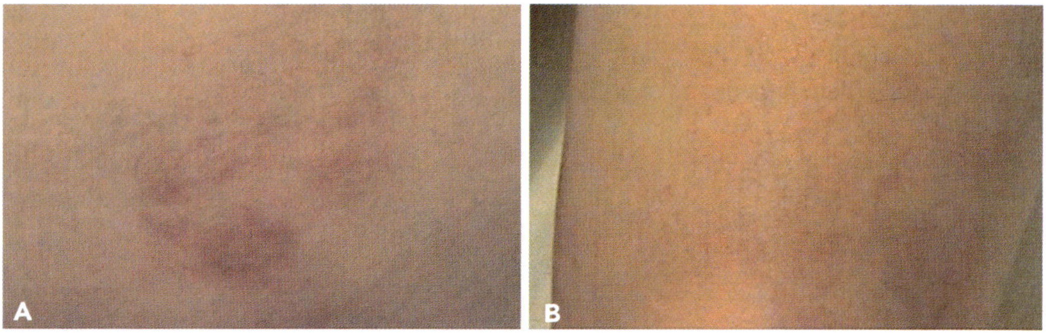

Figure 2 Red telangiectasias: A) before; B) 20 days after 577 nm laser

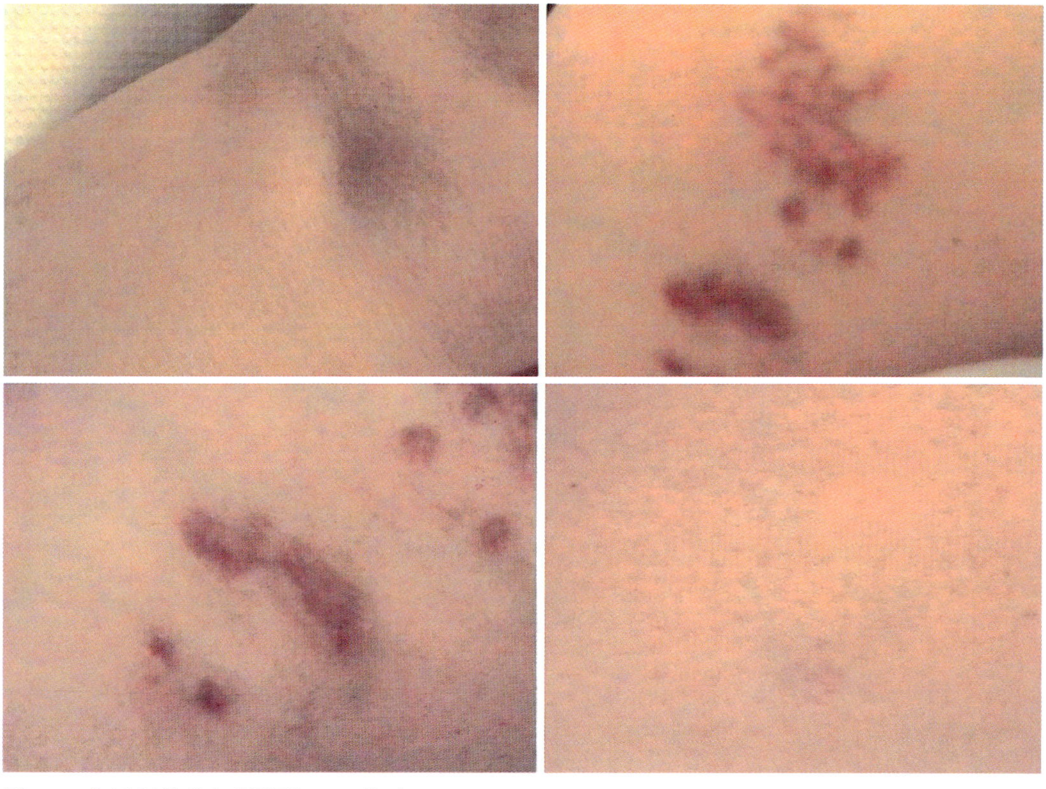

Figure 3 Nd-YAG in TGT lower limbs

TABLE 6 - TELEANGECTASIAS: WHICH CAN BE TREATED BY LASER?

Face	Lower limbs
Always	High flow (red, A/V microfistulae)
	Calibre <2mm
	Recurring

of elimination of telangiectasias using a laser is above all thermal, meaning that it is then necessary to deal with selective superficial burns. But in these cases, the burn is the mechanism of action, not necessarily the side effect, as claimed by colleagues without expertise in laser medicine.

Hypertrichosis and hirsutism

Many problems arise when the removal of steroid-sensitive hairs is claimed to be permanent. It must be remembered that only malformative hairs, which are estimated to grow from no more than 15% of all hair follicles, can be permanently removed.

Steroid-sensitive and constitutional hairs can only be removed temporarily, with the effects lasting months or a few years at most. The advantages of using lasers are the following: the entire body can be treated in each session, without irritating the skin, relatively few sessions are required, and there is little discomfort during treatment.

Hair grows back more sparse, more fragile and colourless (fig. 4). It should also be remembered that the target of irradiation is the hair follicle, not the hair. When the right lasers and/or pulsed light are used with the correct procedures, side effects and complications are absolutely exceptional. Otherwise, all the complications of external surgical irradiation can occur, and they must be treated as such.

Tattoos

A tattoo can only be permanently and successfully erased when the tattooist has failed to do a good job and has left part of the fibro-reticular structure of the dermis, without destroying it with the pigment (fig. 5). This means that the pigment will be gradually eliminated naturally. When it is removed using a laser, the fibro-reticular structure of the dermis rebuilds the normal cyto-architectonics of the tattooed area, leaving no sequelae. If, on the other hand, the tattoo artist has completely destroyed the fibro-reticular structure, whichever method is used to remove the pigment, the epidermal and dermal cells will never arrange themselves according to a precise pattern, but always in a confused manner, so

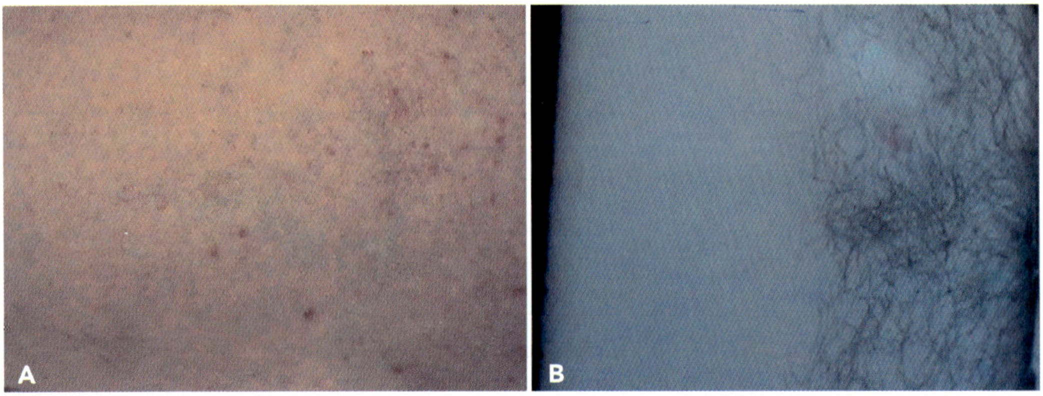

Figure 4 Hair removal: A) hypertrichosis and dyskeratosis; B) after 6 months on half region

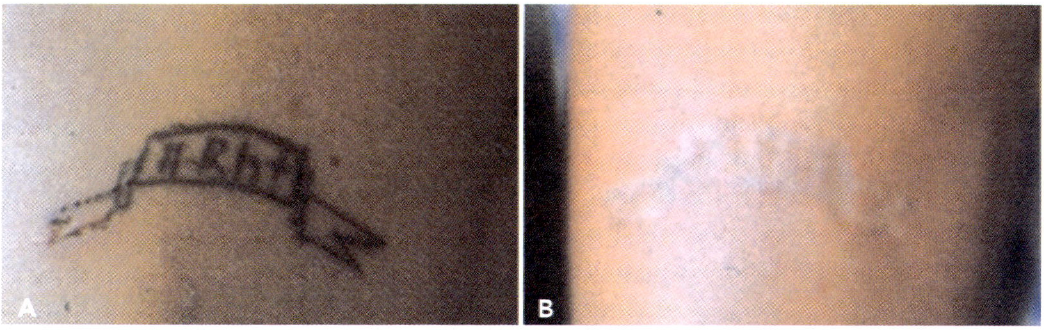

Figure 5 Tattoos: A) before treatment; B) 2 months after treatment. Abrasion with CO_2 laser 30 W SPW 50 Htz Spot/size 1 mm, Fluence 600 mJoule/cm^2

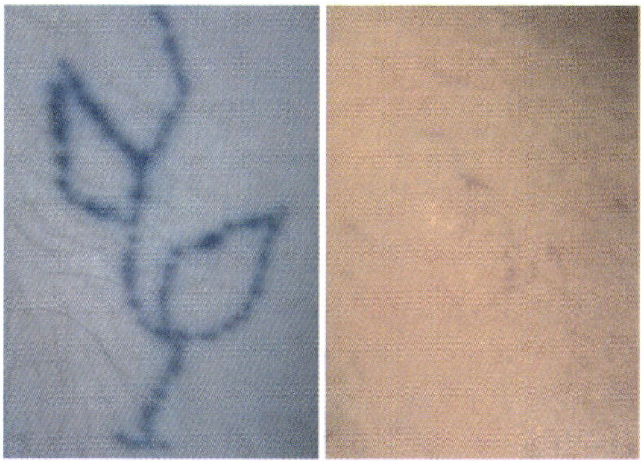

Figure 6 Tattoos

a patch, usually lighter than normal skin, known as a "ghost tattoo" will remain. Legal complications often result if this is not explained to the patient before surgery. Appropriate lasers, with a wavelength complementary to the tattoo, are the method of choice, due to the extent and speed of the results, reduced operative and post-operative stress, and rare incidence of side effects, which are always those of external irradiation with surgical lasers. Before lasers with wavelengths complementary to tattoos existed, when only ablative lasers were available and controlled dermabrasion was performed, the results were poor and often left introflected scars (fig. 6).

Laser resurfacing

This is a controlled selective dermabrasion, which, despite the skill of the surgeon and the correct type of laser and method, can still result in the complications of controlled external irradiation. The immediate post-op phase is particularly important, because the patient and family members have to deal with a very obvious abrasion, without aggravating the lesion. The treatment of any sequelae, complications and side effects is that indicated above. The fractional technique, in which radiation is distributed by a computer in a random spot arrangement over a predetermined area of varying form (square, rectangular, elliptical, etc.), is frequently used today. This system reduces the surgical risk, posed especially when the practitioner has not yet acquired a certain dexterity in the use of the instrument, and saves tissue, so healing should be faster. Nevertheless, it is still a surgical method, despite being improperly termed "non-ablative".

Laser rejuvenation

This is the photobiomodulation of dystrophic and ageing skin which, without any surgical procedure, causes the removal by drainage of old collagen and impurities,

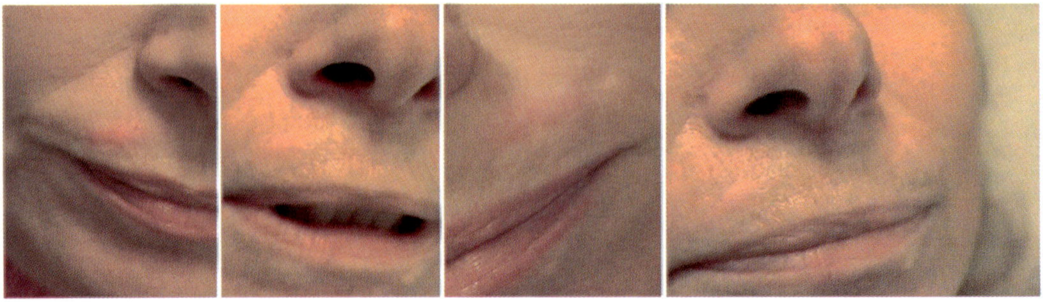

Figure 7 Hypertrophic scars caused by pulsed light, healed with further applications of pulsed light in a different dose

such as dyskeratosis, etc., while stimulating the regeneration of new epithelium and new collagen. Complications, which are very rare, can be those associated with external laser photobiomodulation and almost always heal quickly if the patient agrees to continue photobiomodulation, but at different doses (fig. 7).

Laser and pulsed light for the correction of scars and keloids

There are two methods: rejuvenation and resurfacing. We prefer the former because the results are stable, although it sometimes takes longer, and there are virtually no side effects. Several lasers are used at the same time because they have a different depth of penetration. We start with a standard sub-burn dose, adjusting it according to the clinical response (tabs. 7-8). The surgical procedure, while minimal, localised, selective and gentle, nevertheless lends itself to a high percentage of recurrence, an unpleasant post-operative phase and a real possibility of sequelae and complications.

Case report

We report the case of a model (fig. 8) who had been treated with laser resurfacing to remove very small, introflected acne scars. An unsuitable laser had been combined with a mix of skin cells and nutrients and elastic substances. Fortunately, lasers and

TABLE 7 - POST-TRAUMATIC SCARS - DOSE

DIODE LASER	
Power (W)	30
Wavelength (nm)	808
Emission (Wave)	PW
Fluence (joule/cm^2)	8-10
Rep. Pulse frequency Hertz	3000
Spot size (mm)	3-5 cm
Irradiated points (zones)	Lesion & adjacent tissue
Procedure of irradiation	Fixed point
No. & rhythm of sessions	One session every 20 days

TABLE 8 - POST-TRAUMA HYPERTROPHIC AND KELOID SCARS

Nd-YAG	
Power (W)	5
Wavelength (nm)	1064
Emission (Wave)	PW
Fluence (joule/cm^2)	35 per passage
Pulse Duration (msec)	0.65
Pulse frequency (Hertz)	1
Spot size (mm)	6
Target	Lesion & adjacent tissue
Procedure of irradiation	Fixed point, three passages
No. & rhythm of sessions	Cycle of 3 sessions

Goldman J, 1981; Basford J, 2001; Longo L, 2002

pulsed light in combination with the rejuvenation procedure succeeded in significantly improving the situation, so much so that, after a few years, the patient returned to her job, albeit with some limitations.

Conclusions

In conclusion, the first treatment of side effects and complications is to try to avoid them, acting with prudence, skill and passion (tab. 9). If they do occur, however, it is always possible to try to eliminate them or at least reduce the damage. The conclusions indicated in the last table are key to optimising our work.

TABLE 9 - INDICATIONS FOR OPTIMISING TREATMENT

Continuous practitioner training
The patient must follow the instructions
The instrumentation must be simple
Adequate management of the patient's relatives
Collaboration with other doctors
Attention to patented methods

Bibliography

1. Longo L Terapia Laser, U.S.E.S. ed., Florence, 1986.
2. Longo L. Laser Manual of Medical Technology, OEO Publ, Florence, 2014.
3. Longo L. Non Surgical Laser in Aesthetic Medicine. H. Teixeira Editor, Laser in Medicine and Surgery, Porto, 2017.
4. Longo L. Indicazioni non chirurgiche dei laser in flebologia. In: Mancini S, Compendio di Flebologia, Laris Publisher, Siena, 2009.
5. Longo L. Laser surgery Side effects and complications, "Important issues of modern plastic surgery, emergency medicine and dermatology" International Conference of All Ukrainian Association of Plastic Reconstructive and Aesthetic Surgeons. Ukrainian Society of Aesthetic Medicine, Ukrainian Academy of Dermatology, Odessa, May 28-29, 2015
6. Longo L, Sheykh O. Effetti Collaterali e Complicanze dei laser in medicina estetica , 38° Congresso della Società Italiana di Medicina Estetica, Rome, 12-14 May 2017.

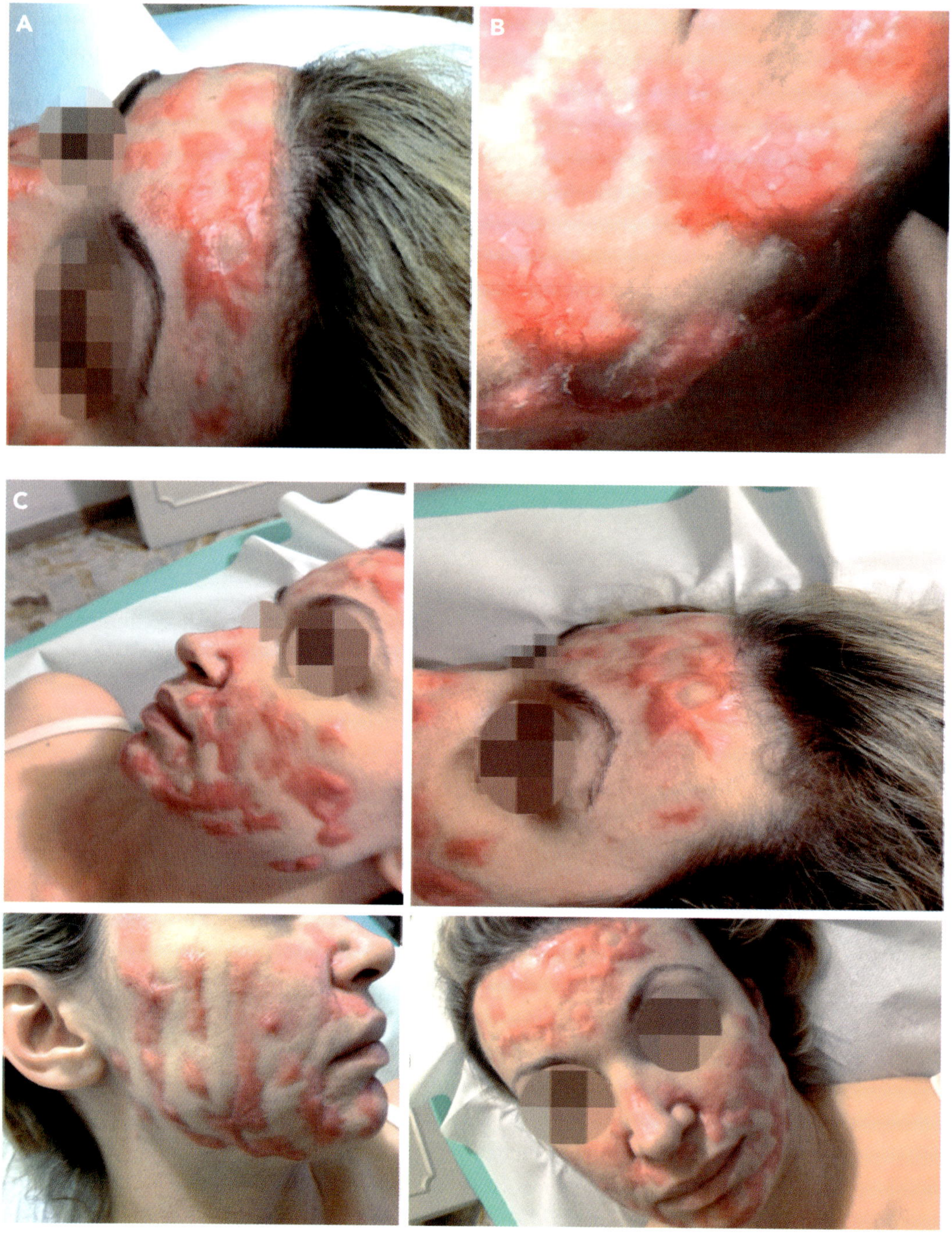
A
B
C

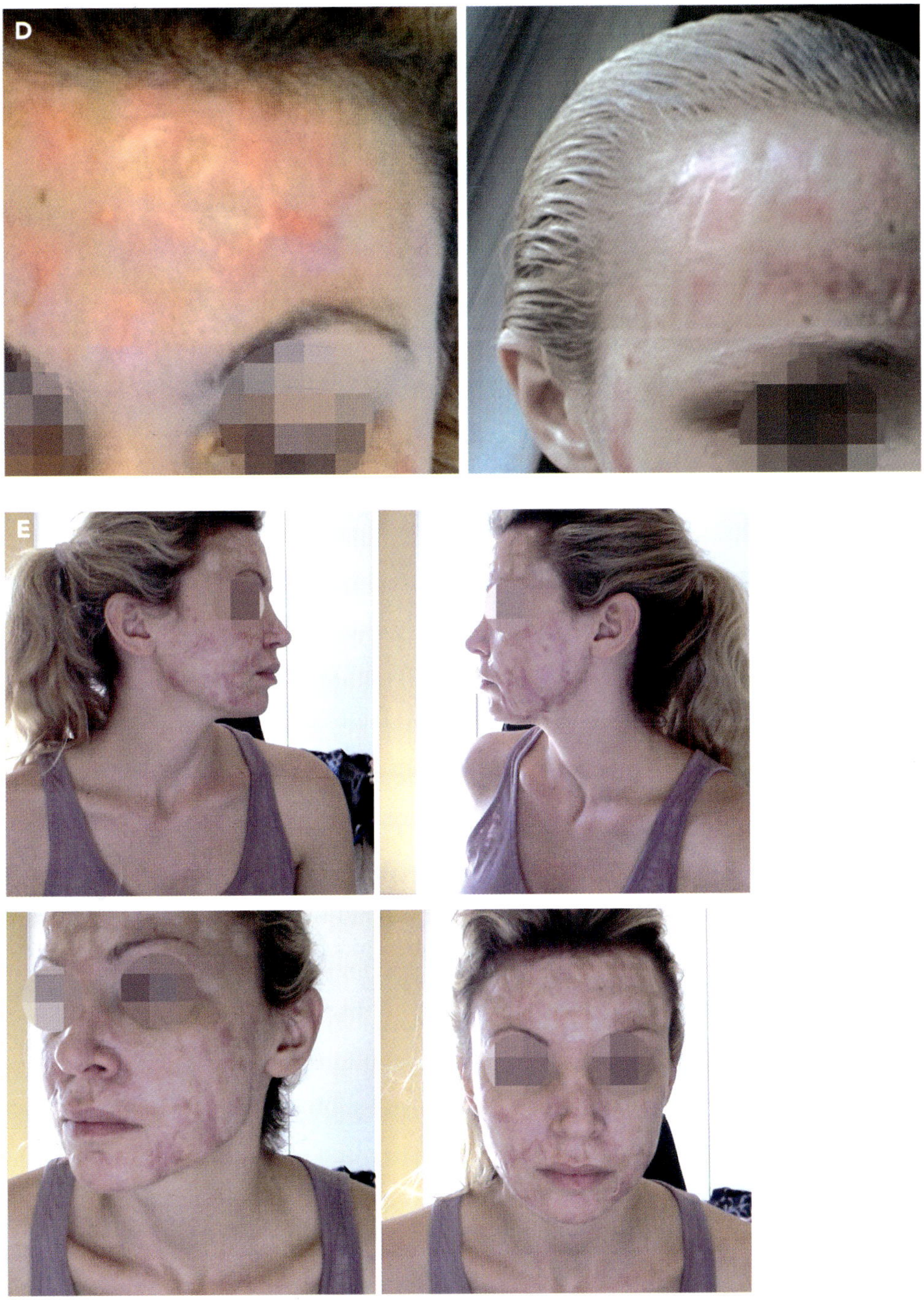

Figure 8 Hypertrophic scars and keloids Post-acne scar surgery performed on 31 January 2012 with "non-ablative" 1470 nm laser in combination with Re-Cell graft. Pre-test 24 May 2012: A) forehead; B) right lower jaw. C) Start of treatment (8 June 2012). D) After 5 sessions (22 September 2012). E) After 20 sessions (29 September 2012).

7

PEELING

HYPERPIGMENTATION: CLASSIFICATION, CAUSES AND TREATMENT

Giuseppe Maria Izzo, Lucia Calvisi

Hyperpigmentation is a darkening of the skin due to a variety of factors. Like most dermatological disorders, it can be extremely disabling for the patient from a psychological point of view, resulting in visits to our clinics requesting lightening treatments.

In terms of classification, skin hyperpigmentations can be divided into:

- endogenous, when the pigment is formed within the body;
- exogenous, when the pigment is applied externally, e.g. tattoos.

The main endogenous pigments that form hyperpigmentation are melanin and haemosiderin.

Melanin hyperpigmentations are multifactorial in origin. They are hard to treat and their main aetiopathogenic factors are an increase in hormone levels (use of contraceptives, pregnancy, thyroid problems, etc.), sun exposure or local inflammation, which lead to an increase in melanin production (fig. 1).

Haemosiderin deposits, on the other hand, can be caused by an increase in hydrostatic pressure (as in the case of chronic venous insufficiency), the processes of vasculitis, ruptured small blood vessels (following sclerotherapy or surgery, post-surgical haematomas, laser therapy or chemical peels).

Determining the nature and measuring the depth of hyperpigmentations are valuable tools for making a correct diagnosis and devising an appropriate treatment programme.

An instrument that is especially dear to us dermatologists is the dermatoscope, which allows us to magnify the lesion in question and establish its depth. Then there is the Wood's lamp, thanks to which we can establish the pigment level and its characteristics (figs. 2-3).

Post-inflammatory hyperpigmentations

Post-inflammatory hyperpigmentations definitely deserve a separate mention as they are among the most frequently occurring complications in aesthetic medicine (figs. 4-5). They are a frequent consequence of trauma or inflammation of the skin following an irritating stimulus (dermatitis or aesthetic medical treatments such as laser or chemical peels), which are statistically more likely to occur in patients with a high Fitzpatrick type (III to VI). It appears as a dark, purplish-brown, irregularly shaped patch at the site of the trauma.

It is a consequence of the stimulation of the production of prostaglandins, leukotrienes and thromboxane by the inflammatory process, resulting in melanocytic hyperplasia and increased melanin production.

Treatment of post-inflammatory hyperpigmentations

Treatment is quite lengthy, difficult and controversial. Combined therapies are those that yield the best results. Various treatments are proposed in literature by different authors, but all agree that resolution, if at all possible, is very slow.

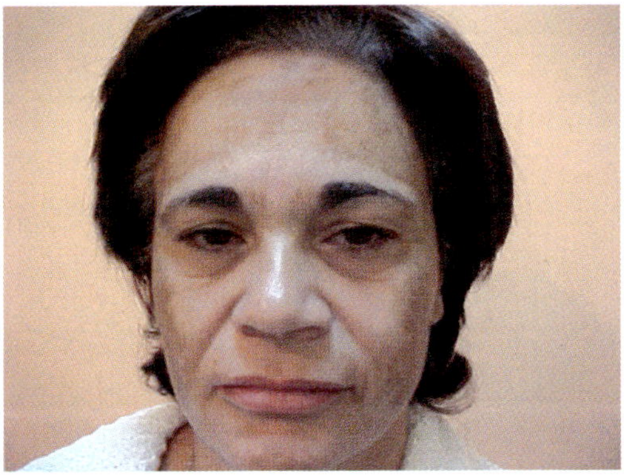

Figure 1 Melasma

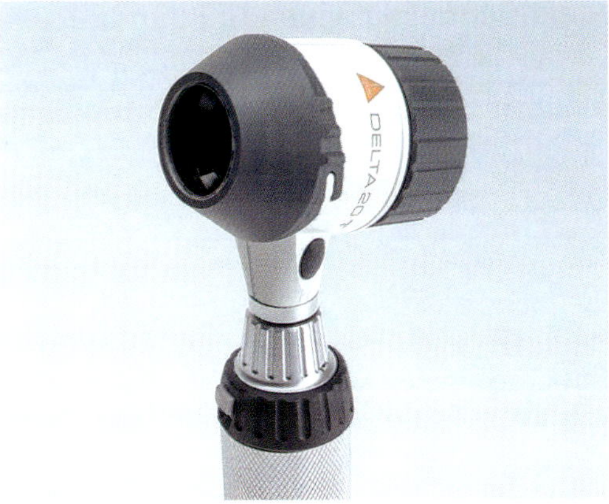

Figure 2 Dermatoscope

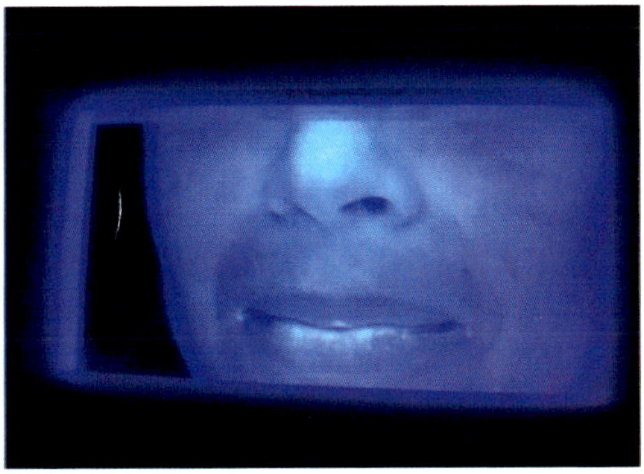

Figure 3 Wood's lamp

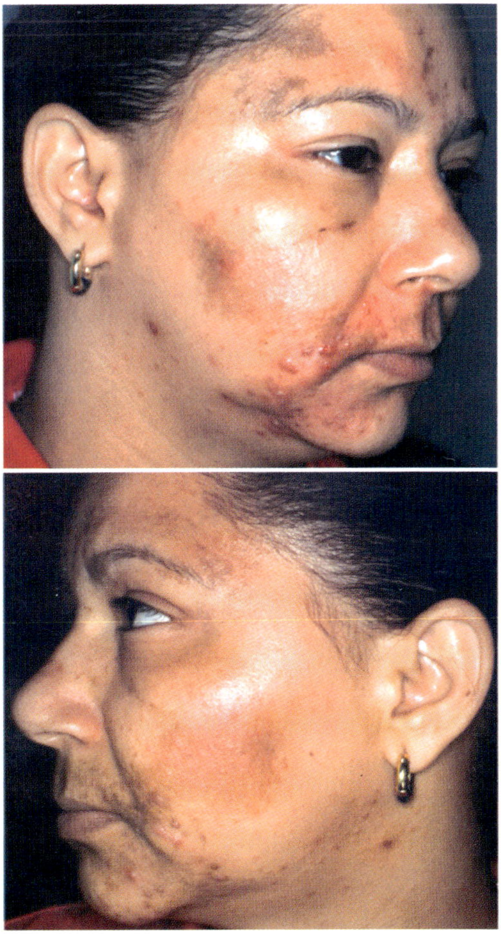

Figure 4 Hyperpigmentation after 70% glycolic in phototype V

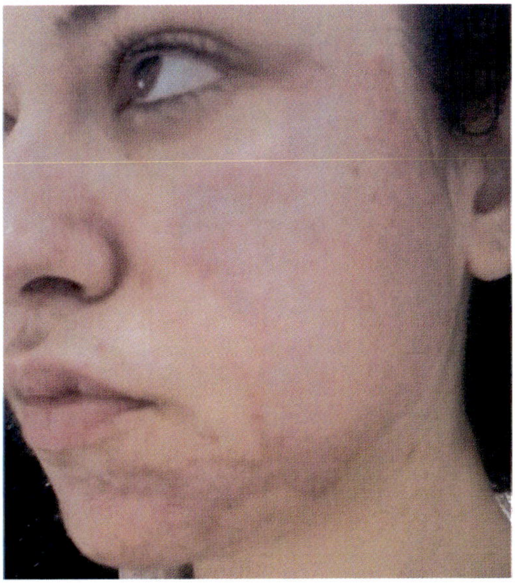

Figure 5 Hyperpigmentation after 35% TCA

Some propose the use of Kligman's formula (2% hydroquinone, 0.025% tretinoin and 0.1% mometasone), which can only be prescribed in Italy as a galenical preparation. In other places in the world, such as Asia, there is a ready-made hydroquinone-based formulation on the market, Triluma (0.01% fluocinolone, 4% hydroquinone, 0.05% tretinoin). Remember that ready-made hydroquinone-based creams have been banned for several years now in Italy, due to problems such as the formation of leukoderma or ochronosis.

Other treatments proposed in literature are azelaic acid, cortisone cream, salicylic acid and retinoids.

Personally, although I have been performing chemical peels for almost twenty years, I have had few post-inflammatory hyperpigmentations in my practice. The few that have occurred have been treated with chemical peels containing salicylic acid at a concentration of 15% (superficial chemical peel) and diligent application of sunscreen.

Bibliography

1. Lipsker D, Lenormand C. Hyperpigmentations [Hyperpigmentation]. Ann Dermatol Venereol. 2019 Oct;146(10):666-682. French.
2. Searle T, Al-Niaimi F, Ali FR. The top 10 cosmeceuticals for facial hyperpigmentation. Dermatol Ther. 2020 Nov;33(6):e14095.
3. Kaufman BP, Aman T, Alexis AF. Postinflammatory Hyperpigmentation: Epidemiology, Clinical Presentation, Pathogenesis and Treatment. Am J Clin Dermatol. 2018 Aug;19(4):489-503.
4. Borelli C, Fischer S. Chemical Peelings zur Behandlung von Melasma, Pigmentstörungen und Hyperpigmentierungen : Indikationen, Effektivität und Risiken [Chemical peeling for treatment of Melasma, pigmentary disorders and hyperpigmentation : Indications, effectivity and risks]. Hautarzt. 2020 Dec;71(12):950-959. German.
5. Nautiyal A, Wairkar S. Management of hyperpigmentation: Current treatments and emerging therapies. Pigment Cell Melanoma Res. 2021 Nov;34(6):1000-1014.
6. Taylor S, Grimes P, Lim J, Im S, Lui H. Postinflammatory hyperpigmentation. J Cutan Med Surg. 2009 Jul-Aug;13(4):183-91. doi: 10.2310/7750.2009.08077. PMID: 19706225.
7. Rigopoulos D, Gregoriou S, Katsambas A. Hyperpigmentation and melasma. J Cosmet Dermatol. 2007 Sep;6(3):195-202.
8. Schalka S. New data on hyperpigmentation disorders. J Eur Acad Dermatol Venereol. 2017 Sep;31 Suppl 5:18-21.
9. Lambert MW. Treatment of Postinflammatory Hyperpigmentation: A Dermatologic Challenge. Skinmed. 2021 Apr 1;19(2):99-102.
10. Pandya AG, Guevara IL. Disorders of hyperpigmentation. Dermatol Clin. 2000 Jan;18(1):91-8, ix.

CHEMICAL PEELS: SIDE EFFECTS AND COMPLICATIONS

Giuseppe Maria Izzo, Lucia Calvisi

Chemical peeling is one of the treatments most frequently practised by aesthetic doctors, dermatologists and plastic surgeons, becoming increasingly popular over the last quarter of a century. In the meantime, companies have continued to make new formulations available to medical users, assembling various molecules in order to maximise the positive effects and limit possible complications related to the procedure. Yet we have witnessed an increase in side effects, often due to a lack of experience or malpractice, generated by an insufficient knowledge of the chemical characteristics of the various peeling agents, superficial preliminary examination of the patient with inadequate diagnostic framing, and poor management of side effects.

The chemicals used offer peels that act at various depths, as far as the mid reticular dermis- They must not go beyond this because they could hinder successful regeneration of the skin due to the destruction of the cutaneous adnexa, where the repair process begins.

Depending on the characteristics of the molecules used, their concentration and pH, and on the application technique or the number of layers applied to the skin, a peel can be [1]:

- very superficial;
- superficial;
- medium;
- deep.

It follows that, very often, the same product can be used to perform a su-

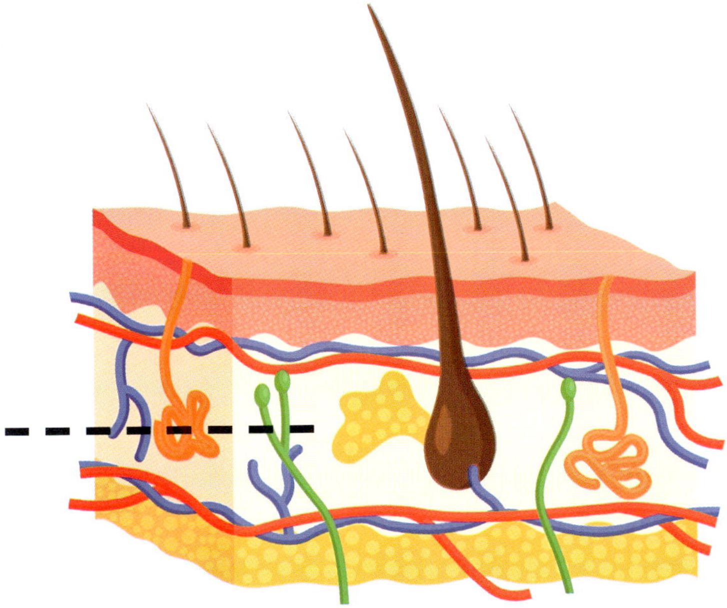

Figure 1 The depth of a peel should go no further than the mid reticular dermis. It must not destroy the cutaneous adnexa, on which the skin's repair process depends

VIDEO 7.1

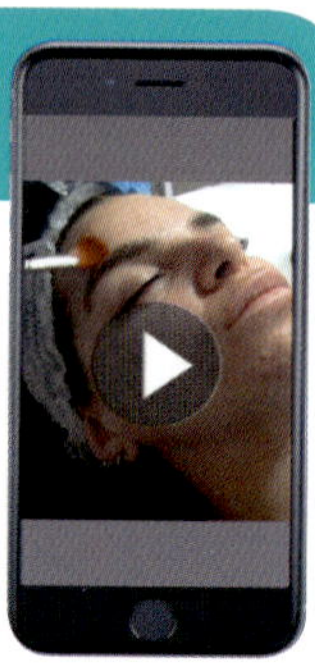

Correct application of a chemical peel

perficial peel or a medium or even medium-deep peel, so classification is not absolute, but relative, depending on a whole series of factors [2]:

- type of substance;
- concentration of the substance;
- number of layers;
- application technique;
- home application or outpatient application;
- skin type;
- area;
- application time.

Correct application of a chemical peel

Having seen how many variables are possible in a chemical peel, it is worthwhile specifying the guidelines for its correct application. In our opinion, the patient should be prescribed a 15-day preparation treatment to be carried out at home. This consists of a cleanser, a different active cream (anti-acne, anti-ageing, lightening, etc.)depending on the type of problem to be treated, and a sun filter with a high protection factor (SPF 50+).

At the outpatient clinic, the patient must be scrupulously cleansed to remove make-up residue, environmental pollutants and sebum, which can hinder the uniform penetration of the active substances. The next step is the application of an acid pH pre-peel to ensure even peeling with no surprises.

Descriptions of how to perform various types of peel are outlined below, bearing in mind that it is advisable to proceed from region to region, starting with the forehead, followed by one cheek, then the other, and finally the perioral area, which is more susceptible to post-inflammation hyperpigmentation. This way of proceeding allows us to assess two things: the possible hypersensitivity of the skin to the peel and the skin's response to the formula in terms of erythema and frost if using a medium-high peel.

Very superficial peel

A very superficial peel (fig. 2) is, in our opinion, highly aesthetic and not very medical, because it determines a corneolysis that makes the skin brighter; it can be used by the practitioner to open up the skin surface for the safe application of another formula for a subsequent and simultaneous superficial or medium peel. These peels often require no neutralisation with a solution of water and bicarbonate of soda because they are self-neutralising, but it is advisable to rinse the face with water.

Superficial peel

Superficial peels (fig. 3) are single-substance peels or are made up of a combination of several agents in order

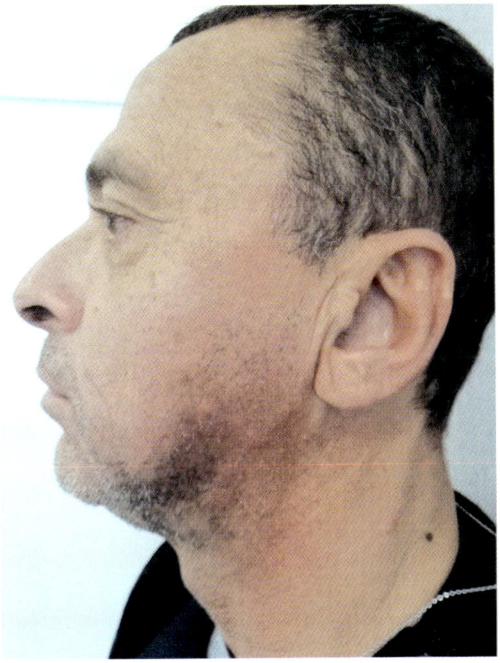

Figure 2 Very superficial peel

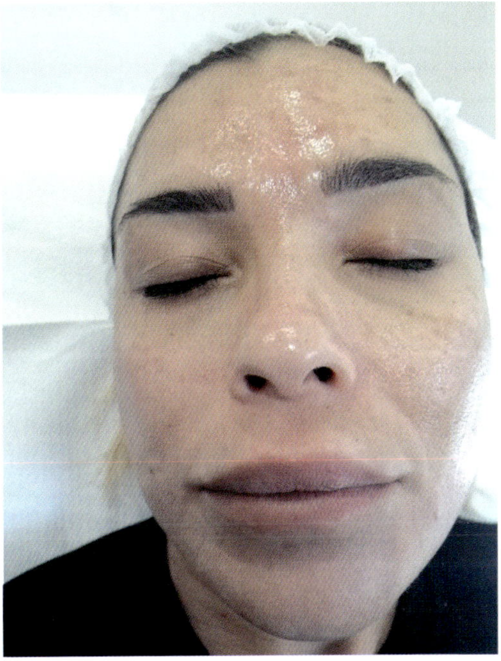

Figure 3 Superficial peel

to achieve a synergistic action with reduced percentages of use, resulting in a lower risk of complications and better correction of the various imperfections. For this type of peel too, manufacturers often tell us that neutralisation is unnecessary, but we always recommend performing it as a precaution. For example, a glycolic acid peeling should always be neutralised with water and bicarbonate because the molecule is very small and can penetrate the dermis, resulting in hyperpigmentation, hypopigmentation and depressed arboriform or hypertrophic scars.

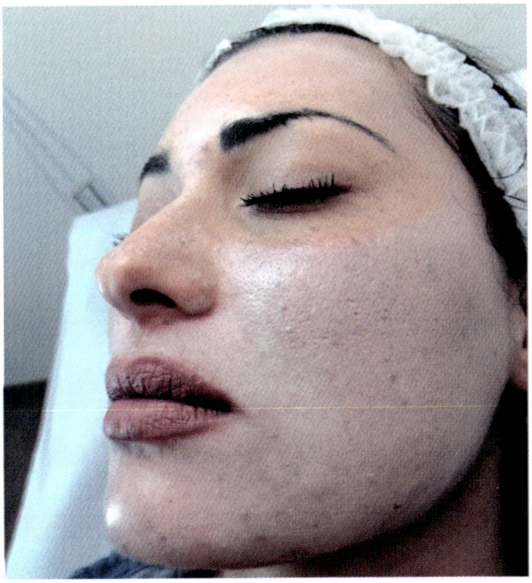

Figure 4 Medium peel

Medium peel

A standard medium peel (fig. 4) is a 15-35% TCA (trichloroacetic acid) peel. Obviously, this peel must be applied region by region, reaching the level of frost desired, either due to use of a higher percentage or multiple layers.

Frost is an expression of the depth reached by the peel and can be of various types (table 1).

TABLE 1 - TYPES OF FROST

Pink frost	Grade 0 Intraepidermal
Milky frost	Grade 1 Papillary dermis
Compact frost	Grade 2 Upper reticular dermis
Compact Frost with erythema	Grade 3 Bordering on the mid reticular

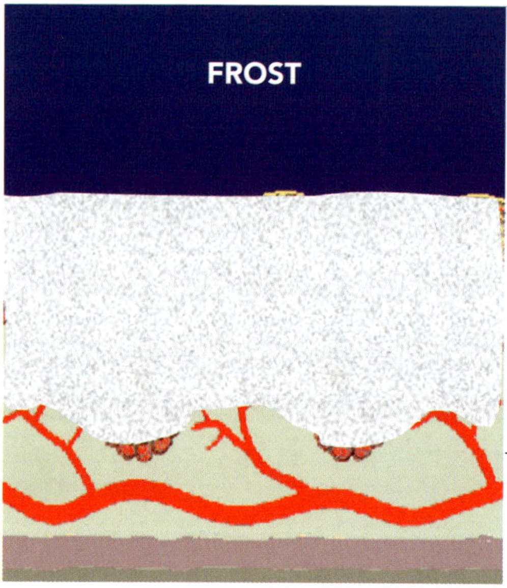

PINK FROST
STRATUM CORNEUM
▼
MILKY FROST
EPIDERMIS
▼
WHITE FROST COMPACT
UPPER RETICULAR DERMIS

Figure 5 Depth of TCA peel. Intensity in direct proportion to the number of cells destroyed

Deep peel

Today, a deep peel (fig. 6) is a phenol peel because 50% TCA is rarely used due to possible complications. Modern phenol peels are not normally used at 88%, like Yoram Fintsi's classic Exoderm, but are between 30 and 60%, often with the addition of 10 or 20% TCA [3].

The correct application of this peel requires a lot of time, because we have to wait 15 minutes between peels to avoid the build-up of phenol in the body, which can cause general complications as it is nephrotoxic, neurotoxic and hepatotoxic, but is quickly metabolised by the body. After completing the phenol peel, which should not be neutralised because it does not cause excessive stinging due to its anaesthetic properties, we can proceed in two ways: if we want a deeper action, we can apply a layer of impermeable occlusive patches for 24 hours, followed by the application of bismuth subgallate powder with a healing and antiseptic action for a week, then removing it with Vaseline; or we can apply the bismuth subgallate powder directly in the same way, obviously with a more superficial action.

Side effects of chemical peels

The side effects of a chemical peel are:
- erythema;
- oedema;
- vesicles;
- blisters.

Erythema is not always considered a

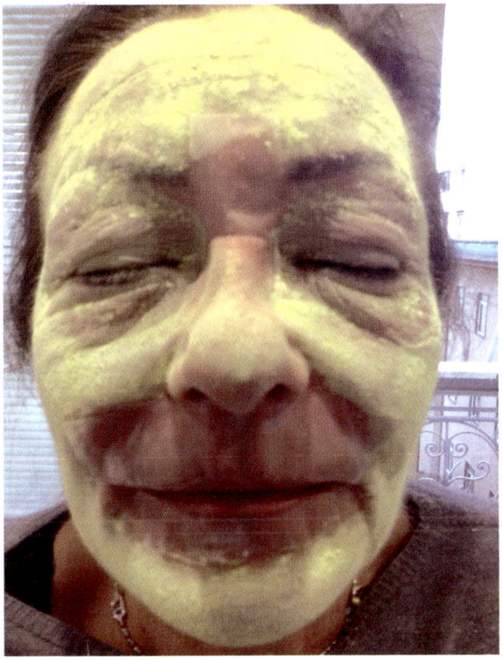

Figure 6 Deep peel

side effect because it is an expression of dermal stimulation induced by the active substance applied. In our opinion, it should be considered a side effect when a hypersensitivity to the molecule applied is evident, arising almost immediately or over time, with the risk of post-inflammatory hyperpigmentation. In the case of erythema, we can use cortisone-based creams alternating with soothing topical products. In more severe cases, perhaps associated with oedema, cortisone is administered by mouth. We prefer Deflazacort due to the less significant and slower side effects of the cortisone.

Oedemas are also generally due to an abnormal sensitivity to the chemical agent and should be treated in the same way as erythema, with a greater emphasis on oral medication, which may also include anti-oedematous drugs.

Vesicles and blisters are also an expression of hypersensitivity; in addition to the oral medication described above, we also recommend the initial application of topical rifamycin in order to avoid bacterial over-infection, and subsequently topical zinc oxide.

Complications of chemical peels

The avoidance of complications is related to the following main variables:

- the type of acid used;
- the characteristics of the patient's skin;
- the quality and condition of the patient's skin;
- exclusion criteria;
- preparation of the skin;
- post-peel treatment.

Complications are also related to the technique used to perform the peel and are related mainly to the following aspects:

- quantity or number of layers of peeling solution applied to the skin;
- observance of the time before completion of the procedure (neutralisation or washing);
- interval between one procedure and the next.

Skin trauma is an intrinsic part of the peeling procedure. The skin's reactivity to acids depends on many variables: some of these are specific to each patient, others depend on the procedure and others are closely related to the type of acid used to perform the peel.

Complications can be divided into immediate and delayed.

Immediate complications occur a few minutes or hours after the outpatient

procedure and include:
- itching, stinging, irritation;
- persistent erythema and oedema;
- epidermolysis;
- ocular and respiratory complications.

Delayed complications occur a few days to weeks after the peel and include:
- infections;
- abnormal healing such as scarring or a change in texture;
- changes in pigmentation, such as hypo-or hyperpigmentation, demarcation lines.

Complications can be summarised as follows:
- hyperpigmentation;
- hypopigmentation;
- persistent erythema;
- telangiectasias;
- rashes;
- hypersensitivity;
- acne-like reactions;
- milia;
- infections;
- scarring.

Hyperpigmentation

Hyperpigmentation is the most frequent complication of any type of chemical peel and can occur for various reasons:
- overly aggressive peeling, especially in patients with a dark phototype;
- as a result of excessive post-peel inflammation which is not properly managed by the practitioner;
- after a harsh peel in patients with melasma;
- sun exposure or tanning lamps with insufficient or no protection during skin recovery after the peel;
- use of photosensitising drugs mainly by mouth;
- improper use of topical products with active substances immediately after the peel [5].

The important thing is that the practitioner knows how to handle hyperpigmentation safely and competently. We believe that topical lightening agents for use at home, possibly containing various molecules with complementary

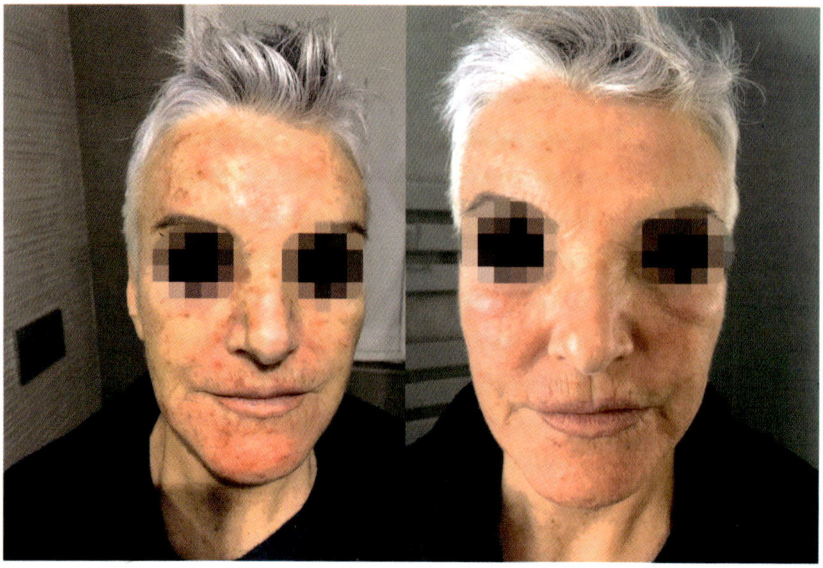

Figure 7
24 hours after 70% glycolic and after 7 days

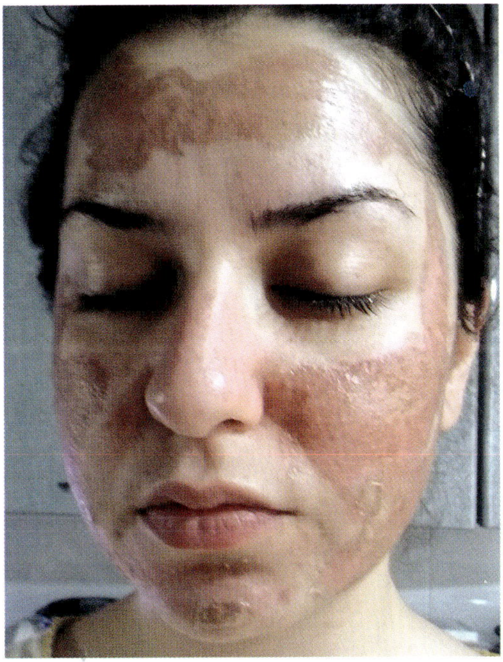

Figure 8 After 50% TCA

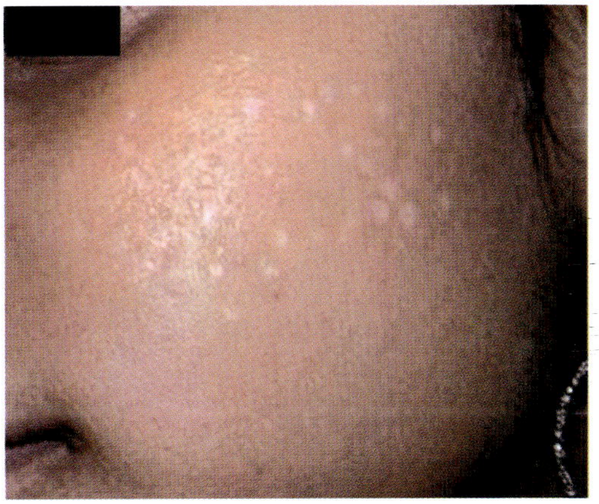

Figure 9 After 25% TCA

actions (tranexamic acid, kojic acid, phytic acid, arbutin, azelaic acid, etc.) together with very high UV protection, as well as mild chemical peels, possibly associated with or followed by LED photobiomodulation, may be useful.

Hypopigmentation

Hypopigmentation is fortunately rarer because it can express:

- a momentary malfunction of the melanocytes, in which case we can prescribe topical agents to stimulate melaninogenesis or normal melanocyte function;
- destruction of the melanocytes, in which case we can try topical agents that attract melanocytes from the surrounding areas.

Persistent erythema

Persistent erythema is a fairly frequent complication of medium to medium-deep peel. It is worrying when it lasts for more than a month/a month and a half, because it is extremely uncomfortable for patients and can lead to significant and persistent post-inflammation hyperpigmentation after a while. In addition to soothing and anti-reddening topical agents, a vascular laser used in fractional mode can help solve the problem safely in just a few sessions.

Telangiectasias

Telangiectasias are the expression of the expansion of the skin capillaries after excessively harsh peeling in patient with phototypes I and II. In this case too, we use a vascular laser, progressively and gently treating individual capillaries, considering the fragility of the patients' skin.

Rashes

Rashes are caused either by hypersensitivity to the molecule applied or by physical urticaria in a patient with diathesis. We recommend oral treatment with corticosteroids and antihistamines.

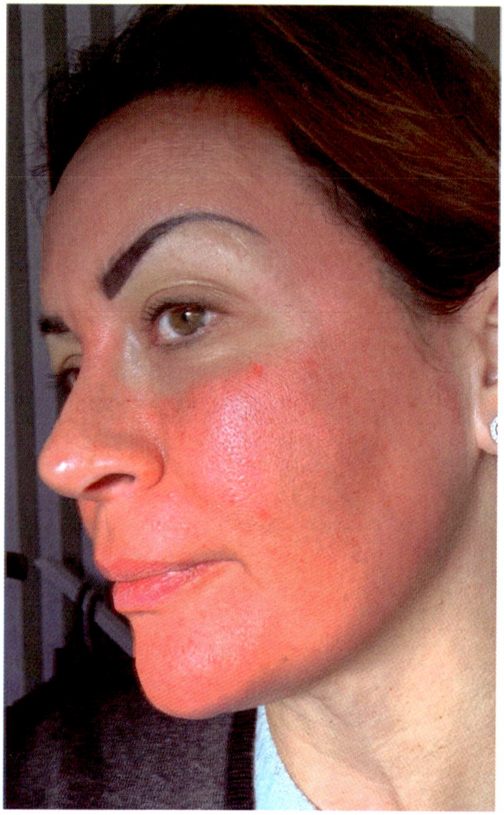

Figure 10 After depigmenting mask

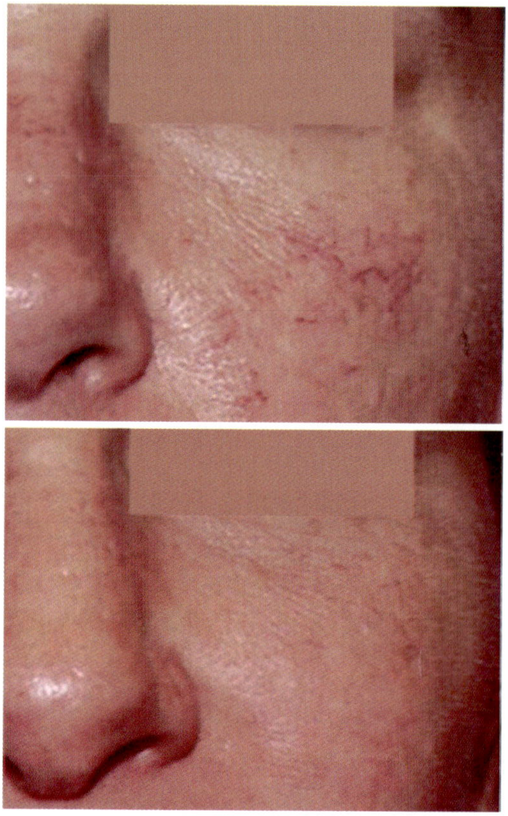

Figure 11 After 25% TCA peel and two 532 laser sessions

Hypersensitivity

Hypersensitivity is manifested in the form of eczema-like dermatitis mainly in diathesis sufferers with a positive history of atopic dermatitis. Oral cortisone treatment is recommended.

Acne-like reactions

Acne-like reactions occur fairly frequently after TCA peeling and are an expression of irritation of the hair follicles and sebaceous glands even in the absence of acne pathology. The prescription of gentle anti-acne topical agents containing low percentages of benzoylperoxide,, combined with topical erythromycin or clindamycin is usually sufficient to solve the problem.

Milia

Milia usually appears after a medium peel [4]. They are sebum retention cysts that often occur following the application of a restructuring and soothing ointment over the days following the peel, which occludes the duct of the hair follicle and sebaceous glans, mainly in thicker and photo-aged scalps. Treatment consists of removing them with a plasma device or a low-power CO_2 laser.

Infections

Infections can occur mainly due to:

- poor patient hygiene
- poor hygiene on the part of the practitioner;

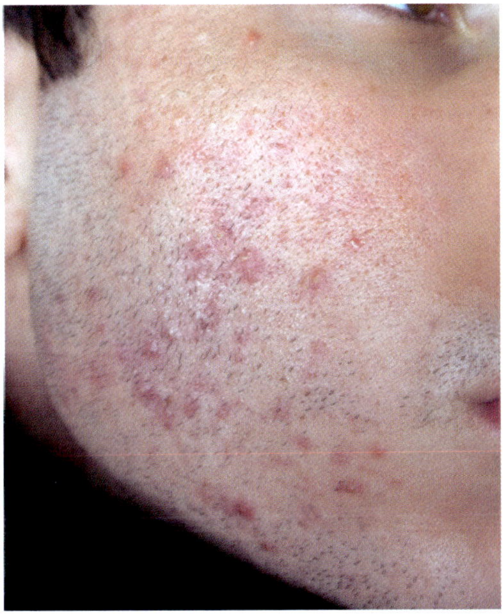

Figure 12 After 25% TCA and water in oil restructuring creams

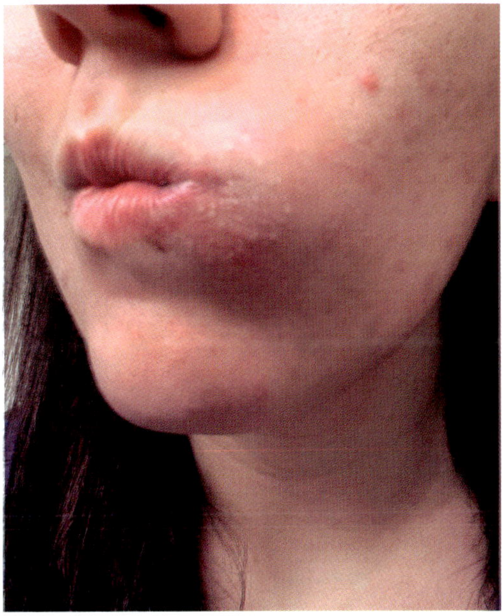

Figure 13 Milia after azelaic acid peel

• both of the above.

Obviously, this concerns bacterial infections, while Candida or Pseudomonas aeruginosa infections are rarer.

Specific oral and topical treatment is necessary; where there is doubt as to the aetiology, an antibiogram culture is helpful. Herpes simplex manifestations are more frequent and can occur after a peel in patients with either a positive or negative history.

Sometimes, due to superficiality or inexperience, the presence of a herpetic manifestation is not detected on the skin, resulting in the widespread manifestation of herpes all over the face in the days following the peel.

Topical and oral anti-herpes agents are necessary. We recommend anti-herpes prophylaxis from two days before the peel to two days afterwards in patients with a positive medical history.

Scarring

Scars are the most severe complication of a chemical peel; they can also occur after a superficial peel, due to excessive reactivity of the patient's skin (pay attention to the anamnesis to ascertain whether the patient has keloid diathesis), but are more frequent after a medium or deep peel, especially after a high-percentage TCA (pay attention to galenical TCAs, due to the frequent instability of their concentration, which can vary over time).

They can be of two types, atrophic or hypertrophic, and sometimes limit the patient's functional and social life (ectropion after high-percentage TCA, limitation of facial movement due to scarring of the neck after high-percentage TCA) [6].

The possible treatments are fractional CO_2 in several sessions without excessively high doses, perhaps alternating

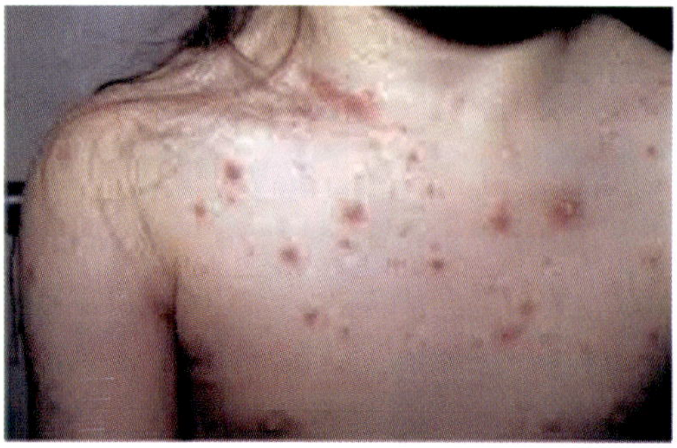

Figure 14 Staphylococcus infection after 70% glycolic

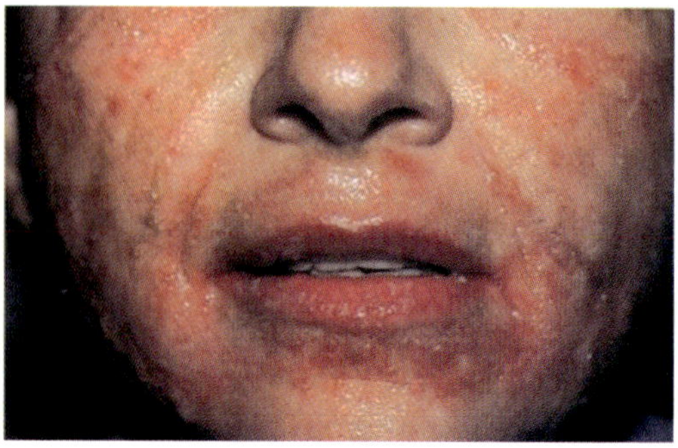

Figure 15 Candidiasis after 50% pyruvic

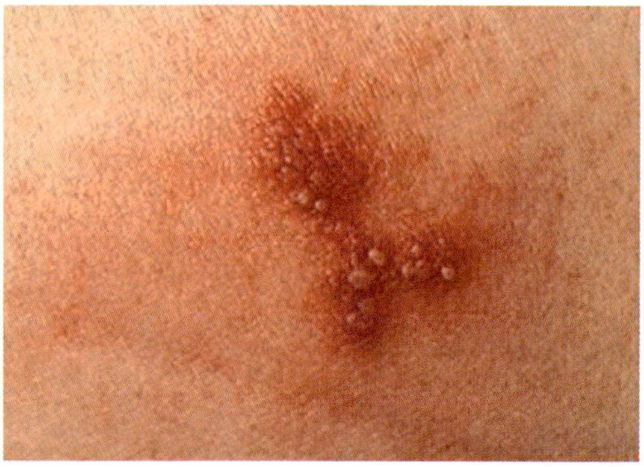

Figure 16 Herpes simplex after 70% glycolic

with vascular laser to reduce the entity of the vascular network, or intralesional infiltrations of diluted triamcinolone, or even plastic surgery, trying not to stimulate the production of new scar tissue.

Bibliography

1. Mark G. Rubin. Procedures in Cosmetic Dermatology Series: Chemical Peel. Elsevier, 2006.
2. Giuseppe Maria Izzo, Lucia Calvisi. I peeling chimici nella pratica clinica. Acta Medica, 2012.
3. Philippe Deprez. Textbook of Chemical Peels: Superficial, Medium, and Deep Peels in Cosmetic Practice. CRC Press, 2016.
4. Nikalji N, Godse K, Sakhiya J, Patil S, Nadkarni N. Complications of medium depth and deep chemical peels. J Cutan Aesthet Surg. 2012;5(4):254-260.
5. Shenoy A, Madan R. Post-Inflammatory Hyperpigmentation: A Review of Treatment Strategies. J Cosmet Dermatol. 2020;19(8):763-768.
6. Costa IMC, Damasceno PS, Costa MC, Gomes KGP. Review in peeling complications. J Cosmet Dermatol. 2017;16(3):319-326.

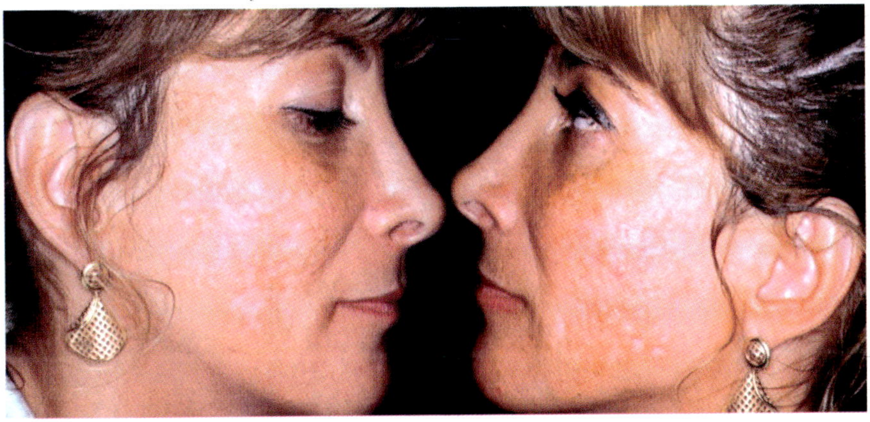

Figure 17 After 70% glycolic left for 30 minutes

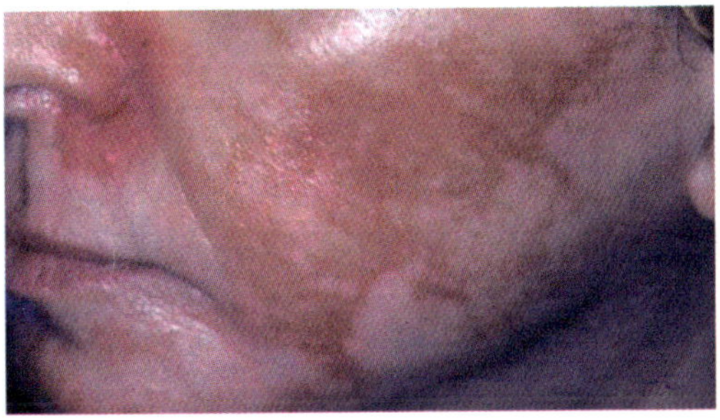

Figure 18 After 35% TCA

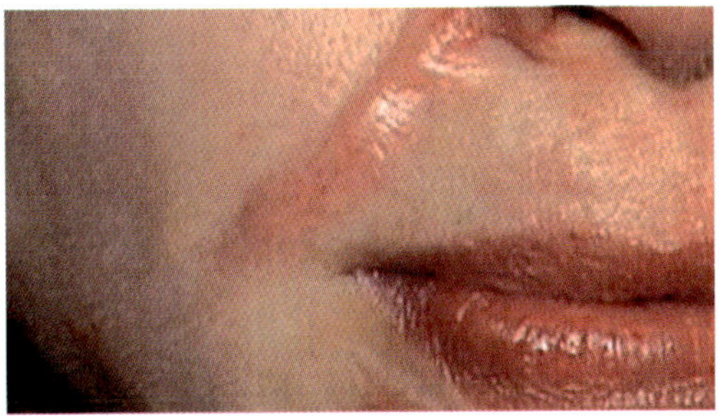

Figure 19 After 35% TCA in patient with keloid diathesis

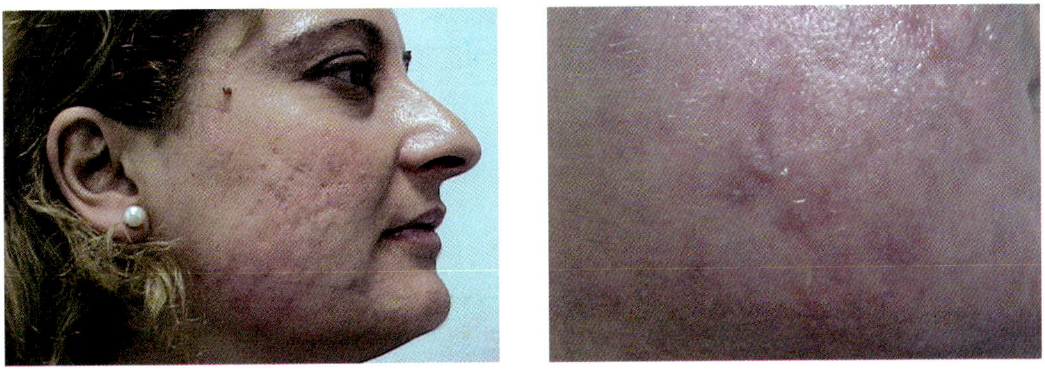

Figure 20 Scar caused by premature removal of flaking skin

8

CARBOXYTHERAPY

THE COMPLICATIONS OF CARBOXYTHERAPY

Lucia Calvisi

Carboxytherapy consists of the subcutaneous administration of medicated carbon dioxide for therapeutic purposes. It is an old method that was first used in France in 1932, when it was discovered that bathing in water rich in carbon dioxide accelerated the wound healing process.

The term carboxytherapy was coined by Luigi Parassoni in 1995 during the 16th congress of the Italian Society of Aesthetic Medicine.

The method is used in cardiology, angiology, to treat metabolic diseases, rheumatology and chronic ulcers, in dermatology and in aesthetic treatments for skin laxity of the face and body, fatty deposits and edematous fibrosclerotic panniculopathy.

Impact on tissues

The aim of carboxytherapy is to improve microcirculation and this is achieved through a hypercapnia mechanism that leads to an increase in oxygen production. This means that the more CO_2 is present in the tissue, the higher the oxygen pressure will be in relation to the percentage of oxygen saturation by haemoglobin.

When carbon dioxide is administered, subcutaneous emphysema is created, and the laxer the tissues are, the more noticeable the subcutaneous emphysema. This is a temporary subcutaneous emphysema; once the insufflation is over, it resolves quickly, and when the treatment has been completed, it is already resolved. Subcutaneous emphysema involves an increase in pressure in the tissues, detected by pressure receptors that activate the release of algogenic molecules: bradykinin, serotonin and catecholamines (adrenalin, noradrenalin). These molecules stimulate the formation of cAMP, a cytosolic messenger that locally activates intradipocyte lipase (local lipolytic effect).

Indications

By virtue of its mechanism of action, carboxytherapy is effective in the treatment of:

- microcirculation disorders and venous insufficiency;
- edematous-fibro-sclerotic panniculopathy;
- fatty deposits;
- skin laxity;
- post-liposuction depressions;
- stretch marks and scars;
- painful and inflammatory conditions;
- certain forms of alopecia;
- diabetic ulcers;
- microangiopathy;
- diabetic and non-diabetic ulcers (as long as they are not infected);
- vaginal atrophy [1-3].

Contraindications

A careful preliminary anamnesis is essential to reduce the risk of complications. All patients with alterations in the organs that determine the disposal of carbon dioxide must clearly be excluded. Exclusion criteria will therefore be cardiac, renal and respiratory failure, circulatory insufficiency, previous heart attack, anaemia, tumours, connective tissue diseases.

A relative contraindication is the treatment of both type I and type II diabetes mellitus. Administering CO_2 could aggravate a condition of systemic acidosis and further lower the blood pH. It is a good idea to have plasma lactic acid assayed in patients taking metformin and to assess systemic ketoacidosis in patients on insulin therapy. A search for ketone bodies in the urine (using Ketostix) may be useful for this purpose.

How to perform a carboxytherapy session

Some useful tips for a successful carboxytherapy session are listed below:

- use only certified and CE-marked

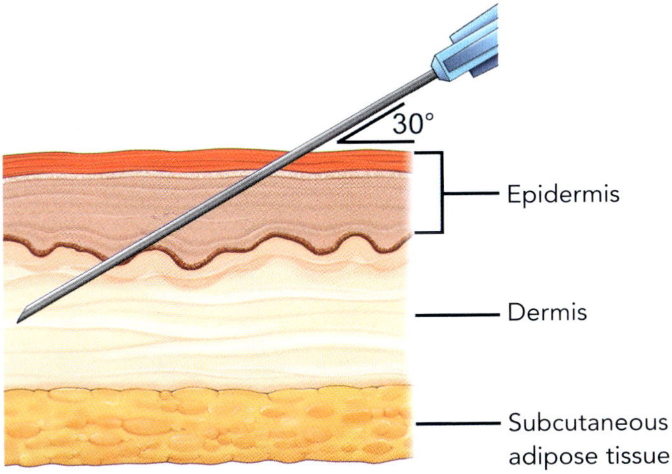

Figure 1
Inclination of the needle by 30°, with the aim of stimulating the elasticity of the area treated

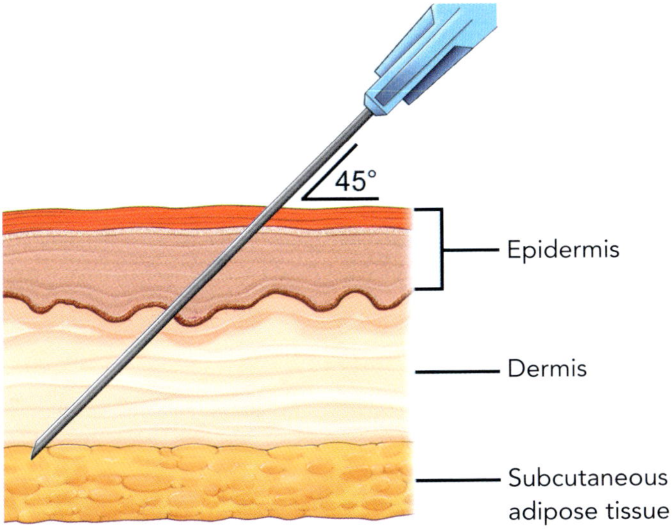

Figure 2
Inclination of the needle by 45°, preferable when treating fatty areas

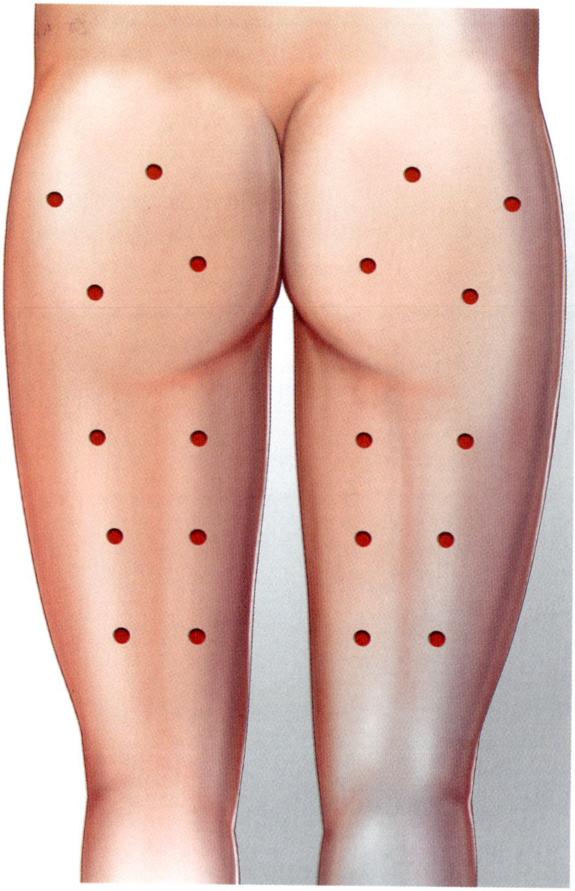

Figure 3 Example of treatment of the back of the thigh

equipment;
- use a disposable sterile tube for each individual patient;
- set the appliance to the correct parameters for the area to be treated;
- have the patient lie down;
- once the area to be treated (face or body) has been identified, proceed with thorough disinfection to avoid the occurrence of bacterial complications;
- the session usually lasts 20-30 minutes.

Depending on how the needle is inclined, we can have different results:
- a needle inclined by 30° generally results in an increase in elasticity and firmness of the area treated (fig. 1);
- a needle inclined by 45° results in a more intense action on fatty tissue, so it is mainly used in areas such as peritrochanteric pads, abdomen and knees (fig. 2).

Side effects

Although carboxytherapy is relatively safe, side effects have been described in literature.

Let us assume that the human body produces 200 mL of CO_2 at rest. This level increases 10-fold during sporting activity. Massive quantities of CO_2

are injected during laparoscopic surgery without any danger to the patient. It can therefore be considered a safe method.

During treatment, the patient experiences a burning sensation, tingling up to the point of pain, depending on the individual degree of sensitivity. As a result of increased microcirculation in the area treated, the local temperature may rise for about 10-20 minutes. After treatment it is normal to feel a prickling sensation in the area due to subcutaneous emphysema. Sometimes, as with all injectable therapies, bruising may occur. These can certainly be considered mild complications.

More severe complications are also reported in literature. Some authors have described cases of lymphangitis and peripheral neuropathy after carboxytherapy. Jamshidian-Tehrania et al. report a case of orbital emphysema following carboxytherapy in the periocular region with the aim of treating periocular wrinkles and reducing dark circles. Emphysema persisted in the upper and lower eyelid ten days after the carboxytherapy treatment (temporary subcutaneous emphysema of the periocular region following treatment is to be considered normal and generally persists for 2-3 hours, after which it reabsorbs spontaneously). In the case described, however, it was necessary to prescribe prednisolone 50 mg by mouth for one week, with resolution of the symptoms.

Couderc et al., on the other hand, reported cases of post-carboxytherapy skin infection and concluded that the problem was probably poor disinfection of the area treated.

Lastly, Calonge et al. report a case of severe abdominal emphysema following carboxytherapy performed to treat "jodhpur thighs", which resolved with antibiotic therapy using amoxicillin plus clavulanic acid.

Bibliography

1. Kołodziejczak A, Podgórna K, Rotsztejn H. Is carboxytherapy a good alternative method in the removal of various skin defects? Dermatol Ther. 2018 Sep;31(5):e12699.

2. Oliveira SMD, Rocha LB, da Cunha MTR, Cintra MMM, Pinheiro NM, Mendonça AC. Effects of carboxytherapy on skin laxity. J Cosmet Dermatol. 2020 Nov;19(11):3007-3013.

3. Lokhande AJ, Mysore V. Striae Distensae Treatment Review and Update. Indian Dermatol Online J. 2019 Jul-Aug;10(4):380-395.

4. Michelle L, Pouldar Foulad D, Ekelem C, Saedi N, Mesinkovska NA. Treatments of Periorbital Hyperpigmentation: A Systematic Review. Dermatol Surg. 2021 Jan 1;47(1):70-74.

5. Ahramiyanpour N, Shafie'ei M, Sarvipour N, Amiri R, Akbari Z. Carboxytherapy in dermatology: A systematic review. J Cosmet Dermatol. 2022 Feb 6.

6. Couderc C, Carbonne A, Thiolet JM, Brossier F, Savey A, Bernet C, Ortmans C, Lecadet-Morin C, Coudière I, Aggoune M, Astagneau P, Coignard B, Cambau E. [Non-tuberculous mycobacterial infections related to esthetic care in France, 2001-2010]. Med Mal Infect. 2011 Jul;41(7):379-83.

9

VASCULAR COMPLICATIONS

ISCHAEMIA, RECOGNISING AND TREATING IT BEFORE NECROSIS

Teresa Lacava, Giuseppe Sito, Silvia Silenzi

Aesthetic medical injection treatments to correct imperfections of the face and body are becoming increasingly popular worldwide. In cosmetic and reconstructive surgery, soft tissue augmentation is performed using different biomaterials [1]. Fillers are classified, based on the duration of their effect, as temporary/biodegradable or permanent/non-biodegradable [2]. Hyaluronic acid (HA), collagen (bovine, porcine and human), poly-L-lactic acid (PLLA), calcium hydroxyapatite (CaHA) and dextran spheres in hyaluronic acid are examples of temporary or biodegradable fillers. Permanent fillers, on the other hand, include polymethylmethacrylate microspheres with bovine collagen, polymethylmethacrylate microspheres suspended in carboxygluconate gel, silicone, saturated hydrocarbons, polymethylmethacrylate silicone suspension, acrylic hydrogel particles suspended in hyaluronic acid, polyacrylamide gel, polyvinyl microspheres suspended in polyacrylamide, e-polytetrafluoroethylene and Gore-Tex [2,3].

Treatment with fillers is considered effective and safe, however the growing use of fillers has inevitably seen an increase in the complications associated with them. The potential complications associated with dermal fillers depend on the type of filler and the site of application. Adverse events caused by dermal gels can be classified, depending on their onset, as: immediate (up to 24 hours after the procedure); early (24 hours to 4 weeks); delayed (more than 4 weeks) [4]. Complications can also be divided depending on their mechanism, into non-ischaemic and ischaemic. The former can be caused by the injection technique and include injection site reactions, uneven contours, inflammatory and infectious reactions. These types of complications normally clear up within 2-7 days. By contrast, ischaemic complications are caused by a vascular, arterial or venous occlusion, resulting in tissue necrosis and, in more severe cases, loss of vision [2].

The incidence of an ischaemic event following the use of dermal fillers has been found to be three cases in every 1,000 injections. In the case of hyaluronic acid injections, this drops slightly to three to nine cases per 10,000 injections [2]. The statistics on vascular events, however, vary from study to study. A study carried out by Alam et al. involving 370 dermatologists reports an incidence of vascular occlusion of one case in 6,410 and one case in 40,882 when using a needle or cannula, respectively [5]. Another publication also found that the relative risk of occurrence of an ischaemic event was twice as high among practitioners in the first five years of practice compared to those with more experience, indicating that injector experience is a significant factor in avoiding vascular occlusion [5].

Dermal filler injections can be risky in any area, but the areas with a higher risk of vascular occlusion are the glabella, forehead, nose, lips, nasolabial fold and temples [2,6]. These complications are technique-dependent and are caused by intravascular injection of the product. Early recognition of a vascular occlusion together with prompt and aggressive treatment are of paramount importance to avoid severe and irreversible consequences.

This chapter discusses the ischaemic complication caused by dermal fillers, explains its aetiology and provides indications for its management to prevent severe consequences such as tissue necrosis.

The causes of ischaemia

Ischaemia is the most severe complication feared by injectors following the use of dermal fillers for aesthetic medical treatments. This is caused by the accidental intravascular injection of a filler. Arterial or venous occlusion can cause tissue necrosis or Nicolau syndrome and, more rarely, loss of vision and stroke [7]. In addition to intravascular injection of the filler, some authors speculate that compression or vascular spasm may result in ischaemic changes in the tissue [2,8]. However, the ischaemic event caused by compression alone is difficult to replicate in animal models [9].

Ischaemia and its effects on tissue can give rise to vasospasm, which occurs due to desensitisation to nitrous oxide and is heightened by the harmful effect of the filler injected into the vessel as a result of the inflammatory reaction [10]. Vasospasm, combined with compression due to extravascular oedema, causes changes in the surrounding tissues. These secondary vascular changes exacerbate ischaemia caused by direct intravascular occlusion. The causes of vascular occlusion and the resulting physiological processes have not yet been fully explained: further investigations detailing the vascular patterns and ischaemic changes caused by the intravascular injection of dermal filler are required. Nevertheless, it is possible to subdivide the ischaemic event into various stages, using skin colour and its state of deterioration as indicators to understand the severity of the complication and to track the time since occurrence of the vascular occlusion.

The stages of vascular occlusion

Obstruction of blood flow caused by intravascular injection leads to a series of changes in the skin which, if recognised and treated in good time, can prevent tissue necrosis. The signs of ischaemia usually occur immediately or within a few hours [11]. Initial symptoms, however, can be variable and are often confused with common post-treatment discomfort [12]. On rare occasions, the onset of ischaemia and the signs that accompany it may occur after a few days. The reason for this has still not been fully clarified at present, but a number of possible explanations have been suggested:

- delayed ischaemic changes may be caused by an ongoing embolism in a small calibre distal arteriole (at the injection site);

TABLE 1 - DESCRIPTION OF THE STAGES OF VASCULAR OCCLUSION AND GUIDELINES FOR WOUND CARE. GUIDELINES DRAWN UP BY THE CMAC (COMPLICATIONS IN MEDICAL AESTHETICS COLLABORATIVE)

Cutaneous ischaemic stages of a vascular occlusion	Pathophysiology	Typical onset and duration
Stage 1: pallor, blanching	Immediate blockage of the vessel or spasm leading to an abrupt interruption of blood flow and tissue perfusion	Immediate, may last a few seconds or persist
Stage 2: *livedo reticularis*	Accumulation of deoxygenated blood within the surrounding venous network	May occur quickly and last 24-36 hours
Stage 3: pustules	Reduction in pH and production of sweat; Metabolic changes allowing the proliferation of *Staphylococcus aureus* as facultative anaerobe	Approximately 72 hours (onset of necrosis)
Stage 4: coagulation* * Coagulation may occur before stage 3, at the same time, or excessive pustule growth may mask the underlying tissue damage. This phase indicates necrotic changes.	The tissue turns black as a result of deteriorating hypoxia, cell lysis and spillage of blood into the tissue; The tissue is hard with preserved architecture due to the coagulative necrotic process	It occurs after a number of days
Stage 5: devitalised tissue - Phase 5a: slough - Phase 5b: eschar	Tissue destruction and accumulation of denatured structural proteins (collagen, fibrin, elastin) and haemoglobin occurs; slough is moist and creamy/yellow or green; eschar is black (dark) and dry	It occurs after a number of days

- if the ischaemic event was caused by a hyaluronic acid filler, the hygroscopic nature of the material could lead to an increase in the size of the injected bolus, resulting in complete occlusion of the vessel or increased compression;
- the bolus of dermal filler causes partial obstruction of the vessel, which is subsequently completed by platelet aggregation [13].

In support of these claims, recent work by Taylor et al. has described patterns of ischaemia in relation to the ophthalmic artery and the corresponding angiosomal region [10]. This study showed how direct venous injection, or the movement of hyaluronic acid embolism through an arteriovenous shunt, could cause a delayed mixed pattern of ischaemia and necrosis.

Regardless of the aetiology of the occlusion or the presence of ischaemic changes, it is of the utmost importance that the practitioner knows how to recognise the clinical signs of ischaemia and is able to treat the patient promptly in order to recover perfusion and avoid severe consequences. To this end, in the absence of regulation in the practice of aesthetic medicine, guidelines have been drawn up by the CMAC (Complications in Medical Aesthetics Collaborative) for the management of vascular occlusion based on skin assessment and to help establish the extent and stage of the ischaemic changes. In fact, occlusion of a vessel leads to a series of relatively standardised events, which can be divided into five different stages as summarised in table 1.

Stage 1 and stage 2: pallor and subsequent livedo reticularis

The blanching of the skin and subsequent *livedo reticularis* (fig. 1A-B) are both common signs of vascular compression. In particular, *livedo reticularis* has a characteristic appearance due to the anatomy and physiology of the skin's microvascular system: the cutaneous arterial flow is made up of numerous ascending arterioles that rise perpendicularly to the skin surface and divide to form a capillary bed on the skin surface. The vascular system is similar to a tree, with the artery representing the central trunk and the arterioles the branches that irrigate the entire surface of the skin. Blockage of the arteriole (or artery) stops or restricts blood flow, causing the skin to turn white almost instantaneously. The pale appearance of the skin will evolve into a marbled appearance, known as *livedo reticularis*. This is a cutaneous manifestation characterised by a mottled discolouration of the skin in which cyanotic purplish or reddish-blue patches, caused by the stasis of deoxygenated blood, take on a net-like pattern and alternate with areas that look normal. It is important to stress that the presence of pallor and *livedo reticularis* does not necessarily indicate that tissue necrosis will occur [4]. In fact, if the vascular obstruction is removed at this stage, with the restoration of blood flow, the ischaemia is likely to clear up without any problems and the tissue will return to its original state. If, on the other hand, the vascular obstruction persists, it progresses to stage 3.

Stage 3 and stage 4: pustules and coagulation

Stages 3 and 4 may occur in order or alternate, but both indicate that tissue necrosis is developing [13]. Pustules seem to appear about three days after vascular occlusion [9]. During an ischaemic event, anaerobic metabolism prevails in the tissue [14]. There is also a dysfunction of the sweat glands, with reduced sweat production, increasing the pH and reducing the amount of salt on the skin.

These factors, combined with the disintegration of the normal cellular architecture, allow both pathogenic bacteria and those normally resident on the skin to penetrate deep into the dermis, where they find an ideal environment in which to multiply.

The stage in which the skin in the ischaemic area turns black, on the other hand, is due to a process called haemorrhagic skin necrosis, which is a manifestation of a thrombotic occlusion of one or more blood vessels that supply the skin.

The red blood cells released from the compromised blood vessels become trapped in the necrotic tissue where, together with the subsequent deoxygenation of haemoglobin, they cause the skin to turn black. In addition to this coagulative process, numerous pro-inflammatory factors such as cytokines are released by the necrotic cells.

The skin surrounding the necrotic area, on the other hand, looks grey-red in colour due to the dilation of the blood vessels adjacent to the ischaemia causing hyperaemia [14].

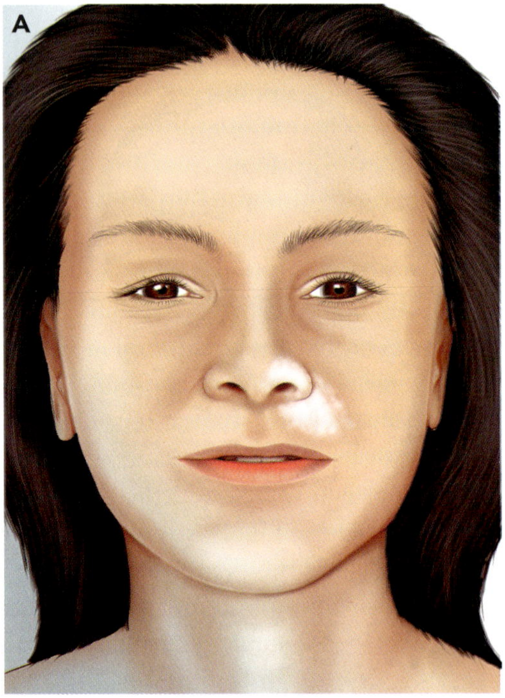

Stage 5: slough and eschar

Stage 5 is characterised by the formation of slough and/or eschar. Both of these indicate tissue necrosis, the extent of which depends on the significance of the occlusion and the state of hydration. Slough may occur before or instead of the development of eschar and represents devitalised tissue containing wound exudate. Slough may emerge as cream-coloured, yellow-green, gelatinous/fibrous material. If the slough is green, it can be taken as a visual indicator of infection.

Eschar, on the other hand, is devitalised tissue made up of dried blood, exudate and denatured proteins, mainly collagen, elastin, fibrin and haemoglobin. The formation of eschar prevents the wound from healing and creates an ideal closed environment for bacterial growth [15]. Regardless of the presence

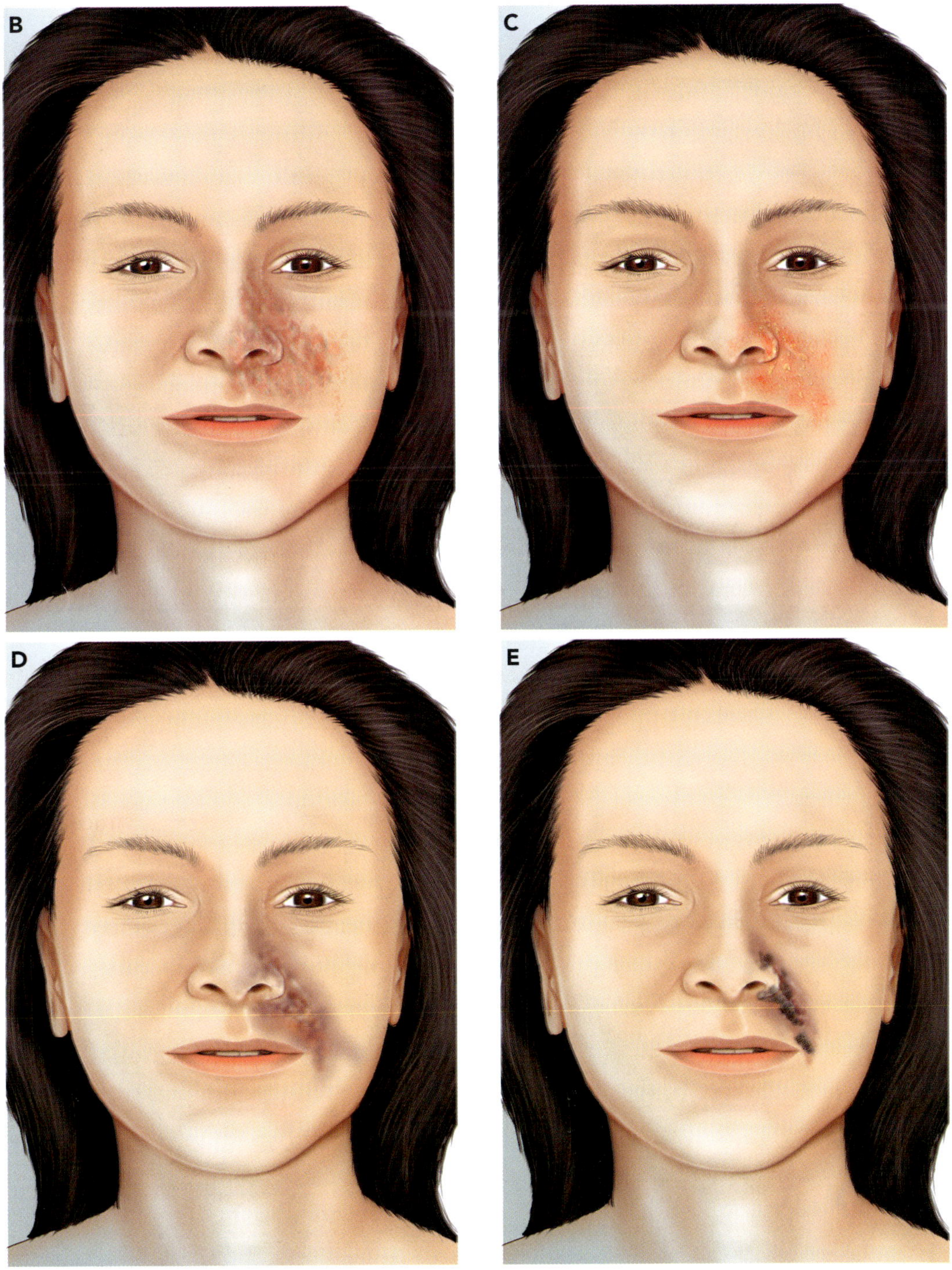

Figure 1 Stages of a vascular occlusion: A) stage 1: pallor, blanching; B) stage 2: *livedo reticularis*; C) stage 3: bacterial proliferation; D) stage 4: coagulation; E) stage 5: eschar formation

of eschar or slough, the wound will need to be managed to prevent infection and promote successful healing, monitored with various follow-ups.

Assessment of a suspected vascular occlusion

Signs of a vascular occlusion may be evident immediately after the aesthetic procedure or occur hours or even days later. However, there are some small steps that an injector can take to enable rapid identification of tissue ischaemia. These include capillary refill time (CRT), pain and skin colour.

Capillary refill time was introduced by Beecher et al. in 1947 as a means of assessing peripheral perfusion. There is some variability between the techniques proposed to perform it, for example: use the thumb or an easily distinguishable instrument, such as the end of a pair of suture scissors, and apply pressure to the area to be analysed for 5-15 seconds. Then record the time it takes for the colour to return to normal (fig. 2). Even the interpretation of normal values is not straightforward, but one approach is to check both sides of the corresponding region of the face, with a CRT value of less than two seconds being considered normal. A CRT > 2 seconds is considered pathological and may indicate a vascular

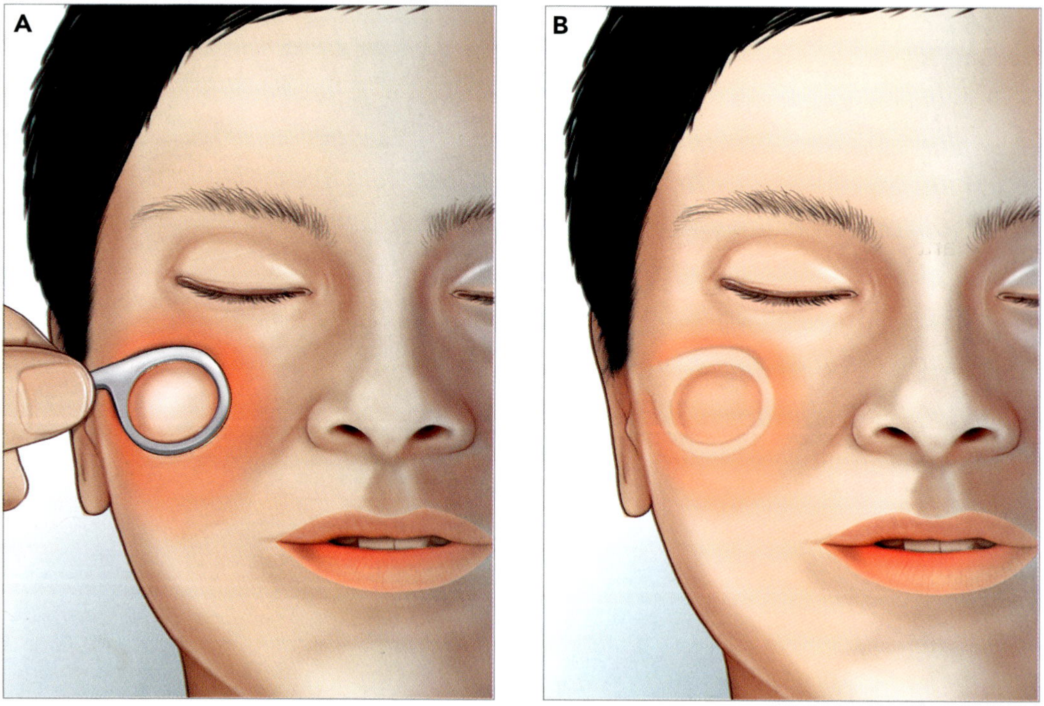

Figure 2 Assessment of capillary filling time. A) To determine the capillary filling time of the skin, it is helpful to use an instrument, such as common suture scissors, to compress the skin. Patterns that are not typical in nature are easier to distinguish. B) The aim of this clinical test is to compare the filling time of the area in question with normal skin, both adjacent to the area and on the opposite side

insufficiency [9,16]. Evaluation of CRT is of paramount importance in cases of suspected occlusion after injection in high-risk areas such as the nose, glabella, lips or forehead. After these treatments, it is advisable to have patients wait 30 to 45 minutes.

Another aspect to be assessed after a procedure is pain. Some discomfort during treatment is normal but if a local anaesthetic has been used, pain should only felt when the anaesthetic wears off. If the patient complains of sudden and increasing pain during treatment, either at the injection site or elsewhere, you should be worried. In these cases, the injection should be stopped immediately and the affected area examined. The patient must also be seen again and examined if they complain of worsening pain after treatment. In the case of vascular occlusion, pain is not always present in the initial stages.

Lastly, the assessment of skin colour is important in cases of suspected vascular occlusion. This is an important indicator of ischaemic changes. As mentioned earlier, skin signs can be grouped into five different phases (fig. 1). Careful observation of the skin can help predict and prevent tissue necrosis. In the case of restricted or interrupted blood supply, the tissue may blanch instantly. However, skin pallor is a passing phase, which is soon replaced by *livedo reticularis*, a skin manifestation characterised by a mottled purple skin pattern caused by the accumulation of deoxygenated blood [9]. In these cases, it is important to carefully assess the treated area, especially along the course of the artery and communicating vessels, as the filler injected may travel in branches remote from the injection site. The observation of these two early aspects in skin colour changes requires prompt intervention to restore blood flow and limit progression to tissue necrosis. The ischaemic skin changes of pallor and mottling do not indicate inevitable necrosis [17]. In fact, all tissues can withstand varying periods of ischaemia, depending on the tissue type: tissue damage will depend on the size and duration of the occlusion, the underlying anatomy, overall vascular integrity, healing capacity and the presence of infection. If recognised in time and treated promptly, ischaemia requires minimal support and the area will soon return to normal (stages 1 to 3), while if it is treated late, when necrosis is established (stages 4 and 5), it will require more intensive treatment and more frequent visits.

Treatment of a vascular occlusion caused by hyaluronic acid dermal fillers

Although ischaemic events are rare, it is very important to have a clear and simple protocol for their management. All the necessary materials should always be on hand and staff should be trained to remain calm and help with the treatment of the patient and the organisation of the outpatient clinic. Since the adverse event is likely to occur outside the hospital setting, it is necessary to inform the patient and their family of the currently available and CMAC-recommended protocol for the management of a vascular oc-

TABLE 2 - MANAGEMENT OF A VASCULAR OCCLUSION CAUSED BY AN HA-BASED FILLER CROSS-LINKED WITH HYALURONIDASE [13]

Phases in the management of a vascular occlusion caused by HA
1. Examine the area treated and the untreated side as a control for the assessment of CRT along the entire path of the affected artery: a value > 2 seconds is considered pathological
2. Disinfect the skin and outline the entire ischaemic area
3. The CMAC recommends reconstituting 1,500 UI of hyaluronidase with 1 ml of bacteriostatic NaCl with 0.9-2% lidocaine
4. Infiltrate 1,500 UI of hyaluronidase with a needle or cannula (if appropriate) along the course of the affected artery and into the larger ischaemic area. Use more than one ampoule at a time if the area affected is significant
5. Apply warm compresses to increase vasodilatation and massage the affected area vigorously to encourage diffusion of the hyaluronidase and the mechanical breakage of the HA molecule bonds
6. Re-assess the CRT and if it is still delayed repeat the treatment* *The process can be performed hourly (at least)

clusion based on the collective experience of various authors in treating hundreds of vascular occlusions over the past eight years (tab. 2) [13].

We propose a protocol divided into three phases: identification, treatment and assessment of the patient with follow-up. If, as in this case, the dermal filler used is hyaluronic acid (HA), pharmacological treatment consists in the injection of hyaluronidase into the affected area. The following materials should always be available in the doctor's surgery:

- 1,500 UI ampoules of freeze-dried hyaluronidase (it is advisable to have three ampoules plus one reserve);
- lidocaine or another anaesthetic;
- acetylsalicylic acid (500 mg tablets);
- antibiotics;
- nitro-glycerine-based transdermal patches;
- soothing arnica cream;
- injection material and cannulas;
- drugs for the treatment of anaphylaxis associated with hyaluronidase:
  - methylprednisolone
  - adrenaline
  - minimum respiratory support material.

Case report

In October 2019, a 25-year-old patient was treated with cross-linked hyaluronic acid (HA) for volumetric lip augmentation. The patient had previously undergone other hyaluronic acid treatments without any side effects. Immediately after treatment, the area treated showed signs of pallor in the columella and left cheek area (fig. 3A). The treatment was immediately suspended because a vascular occlusion was suspected. The patient was in-

formed of the problem and tests were promptly run to confirm the suspected ischaemia. First of all, the CRT test was performed, both on the blanched area and on the opposite side of the face as a control. The CRT value recorded in the area treated was more than two seconds and, as a delayed CRT indicates arterial impairment, the protocol for the management of a vascular occlusion was activated. Before proceeding with the infiltration of hyaluronidase, a warm compress was applied to the affected area to encourage vasodilatation. The area was also massaged vigorously to encourage the breakdown of cross-links between the hyaluronic acid molecules. As the situation showed no signs of improvement, the vascular occlusion management procedure was applied.
The treatment of ischaemia involves the infusion of high doses of hyaluronidase at frequent intervals and continuous monitoring of the patient's health to assess the evolution of the lesions due to the ischaemic event. Three separate injections of hyaluronidase were administered on the same day as the treatment: 900 UI immediately after the onset of skin pallor and, two injections of 300 UI each two hours later. After the first day of infiltration with 1,500 UI of hyaluronidase, the area treated looked cyanotic (fig. 3B).
On the second day after treatment, the CRT test was performed again and, as the perfusion time was still delayed (video 9.1), three separate infiltrations with 300 UI of hyaluronidase were injected at two-hour intervals.
During the clinical check-up on the third day, despite the protocol in place, the patient complained of gingival pain and the area treated showed signs of skin distress with the presence of pustules (fig. 3C).
On the fourth day after treatment, a single injection of 100 UI of hyaluronidase was performed only in the hard and painful spots: the situation was gradually improving (fig. 3D).
On the following day, 30 UI of hyaluronidase was injected into the only spot that was still hard and painful at the root of the nose (fig. 3E).
The patient in question suffered from allergies, so before each infiltration with hyaluronidase, she was given intravenous cortisone. The patient also received the following adjuvant therapy: salicylic acid 400 mg/ 24h for 10 days; antibiotic therapy based on levofloxacin 500 mg/ 24h for 5 days and clarithromycin 500 mg/12h for 7 days; furosemide 100 mg/24h for 2 days (on the second and third days after treatment); warm compresses and arnica cream.
There are currently no standardised guidelines for the management of severe complications following hyaluronic acid filler injections. The protocol proposed in this study is based on the use of high doses of hyaluronidase a few hours apart.
The result achieved was excellent: complete resolution of the ischaemic complication within 14 days (fig. 3F). This procedure could represent a valid reference to be followed in the event of a complication related to vascular occlusion.

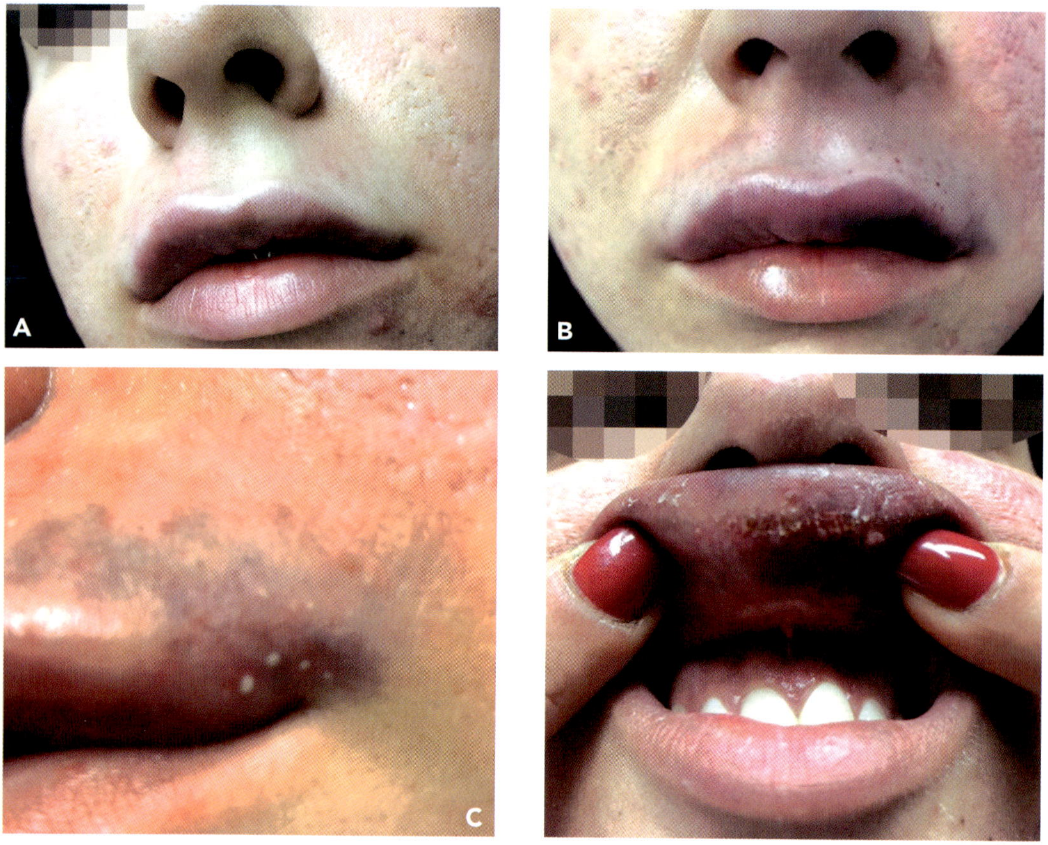

Bibliography

1. Park K, Nishiwaki F, Kabashima K, Miyachi Y. A case of foreign-body granuloma of the glabella due to polyacrylamide filler and an intractable ulcer after skin biopsy: An immunohistochemical evaluation of inflammatory changes. Case Rep Dermatol. 2013;5(2):181-185.
2. Witmanowski H, Błochowiak K. Another face of dermal fillers. Postep Dermatologii i Alergol. 2020;37(5).
3. Jordan DR, Stoica B. Filler Migration: A Number of Mechanisms to Consider. Ophthal Plast Reconstr Surg. 2015;31(4).
4. Urdiales-Gálvez F, Delgado NE, Figueiredo V, et al. Treatment of Soft Tissue Filler Complications: Expert Consensus Recommendations. Aesthetic Plast Surg. 2018;42(2).
5. Alam M, Kakar R, Dover JS, et al. Rates of Vascular Occlusion Associated with Using Needles vs Cannulas for Filler Injection. JAMA Dermatology. 2021;157(2).
6. Chatrath V, Banerjee PS, Goodman GJ, Rahman E. Soft-tissue Filler-associated Blindness: A Systematic Review of Case Reports and Case Series. Plast Reconstr Surg - Glob Open. 2019;7(4).
7. Vargas-Laguna E, García-Gavín J, Bárcena-Ruiz E. Safety in Dermatologic Procedures: Vascular Occlusion by Filling Materials. Actas Dermosi-

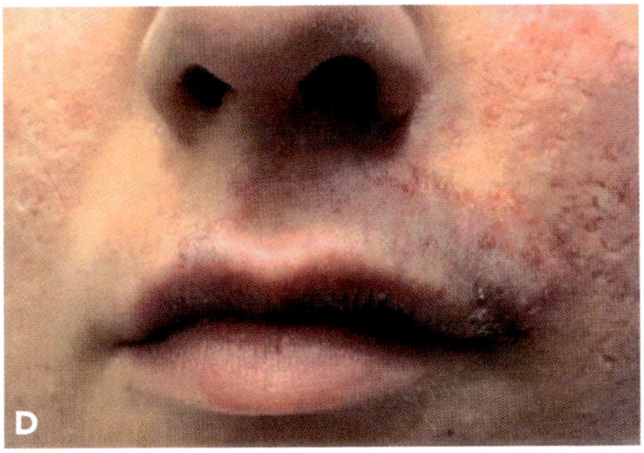

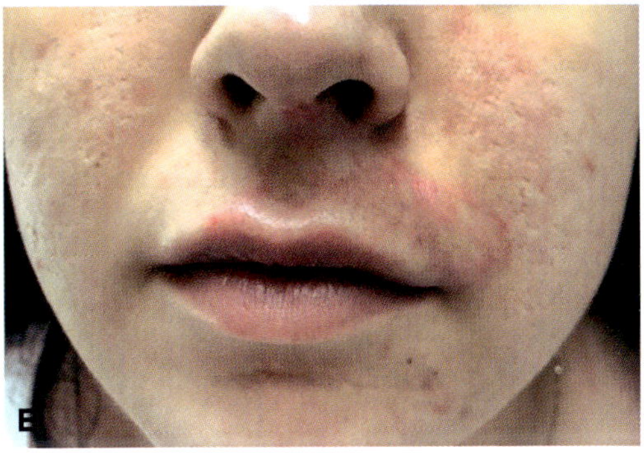

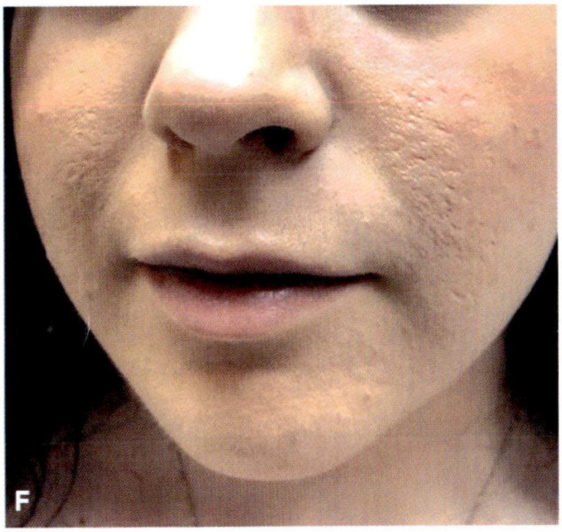

VIDEO 9.1

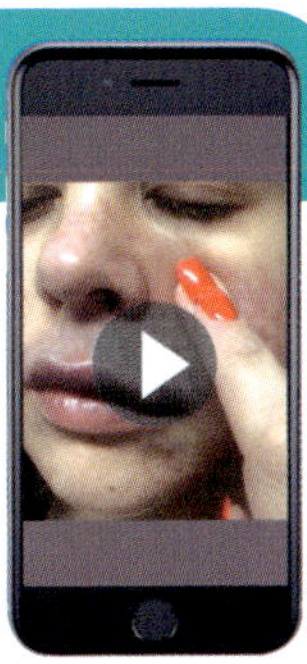

CRT test performed on the second day after treatment

Figure 3
Case report. A) 25-year-old patient with visible skin pallor on the columella, which appeared immediately after HA-based filler treatment for volumetric lip augmentation. B) Visible skin distress after HA treatment. First day after treatment, after infiltration of 900 UI of hyaluronidase. The cyanotic area is clearly visible. C) Third day after treatment: the skin shows symptoms of distress with pustules in the erythematous, oedematous area with well-defined painful patches. D) Fourth day after treatment: an injection of hyaluronidase was performed only in the hard and painful spot at the root of the nose. E) Fifth day after treatment: the patient received an injection of 30 UI of hyaluronidase at the root of the nose. The symptoms are almost gone. F) 14 days after treatment: the ischaemic symptoms have completely cleared up without consequences

filiogr. 2021;112(9).
8. Bravo BSF, Balassiano LKDA, Da Rocha CRM, et al. Delayed-type necrosis after soft-tissue augmentation with hyaluronic acid. J Clin Aesthet Dermatol. 2015;8(12).
9. DeLorenzi C. New high dose pulsed hyaluronidase protocol for hyaluronic acid filler vascular adverse events. Aesthetic Surg J. 2017;37(7).
10. Taylor GI, Shoukath S, Gascoigne A, Corlett RJ, Ashton MW. The functional anatomy of the ophthalmic angiosome and its implications in

blindness as a complication of cosmetic facial filler procedures. Plast Reconstr Surg. Published online 2020.

11. Tobalem S, Schutz JS, Chronopoulos A. Central retinal artery occlusion-rethinking retinal survival time. BMC Ophthalmol. 2018;18(1).
12. Hong JY, Seok J, Ahn GR, Jang YJ, Li K, Kim BJ. Impending skin necrosis after dermal filler injection: A "golden time" for first-aid intervention. Dermatol Ther. 2017;30(2).
13. Murray G, Convery C, Walker L, Davies E. Guideline for the management of hyaluronic acid filler-induced vascular occlusion. J Clin Aesthet Dermatol. 2021;14(5).
14. Gibbs MB, English JC, Zirwas MJ. Livedo reticularis: An update. J Am Acad Dermatol. 2005;52(6).
15. Thomas AM, Harding KG, Moore K. The structure and composition of chronic wound eschar. J Wound Care. 1999;8(6).
16. Mrgan M, Rytter D, Brabrand. M. Capillary refill time is a predictor of short-term mortality for adult patients admitted to a medical department: An observational cohort study. Emerg Med J. 2014;31(12).
17. Kalogeris T, Baines CP, Krenz M, Korthuis RJ. Cell Biology of Ischemia/Reperfusion Injury. In: International Review of Cell and Molecular Biology. Vol 298; 2012.

NEOVASCULARISATION AND THE TYNDALL EFFECT

Lucia Calvisi

Dermal fillers represent an aesthetic medical procedure that has becoming increasingly popular in recent years, second in frequency only to botulinum toxin. While the incidence of complications is not high and most of them are mild, it is the very increase in the number of procedures that is causing an increase in the occurrence of complications.

One of the complications that can occur is neovascularisation. The tissue trauma caused by the injection, especially in certain areas of the face, such as the perioral or periocular area, in patients with a specific predisposition, who may have signs of rosacea or thin skin, may lead to the appearance of new blood vessels at the site of venepuncture. Excessively vigorous massage after treatment or the injection of excessive amounts of filler seems to favour the occurrence of this type of complication. New blood vessels can occur from a few days after treatment to a few weeks (Fig. 1).

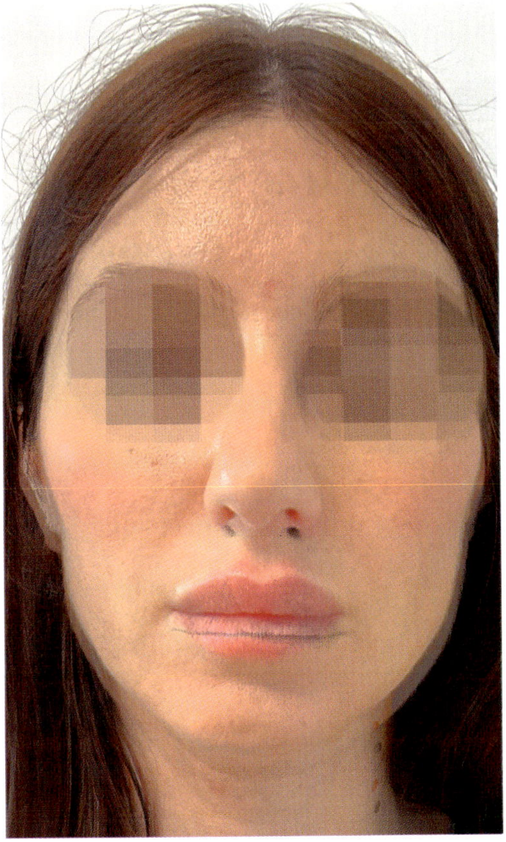

Figure 1 Neovascularisation at the injection site (upper lip)

From a psychological point of view, they can be a considerable problem, especially in fair-skinned or psychologically unstable patients: in fact, the patient complains that they have come to our surgery with the aim of improving their physical appearance and then find themselves with telangiectasias where they did not exist before. The injecting doctor's task will therefore be to reassure the patient that these capillaries often reabsorb by themselves or, alternatively, that the problem can be solved very easily using a vascular laser such as the 532 KTP laser or IPL (Intense Pulsed Light) to close them permanently.

Tyndall Effect

The Tyndall effect is a technical error due to implantation of the filler too close to the surface, to the choice of an unsuitable filler for the region being treated, to the presence of very thin skin, which perhaps required hyaluronic acid with a lower molecular weight, or even to the injection of excessive amounts of product in the same site. This leads to the appearance of a blue-greyish discol-

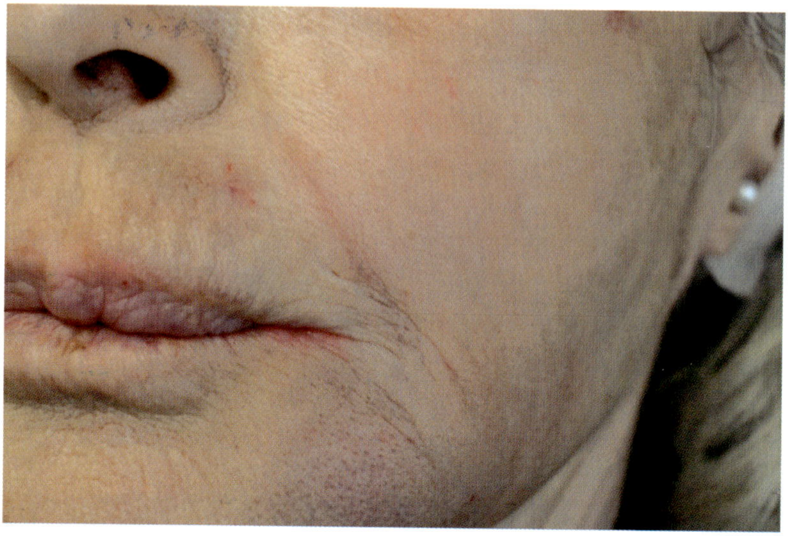

Figure 2 Tyndall effect at naso-labial level

ouration due to the particular reflection of light on the skin where the hyaluronic acid is present.

Areas particularly at risk of developing the Tyndall effect are the nasolabial folds, the nasal spine, the tear trough (mainly due to inappropriate product choice) and fine perioral wrinkles.

Once discolouration is present, the only way to eliminate it is to use hyaluronidase (remember that in Italy the use of hyaluronidase injections is off-label); an alternative in the periocular area may be topical hyaluronidase, which is, however, slower in terms of results.

The Tyndall effect was mainly observed in the past, when only a few types of filler were available in the aesthetic medical toolkit and had to be used to treat all areas of the face. But this was a long time ago. There was no choice of hyaluronic acids with an adequate molecular weight and G', so discolouration of the skin was seen much more frequently. Today, this type of complication is mainly attributable to malpractice.

During the preliminary examination of the patient and when explaining the corrective treatment that we are going to perform, it is essential to explain that, following the breakdown of the hyaluronic acid dissolved by the hyaluronidase, the area treated may almost look worse, hollowed-out and different to what they are used to. This is especially true in the tear trough area, where, paradoxically, patients who are used to having a "full" appearance of the area, complain of the appearance of dark circles when the product is dissolved (fig. 3). Consequently, after treatment of this region with hyaluronidase, it is necessary to correct the "hollow" appearance of the area again.

Bibliography

1. Funt D, Pavicic T. Dermal fillers in aesthetics: an overview of adverse events and treatment approaches. Clin Cosmet Investig Dermatol.

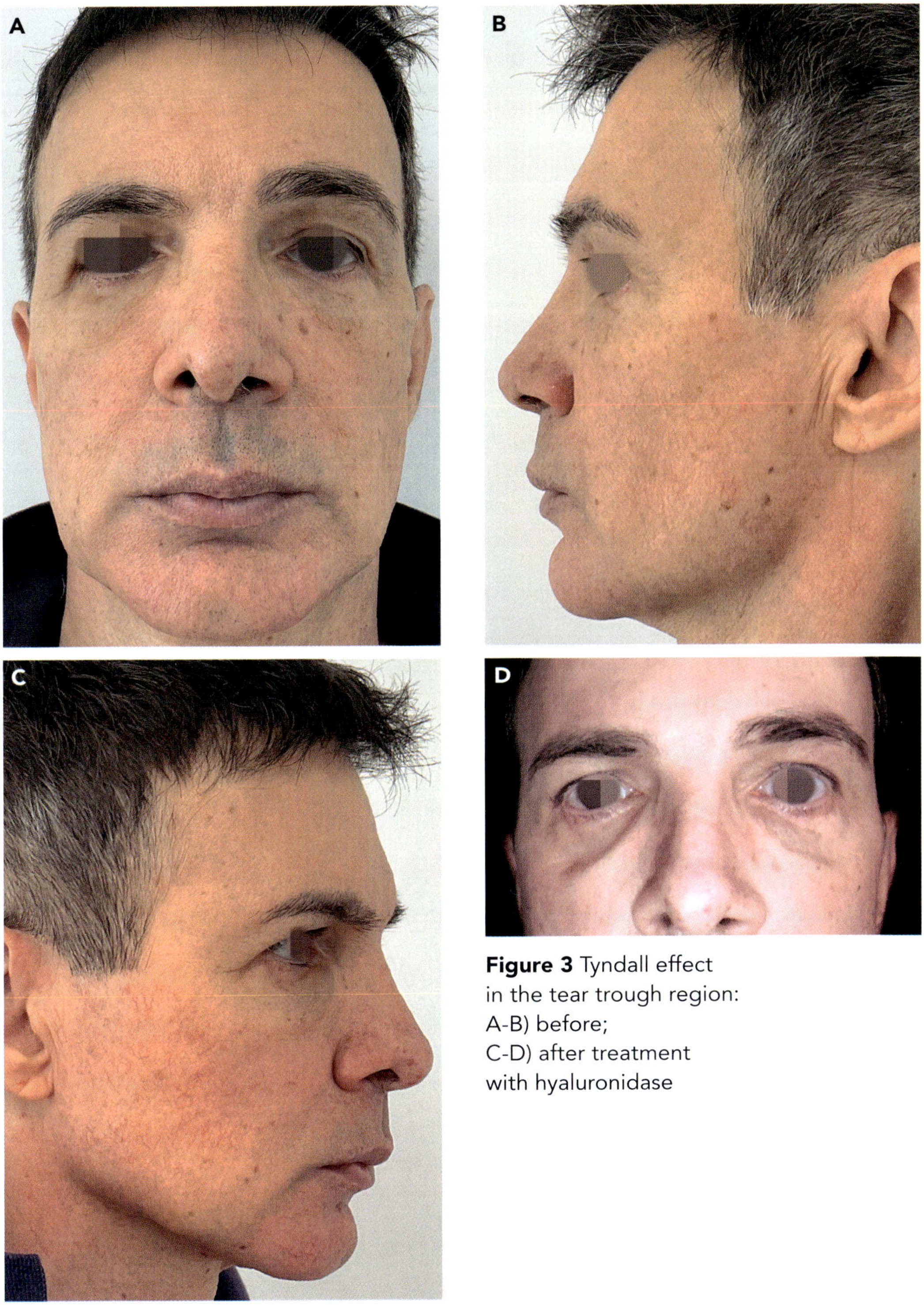

Figure 3 Tyndall effect in the tear trough region: A-B) before; C-D) after treatment with hyaluronidase

2013 Dec 12;6:295-316.
2. Urdiales-Gálvez F, Delgado NE, Figueiredo V, Lajo-Plaza JV, Mira M, Moreno A, Ortíz-Martí F, Del Rio-Reyes R, Romero-Álvarez N, Del Cueto SR, Segurado MA, Rebenaque CV. Treatment of Soft Tissue Filler Complications: Expert Consensus Recommendations. Aesthetic Plast Surg. 2018 Apr;42(2):498-510.
3. Urdiales-Gálvez F, Delgado NE, Figueiredo V, Lajo-Plaza JV, Mira M, Ortíz- Martí F, Del Rio-Reyes R, Romero-Álvarez N, Del Cueto SR, Segurado MA, Rebenaque CV. Preventing the Complications Associated with the Use of Dermal Fillers in Facial Aesthetic Procedures: An Expert Group Consensus Report. Aesthetic Plast Surg. 2017 Jun;41(3):667-677.
4. Witmanowski H, Błochowiak K. Another face of dermal fillers. Postepy Dermatol Alergol. 2020 Oct;37(5):651-659.
5. Heydenrych I, De Boulle K, Kapoor KM, Bertossi D. The 10-Point Plan 2021: Updated Concepts for Improved Procedural Safety During Facial Filler Treatments. Clin Cosmet Investig Dermatol. 2021 Jul 6;14:779-814.
6. Engelman DE, Bloom B, Goldberg DJ. Dermal fillers: complications and informed consent. J Cosmet Laser Ther. 2005 Mar;7(1):29-32.
7. Sclafani AP, Fagien S. Treatment of injectable soft tissue filler complications. Dermatol Surg. 2009 Oct;35 Suppl 2:1672-80.
8. Ortiz AE, et al. Analysis of U.S. Food and Drug Administration Data on Soft-Tissue Filler Complications. Dermatol Surg. 2020 Jul;46(7): 958-961.

RETINAL ISCHAEMIA

Alberto Diaspro, Luigi Emanuelli

The term ischaemia defines the reduced or absent blood flow, i.e. exchange between blood oxygen and tissue carbon dioxide, in a given anatomical region; retinal ischaemia is one of the leading causes of irreversible blindness in the western world.
The increasingly widespread use of filler injections for facial rejuvenation coincides with a non-linear increase in the number of reports of complications and even serious adverse events, of which amaurosis is the most significant: in the five years following the first documented cases in 2015, there was a 50% increase in the number of cases reported in literature alone [1].
The retina is a neuro-vascular area of diencephalic origin so, like brain tissue, it is highly dependent on normal and constant oxyaemia levels, ensured by an efficient vascular system, because it is the tissue that consumes the most oxygen in the whole body (13 mL\100g\min).
The main causes of retinal ischaemia are occlusions, the embolic blockage of a central arterial or venous vessel or of a branch: central arterial occlusions have an incidence of 8.5 / 100,000, with 92% of cases losing the use of the affected eye and 8% showing variable recovery.
The incidence of the rare but devastating complication of iatrogenic vascular occlusion after the injection of filler is estimated to be 0.001%, however this is presumably higher in view of the limited reliability of the number of cases reported in literature, which is probably lower than the cases that actually occurred: in all cases it can cause irreversible loss of vision within a few minutes [2].

Anatomy

There are two opposing theories as to the nature of arterial occlusion. According to one, it would either be secondary to spasm with vasoconstriction of both the damaged primary artery and its tributary circulations due to the injection of the filler into the tissue, and according to the other, it would be die to authentic embolisation, i.e. the movement of injected product particles into the vessel lumen up to the critical diameter which, when reached, does not allow further progression and determines the consequent interruption of distal blood flow.
Whether it is due to direct intravascular injection or perivascular compression, or even both, the outcome may be the same, and as such the aetiopathogenetic distinction plays a secondary role with respect to the indication for prevention and prompt treatment.
The local-regional arteries at risk are the superficial temporal artery, which has some anastomoses with intraorbital vessels, the supraorbital and supratrochlear arteries, which are directly anastomosed with the ophthalmic artery, and the angular artery of the nose, the distal portion of the facial artery.
The most important and most dangerous anastomoses with regard to loss of

vision are those between the facial (angular) artery and the ophthalmic artery; there are also small interconnections between the intra orbital and infratrochlear arteries and the facial (angular) artery. These have been shown to be the main causes of occlusion of the central retinal artery (ACR).
The presence of the cilioretinal artery can partially alleviate acute obstruction of the local circulation in about a lucky 10% of patients.
In general, occlusion of only one branch of the retinal artery has a more favourable prognosis than occlusion of the common truncus arteriosus, sparing an upper or lower visual hemicampus associated with the maintenance of partial distinct vision.
The nose and glabella regions in particular are involved, with implication of the arterial region of the ophthalmic artery, with its cutaneous terminal branches, the supraorbital and supratrochlear arteries, that of the central retinal artery and the naso-ciliary artery.
In these cases, the filler presumably travels in the opposite direction to the blood flow [3,4].
Please see the relevant texts for the details of the vascular anatomy mentioned, which is not the subject of this chapter.

Injection areas at risk

The injection areas most at risk of retinal ischaemia due to vascular occlusion secondary to injection of fillers seem to be the nose, reported as the injected area in 56.3% of reported cases (previously 41%), followed by the glabellar region, in 27.1% of reported cases (previously 44%). Next are the periocular area (18.8%, previously 9%) and fronto-temporal region (14.6%, previously 11%) [1,2,5].
It is significant to point out that nose and glabella were already the two areas most at risk in the past, but with a clear prevalence of the latter, as indicated in the percentages in brackets: in more recent years, nose reshaping using injectable fillers has become a widely used and very fashionable technique, but it is burdened by a significant series of complications, some of which severe, which have become more frequent (see the chapter on complications from fillers in the middle third).
The periocular area has also seen rates double, definitely due to the same increase in interest over the years [6], although retinal ischaemia is not among the most frequent complications reported in this area (see the chapter on eyelid complications).
The nasal spine, glabella and internal canthus in particular are the most risky injection sites, because in these areas the branches of the ophthalmic artery are anchored to the bony rim when they exit, and there are arteriovenous connections between the ophthalmic and facial veins that allow bidirectional flow, as they have no valves within their lumen.
Lastly, there are ipsi- and contra-lateral anastomotic circles between the facial and ophthalmic arteries that allow distant embolisation, and small-calibre anastomoses between the posterior and anterior ciliary vessels running to the choroid and extrinsic ocular muscles, which may react with spasms in response to ophthalmic artery embolism to limit hypoxic damage [7].

Semeiotics

Arterial occlusion results in extremely intense pain at the injection site, possible erythema and local oedema, the appearance of eyelid ptosis and ophthalmoplegia (deficit of eye movement due to partial or complete paralysis of extrinsic oculomotor muscles). These four signs may all be present or only partially present, but their absence does not determine lesser severity [8].

The latter may all recover, but the most dramatic and important sign is the decline in visual acuity to amaurosis, complete blindness.

The signs and symptoms are often immediate and concurrent with the injection; otherwise they may occur even later. Diagnosis must be immediate, just the time it takes to refer the patient to a second level emergency room: the immediate decline in sight and subsequent deficit are associated with afferent pupillary defect with failure to respond in miosis due to alteration of the oculomotor reflex and pallor upon examination of the retinal fundus.

Prevention

General rules of good clinical practice with respect to this complication are of paramount importance.

It is important to modulate the pressure exerted on the syringe plunger, because if it exceeds the systolic pressure, it may facilitate the onset of embolism by accidental intravascular injection due to spasm triggered by the mechanical stress placed on the vessels by the suddenly expanded tissues.

It is also likely that, if modulated gently during injection, the pressure will be dispersed to multiple vessels rather than transmitted to just one. The average injection pressure required to embolise the ophthalmic artery is 166.7 mmHg [9].

The product must always be injected in a limited quantity in order to occlude the branches of the ophthalmic artery, compared to its calibre this is very minimal: the study of the internal volumes of some facial vessels has found values between 0.04-0.12 ml (0.085 ml average volume) for the portion of arteries such as the supratrochlear from the glabella to the orbital apex and the injection volume must therefore not exceed these critical values at the injection sites [4].

Injection of too much product under excessive pressure into one of these vessels can result in a retrograde iatrogenic flow pushed centripetally past the ophthalmic artery. When this ceases, the systolic pressure allows the product to be pushed physiologically in a centrifugal direction and enter from the ophthalmic artery into the central retinal artery, resulting in occlusion of the latter by embolisation [2].

Treatment

As retinal tissue must be considered an extension of the brain, its susceptibility to anoxia is greatest with an ischaemic survival time of minutes, allowing a very limited time of action, less than an hour from the onset of symptoms. Consequently, management of time to action is critical to any chance of restoring sight. If hyaluronic acid has been injected it can potentially be dissolved, but there is currently no consensus on the optimal therapy [10,11].

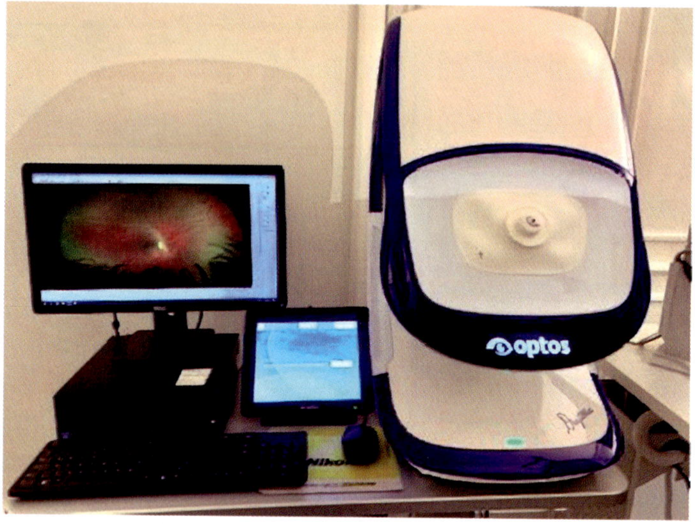

Figure 1 Non-mydriatic wide field retinograph. Courtesy of Dr. L. Emanuelli

The repeated peri-bulbar injection of high doses of hyaluronidase, followed by retro-bulbar injection, has long been the accepted standard of care, considering its ability to diffuse through the vessel wall, but this is now a matter of debate. Its benefit must also be weighed against the technical difficulty and potential risks [12,13].

This is an ophthalmic and potentially neurological emergency that must be investigated in a multi-specialist setting by an ophthalmologist. The investigation should involve the performance of an ophthalmoscopy with retinography (figs. 1-2), measurement of the ocular tone and possible paracentesis of the anterior chamber, passing through the cornea with a dedicated scalpel in order to reduce the endocular pressure, allow the dilation of the obstructed vessel and facilitate the flow that is still possible. Certainty in the diagnosis can then be established by performing ocular coherence tomography (OCT) (fig. 3) or magnetic resonance imaging with contrast medium (angio-RMN), with a neurological consultation if necessary.

Contemporary medicine envisages interdisciplinarity with respect to expertise, which is why a doctor who is not specialised in ophthalmology must obviously undertake the relative diagnostic-therapeutic manoeuvres, delegating advanced therapies to the specialist: eye movements, visual acuity and light perception must be tested.

The prompt administration of hyaluronidase should be considered as soon as possible after the onset of symptoms, after immediately stopping the injection, especially if there is concomitant blanching or skin ischaemia in the injection area. The use of hyaluronidase to dissolve cross-linked hyaluronic acid is highly effective and has been shown to prevent tissue necrosis. Rapid use could save threatened tissues. The authors recommend using 1,500 units per 1 ml with 1% lidocaine or 2% lidocaine without adrena-

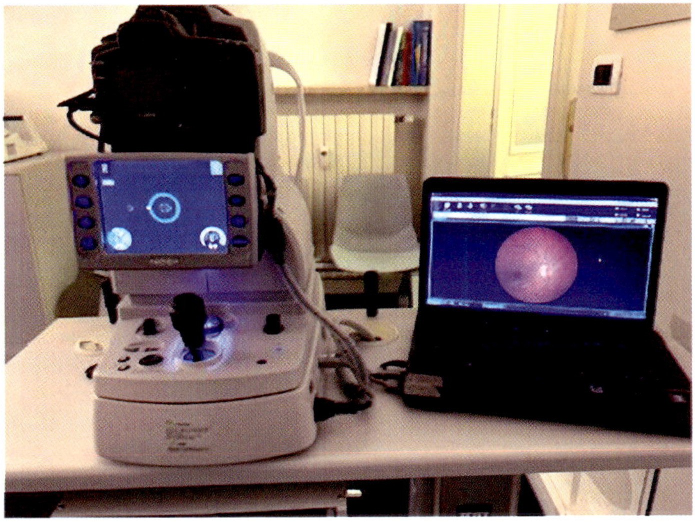

Figure 2 White light retinography. Courtesy of Dr. L. Emanuelli

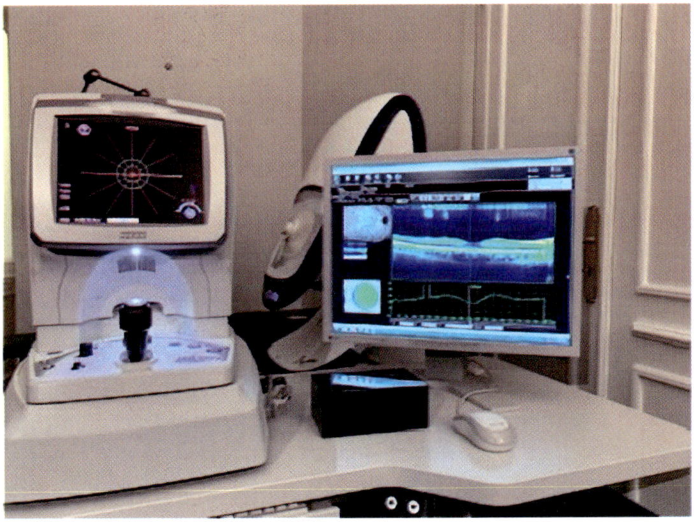

Figure 3 Ocular coherence tomograph (OCT). Courtesy of Dr. L. Emanuelli

line, employing a high-dose pulsed dosing pattern repeated up to four times.
Hyaluronidase can potentially indirectly dissolve and improve perfusion, which is why it should be injected at high doses and repeated, having a local-regional action with respect to retinal ischaemia; however, its role in filler-associated blindness has yet to be determined [14].
Reduce intraocular pressure by administering one drop of 0.5% timolol eye drops, if available, into the affected eye while waiting for transfer to hospital. The authors recommend that timolol be part of a sight loss kit readily available at the doctor's surgery [15].

The administration of local hypotonic agents, beta-blockers and acetazolamide, and steroids (betamethasone 4 mg x 2 in a single dose or analogue) reduces retinal oedema.
300 mg aspirin is appropriate; there is no direct evidence that aspirin prevents platelet aggregation in hyaluronic acid-related occlusion; however, it is reasonable, based on extrapolation of the evidence from acute coronary syndrome, to prescribe 300 mg as an immediate dose with 75 mg daily until the occlusion dissolves and vision is restored. Safety must be considered within the context of the individual patient, and if the patient is allergic to aspirin, clopidogrel at a dose of 300 mg can be used immediately with 75 mg daily [14].
If the patient has no medical contraindications, the use of sublingual glycerol trinitrate is a quick and effective method of increasing vasodilation.
Instruct the patient to breathe into a paper bag for about 10 minutes every half hour so that the increase in carbon dioxide promotes dilation of the arterioles [16].
The ophthalmic specialist tests the relative afferent pupillary defect (RAPD), which is an objective measurement of relative optic nerve damage by means of the "oscillating light test", which assesses pupillary constriction upon exposure to light, extra-ocular muscle movement for ophthalmoplegia and ptosis, including measurement of marginal reflex distance [17].
The dose of acetazolamide (Diamox) and topical ocular antihypertensives is then increased to reduce intraocular pressure [18]. This is followed by anterior chamber paracentesis to induce pressure shock on the occluded retinal vessel in order to at least partially restore its patency [19,20].
The doctor then considers retro-bulbar injection therapy with 1,500 UI in 4 ml of saline with a 25 G retro-bulbar needle, considering that the success rates reported in the literature are just over 10% and must be weighed against the iatrogenic risks of the procedure even in experienced hands [21-24].
Hyperbaric therapy (Hyperbaric Oxygen Therapy - HOT) must be considered with respect to the guidelines and the relevant contraindications, as its rationale is based on the assumption that the administration of hyperbaric oxygen can induce regression of hypoxic hypoperfusion damage [25,26]. While waiting for access to HOT, the patient starts oxygen treatment as soon as possible in an oro-facial mask with a reservoir, with a total of 60 minutes of O_2 at pressure, for 20-30 treatments, depending on clinical evolution and the degree of macular engagement. The fundus oculi examination is performed to assess the involvement of the area of oedema and modulate the dosage of acetazolamide and any anticoagulant and fibrinolytic therapies. Fluorangiography highlights the ischaemic area, the degree of occlusion present and the countermeasures still applicable [27-30].

Conclusions

Loss of sight is a very severe and feared complication of facial filler treatments. It is caused by the injection of fillers into vessels that anastomise with branches of the ophthalmic arteries.

There is currently no internationally accepted consensus on the immediate management of soft tissue filler-induced vision loss. The therapeutic choices indicated are aimed at supporting retinal perfusion, reducing intraocular pressure and retinal oedema, promoting lysis of the hyaluronic acid embolus and so restoring sight loss [31,32]. It is essential for some appropriate therapeutic manoeuvre to be promptly implemented, because literature confirms that all patients with amaurosis that has regressed completely or partially received one of therapies indicated [33-35].

Bibliography

1. Beleznay K, Carruthers JDA, Humphrey S, et al. Update on avoiding and treating blindness from fillers: a recent review of the world literature. Aesthet Surg J. 2019;39:662-674.
2. Goodman GJ, Magnusson MR, Callan P, Roberts S, et al. A Consensus on Minimizing the Risk of Hyaluronic Acid Embolic Visual Loss and Suggestions for Immediate Bedside Management. Aesthet Surg J. 2020;40(9):1009-1021.
3. Taylor GI, Shoukath S, Gascoigne A, Corlett RJ, Ashton MW. The Functional Anatomy of the Ophthalmic Angiosome and Its Implications in Blindness as a Complication of Cosmetic Facial Filler Procedures. Plast Reconstr Surg. 2020 Oct;146(4):745.
4. Khan TT, Colon-Acevedo B, Mettu P, et al. An Anatomical Analysis of the Supratrochlear Artery: Considerations in Facial Filler Injections and Preventing Vision Loss. Aesthet Surg J. 2017;37(2):203-208.
5. Sito G, Manzoni V, Sommariva R. Vascular Complications after Facial Filler Injection: A Literature Review and Meta-analysis. J Clin Aesthet Dermatol. 2019 Jun;12(6):E65-E72.
6. Diaspro A, Sito G. Hyaluronic acid for lower eyelid and tear trough rejuvenation: review of the literature. Plast Aesthet Res 2020;7:62.
7. Taylor GI, Shoukath S, Gascoigne A, Corlett RJ, Ashton MW. The Functional Anatomy of the Ophthalmic Angiosome and Its Implications in Blindness as a Complication of Cosmetic Facial Filler Procedures. Plast Reconstr Surg. 2020 Oct;146(4):745.
8. Myung Y, Yim S, Jeong JH, Kim BK, Heo CY, Baek RM, Pak CS. The Classification and Prognosis of Periocular Complications Related to Blindness following Cosmetic Filler Injection. Plast Reconstr Surg. 2017 Jul;140(1):61-64.
9. Cho KH, Dalla Pozza E, Toth G, et al. Pathophysiology Study of Filler-Induced Blindness. Aesthet Surg J. 2019;39(1):96-106.
10. Sharma RA, Newman NJ, Biousse V. Conservative treatments for acute nonarteritic central retinal artery occlusion: Do they work? Taiwan J Ophthalmol. 2021;11(1):16.
11. DeLorenzi C. Commentary on: Blindness After Facial Filler Injections: The Role of Extravascular Hyaluronidase on Intravascular Hyaluronic Acid Embolism in the Rabbit Experimental Model. Aesthetic Surg J. 2020:40(3):327-329.
12. Zhu GZ, Sun ZS, Liao WX, Cai B, Chen CL, Zheng HH, Zeng L, Luo SK. Efficacy of Retrobulbar Hyaluro-

nidase Injection for Vision Loss Resulting from Hyaluronic Acid Filler Embolization. Aesthet Surg J. 2017 Dec 13;38(1):12-22.
13. Rudraprasad D, Gagan S, Joseph J, Vasanthapuram VH, Naik MN. Retrobulbar Hyaluronidase Injection: Does It Reach the Eye? Ophthalmic Plast Reconstr Surg. 2022 Mar-Apr 01;38(2):176-179.
14. Murray G, Convery C, Walker L, Davies E. Guideline for the Management of Hyaluronic Acid Filler-induced Vascular Occlusion. J Clin Aesthet Dermatol. 2021;14(5):E61–E69.
15. Barbarino S, Banker T, Fezza J. Standardized approach to treatment of retinal artery occlusion after intraarterial injection of soft tissue fillers: EYE-CODE. J Am Acad Dermatol. 2022 May;86(5):1102-1108.
16. Frayser R, Hickham JB. Retinal vascular response to breathing increased carbon dioxide and oxygen concentrations. Invest Ophthalmol.1964;3:427-431.
17. Arlette JP, Ashenhurst M, Hill V, Jiang K. Prevention and Management of Filler Induced Iatrogenic Stroke of the Eye [Formula: see text]. J Cutan Med Surg. 2021 Sep;25(5):543-552.
18. Navarro-Hernandez E, Pérez-López M. Effectiveness of retrobulbar hyaluronidase in the treatment of visual loss caused by periocular hyaluronic acid injection. A systematic review. Arch Soc Esp Oftalmol (Engl Ed). 2022 Jul 1:S2173-5794(22)00089-5.
19. Graue G, Ochoa Araujo DA, et al. The M.A.STE.R.S algorithm for acute visual loss management after facial filler injection. J Cosmet Dermatol. 2020;19:2859-2866.
20. Ffytche TJ. A rationalization of treatment of central retinal artery occlusion. Trans Ophthalmol Soc UK (1962). 1974 Jul;94(2):468-79.
21. Sorensen EP, Council ML. Update in Soft-Tissue Filler-Associated Blindness. Dermatol Surg. 2020 May;46(5):671-677.
22. Sharudin SN, Ismail MF, Mohamad NF, Vasudevan SK. Complete recovery of filler-induced visual loss following subcutaneous hyaluronidase injection. Neuroophthalmology. 2018 Jul 13;43(2):102-106.
23. Wibowo A, Kapoor KM, Philipp-Dormston WG. Reversal of Post-filler Vision Loss and Skin Ischaemia with High-Dose Pulsed Hyaluronidase Injections. Aesthetic Plast Surg. 2019 Oct;43(5):1337-1344.
24. Chesnut C. Restoration of Visual Loss With Retrobulbar Hyaluronidase Injection After Hyaluronic Acid Filler. Dermatol Surg. 2018 Mar;44(3):435-437.
25. Linee guida S.I.M.S.I. (Società Italiana di Medicina Subacquea e Iperbarica) sulle indicazioni all'ossigenoterapia iperbarica, II ed. (2015). https://simsi.it/wp-content/uploads/2019/04/lineeguida_2015.pdf
26. Linea Guida Ossigenoterapia Iperbarica (OTI): controindicazioni ed effetti collaterali (01 ottobre 2018). https://simsi.it/wp-content/uploads/2019/04/Linea_Guida_controindicazioni_OTI_27.09.18.pdf
27. Butler FK Jr, Hagan C, Murphy-Lavoie H. Hyperbaric oxygen therapy and the eye. Undersea Hyperb Med. 2008 Sep-Oct;35(5):333-87.

28. Oguz H, Sobaci G. The use of hyperbaric oxygen therapy in ophthalmology. Surv Ophthalmol. 2008 Mar-Apr;53(2):112-20.
29. Oguz H, Sobaci G. The use of hyperbaric oxygen therapy in ophthalmology. Surv Ophthalmol. 2008 Mar-Apr;53(2):112-20.
30. Weinberger AW, Siekmann UP, Wolf S, Rossaint R, Kirchhof B, Schrage NF. Treatment of Acute Central Retinal Artery Occlusion (CRAO) by Hyperbaric Oxygenation Therapy (HBO)--Pilot study with 21 patients. Klin Monbl Augenheilkd. 2002 Oct;219(10):728-34. German.
31. Jones DH, Fitzgerald R, Cox SE, et al. Preventing and Treating Adverse Events of Injectable Fillers: Evidence-Based Recommendations From the American Society for Dermatologic Surgery Multidisciplinary Task Force. Dermatol Surg. 2021;47(2):214-226.
32. Walker L, et al. Consensus Opinion for The Management of Soft Tissue Filler Induced Vision Loss. J Clin Aesthet Dermatol. 2021 Dec;14(12):E84-E94.
33. Kapoor KM, Kapoor P, Heydenrych I, Bertossi D. Vision Loss Associated with Hyaluronic Acid Fillers: A Systematic Review of Literature. Aesthetic Plast Surg. 2020 Jun;44(3):929-944.
34. Hadanny A, Maliar A, Fishlev G, Bechor Y, Bergan J, Friedman M, Avni I, Efrati S. Reversibility of retinal ischemia due to central retinal artery occlusion by hyperbaric oxygen. Clin Ophthalmol. 2016 Dec 29;11:115-125.
35. Mac Grory B, Schrag M, Biousse V, Furie KL, Gerhard-Herman M, Lavin PJ, Sobrin L, Tjoumakaris SI, Weyand CM, Yaghi S; American Heart Association Stroke Council; Council on Arteriosclerosis, Thrombosis and Vascular Biology; Council on Hypertension; and Council on Peripheral Vascular Disease. Management of Central Retinal Artery Occlusion: A Scientific Statement From the American Heart Association. Stroke. 2021 Jun;52(6):e282-e294.

10

SPECIAL REGIONS

EYELID COMPLICATIONS

Alberto Diaspro, Luigi Emanuelli, Francesco Romeo

The treatment of periocular ageing plays a crucial role among facial rejuvenation procedures.

The youthful appearance of the eye includes a well-defined upper eyelid crease, with the pre-tarsal skin visible from the medial to the lateral canthus and the presence of adequate volume at pre-septal skin level, with fullness tapering into the skin of the supra-ciliary region. There must be a medial concavity where the nasal fat compartment projects and from where this ends an increasing convexity to the far side of the eyelid.

Excessive groove depth due to loss of volume (sunken eye) and the presence of excess skin (dermatochalasis) are both associated with an ageing appearance.

A youthful appearance of the lower eyelid is defined by the absence of discontinuities in the junction between the lower eyelid and cheek and the absence of visible "bags", furrows or excess skin.

Eyelid rejuvenation has become a topic of great interest because not all patients request or need surgical blepharoplasty, and the treatment of selected imperfections secondary to the ageing of this region has been possible since 2004 with very satisfactory results [1-3].

Anatomy

The eyelids are considered to be difficult sites to inject, yet the production of scientific articles focusing on the anatomy of this area with respect to non-surgical rejuvenation procedures is of relative significance when compared with the numerous articles dealing with the anatomical details of this area with respect to blepharoplasty techniques.

Only two studies have been published on the lower eyelid, and this was seven years after the technique was introduced. Subsequently, the anatomy and the ageing process of this region began to be considered strongly related to that of the mid-facial region and not treated as separate [1].

Literature on the upper eyelid, on the other hand, is different, as its non-surgical rejuvenation techniques were published later than those of the lower eyelid [3], and are still being studied in depth [4]. Please see the articles mentioned and the corresponding publications for further reading.

Indications

The critical issues to be addressed are related to careful clinical assessment and planning of treatment. This will leave room for complications of unknown origin alone.

Upper eyelid

It is usually necessary to add volume to the sunken eye, where volume is congenitally deficient, in the hollow eye without or with modest eyelid folds, and in the rare cases of a full eye with modest eyelid folds.

In the sunken eye, an important distinction must be made between young and adult patients. As it is a condition that is strongly linked to family history, the clinical evidence can become visible very early on, even in the immediate post-adolescent period. Making an early diagnosis means offering the chance of a truly effective treatment that can transform a sunken eye into a regular, pleasantly full eye. When choosing the technique, the principles are those of the hollow eye.

The filler approach alone is indicated in the hollow eye with no or moderate presence of eyelid folds. Deciding whether to treat the hollow eye with the lipofilling technique or hyaluronic acid depends entirely on convenience. The undeniable regenerative capacity of fat leans undoubtedly in favour of the former. Lower costs and its repeatability and precision of symmetry definitely lean towards hyaluronic acid. Hyaluronic acid is also easy to inject, if only for the reason that the material is ready-made, all we have to do is to make a careful choice with a moderate prevalence of elasticity as opposed to viscosity and no local anaesthetic if possible, in order to avoid probable, albeit brief and transitory, eyelid ptosis. The efficacy is equal and the results pleasing in both approaches. Both techniques are operator-dependent; the experience of the specialist is the basis for success.

In the hollow eye with dermatochalasis, a dual approach of resection and filler must be planned. The timing is easily defined.

If we approach with surgical resection first, we can simultaneously proceed with fat grafting to fill the hollow. Then, after three months, we reassess the case and decide whether we are satisfied or whether to proceed with a further session or supplement any deficit with hyaluronic acid.

If, after resection, we proceed with an increase in volume, we wait two months and usually achieve complete resolution with a single injection of hyaluronic acid.

If we increase the volume first, the suggested rule for the treatment of dermatochalasis is the performance of surgical resection after two months if the volume is added using hyaluronic acid filler and after three months if the volume is added with a fat graft.

In my experience, this is only theoretical, as patient satisfaction after treatment with filler alone often causes the delay of resection, even for years, as the increase in volume results in "recovery" from dermatochalasis.

The total volume injected on each side is 0.35 mL +/- 0.15 mL (range 0.1-0.5 mL). The injection technique involves use of a microcannula (25 or 27 G, 40 mm): after pricking the skin with the needle and crossing the muscle plane, the microcannula advances medially in the suborbicular plane known as ROOF (retroorbicularis oculi fat), and, upon reaching the orbicularis retaining ligament (ORL), enters the retro-septal space where the lateral compartment of the nasal fat pad is located [3,5].

Lower eyelid

The injection of hyaluronic acid for the rejuvenation of the lower eyelid has been shown to be most effective and should, therefore, be ideally indicated in patients between 30 and 40 years of age, although it presents noticeable benefits in patients up to the age of 50. Afterwards, it should no longer be the treatment of choice given the ptosis of

the retro-orbicular and medial cheek fat, which is responsible for its deterioration and the tension action on the orbicular ligament, limiting the correction that can be achieved with the injection of hyaluronic acid alone.
There are numerous classifications, which is why there is still no agreement as to the indications for treatment with respect to the morphology of the blemish, other than the age of the patient.
The total volume injected on each side is usually 0.35 ± 0.1 mL (range 0.2-0.65 mL): using the needle, it is necessary to identify and protect the infraorbital foramen with gentle finger pressure, followed by insertion of a 30 G 13 mm needle into the deepest part of the tear trough, which is always treated first with injection of a single bolus on the bony surface. The area injected is then gently massaged to create a natural shape and then the result is assessed for further injection, if necessary.
When the cannula is preferred, the point of entry is at the intersection of the vertical line passing through the outer canthus and the line marked by the palpebromalar groove, a continuation of the tear trough. Once inserted, it is necessary to cross the orbicularis muscle and advance until it reaches the bony crest of the orbital rim, to slide medially towards the inner canthus injecting a bolus of hyaluronic acid at the point of greatest skin depression and avoiding linear deposits often visible after treatment. The infraorbital foramen will then be located more caudally and deeply than the injection plane.
The first bolus can be supplemented with additional amounts if the result is unsatisfactory; in this case too, gentle massage is recommended [6].

Dermatochalasis and rhytidosis of the lower eyelid

When the decision is made to opt for non-surgical treatment of upper and/or lower eyelid rhytidosis using plasma or laser EBD, these must be assessed using the same diagnostic approach as for surgical resection [7,8].
The reported outcomes can be satisfactory when the correct indications and details of technique are followed. These are not, however, the subject of this chapter, so please see the relevant publications for further details, but they are not always free of complications as presented in the section of the chapter.

Complications

The first articles focused on complications resulting from hyaluronic acid treatment of the lower eyelid were published in 2012 [1], whereas the first reports of complications in the upper eyelid were initially reported secondary to adipose tissue grafting procedures [9] and only later after hyaluronic acid injection [10].
The most commonly reported complications include [1,5,6,9,10]:

- reactive oedema due to attraction of interstitial liquids in the case of very superficial injection for skin biostimulation (fig. 1);
- Tyndall effect, a blue-grey discolouration, in 30.5% of cases of injection with hyaluronic acid (fig. 2);
- irregular contours, ranging from 4.25% to 30.5% of cases (fig. 3);
- chronic oedema, reported in up to 11% of cases, even with fatty tissue

grafting (figs. 4-6).

Complications from hyaluronic acid implantation in the upper eyelid are basically related to superficial filler injection, i.e. into subcutaneous or relatively deep retro-orbicular planes (figs. 7-9). The hyaluronic acid is visible on the surface and create permanent Tyndall effect, well beyond the duration of the filler itself. In relative depth, in the retro-muscular and therefore pre-septal space, it is subject to easy migration, particularly medially, creating a convex deformity where a pleasant concavity is present in nature.

Rarely reported complications secondary to hyaluronic acid injections into the eyelids are:

- formation of granulomas, both after injection of hyaluronic acid and fat graft;
- cellulitis and migraine;
- diplopia;
- eyelid skin reactions similar to xanthelasmas;
- tear duct obstruction.

The injection of an adequate dose of hyaluronidase has always been considered the best treatment (figs. 10-11). In the case of chronic oedema, early manual lymphatic drainage on a weekly basis for the first two months after onset is useful. In order to avoid complications from lymph stasis, it is preferable to carry out treatments of the peri-oculo-palpebral area at least thirty days apart, especially botulinum toxin and traction

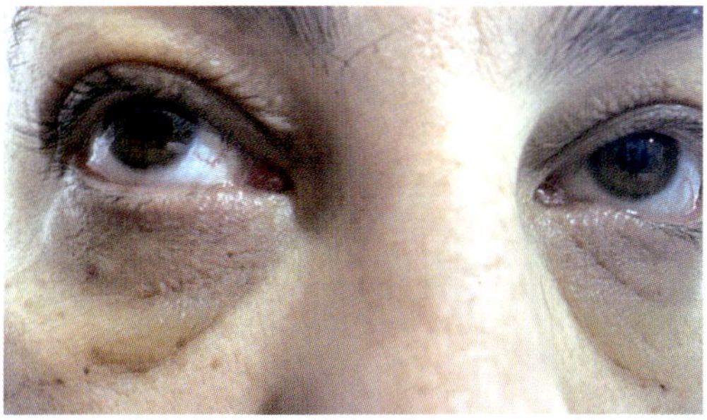

Figure 1 Iatrogenic interstitial oedema after excessively superficial injection of hyaluronic acid for skin biostimulation

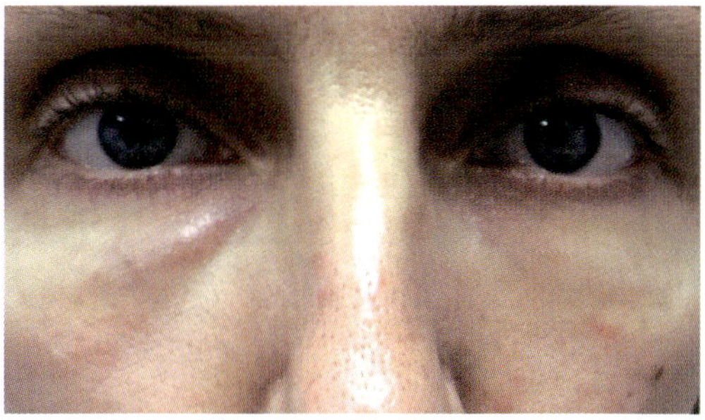

Figure 2 Tyndall effect after excessively superficial injection into the right tear trough

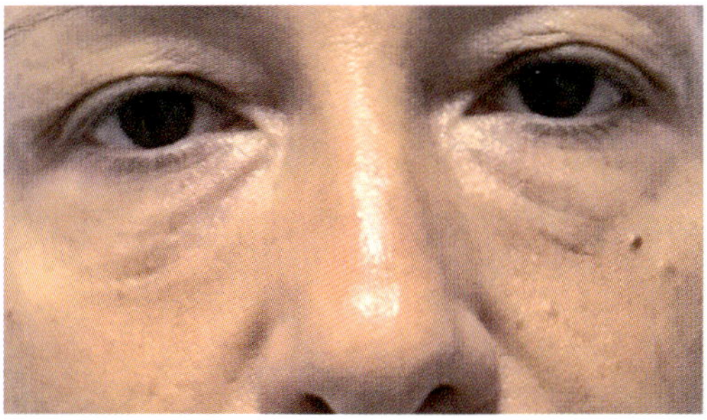

Figure 3 Irregular contour of the lower eyelids: excess product injected too close to the surface

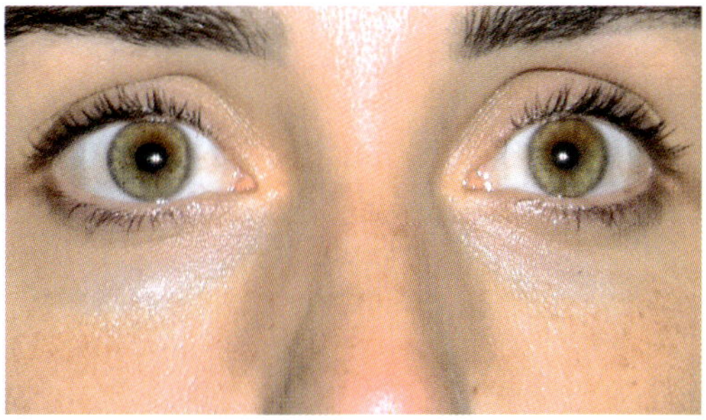

Figure 4 Chronic oedema of the right lower eyelid which appeared approximately one year after implantation, frontal view

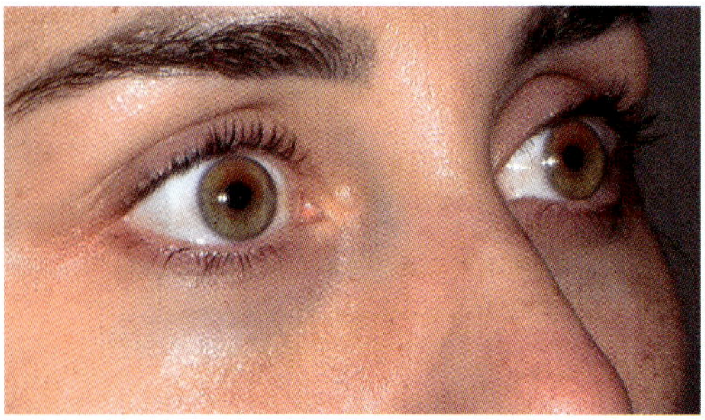

Figure 5 Chronic oedema of the right lower eyelid which appeared approximately one year after implantation, oblique view

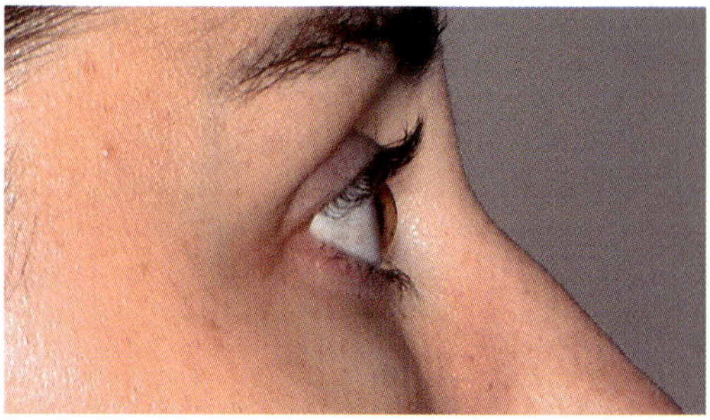

Figure 6 Chronic oedema of the right lower eyelid which appeared approximately one year after implantation, side view

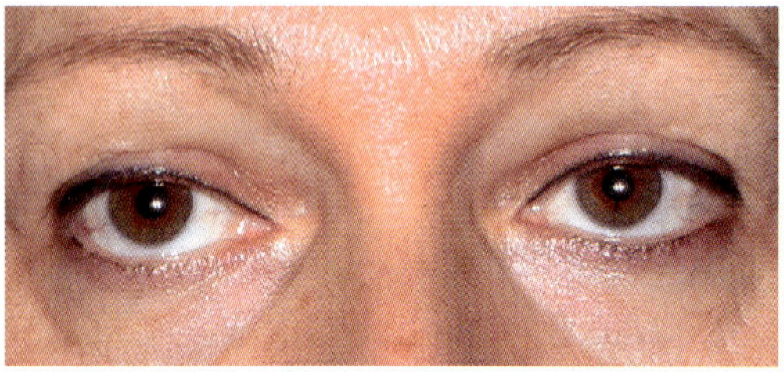

Figure 7 Irregular contour of the upper eyelids, excess product injected too close to the surface: front view, eyes open

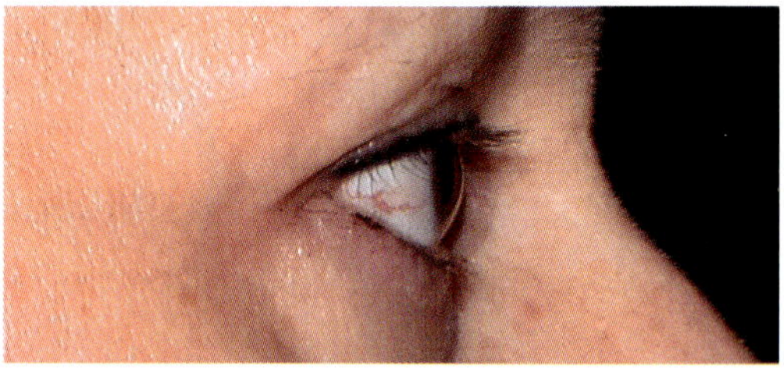

Figure 8 Irregular contour of the upper eyelids, excess product injected too close to the surface: side view

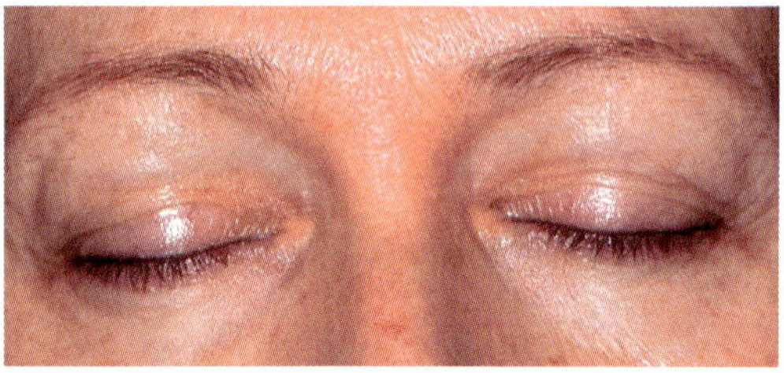

Figure 9 Irregular contour of the upper eyelids, excess product injected too close to the surface: front view, eyes closed

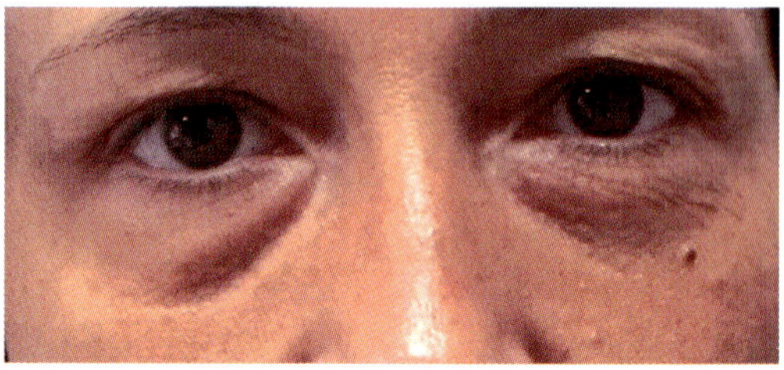

Figure 10 Hyaluronidase treatment of contour irregularities (see fig. 3): restoration of the natural contour of the lower eyelids

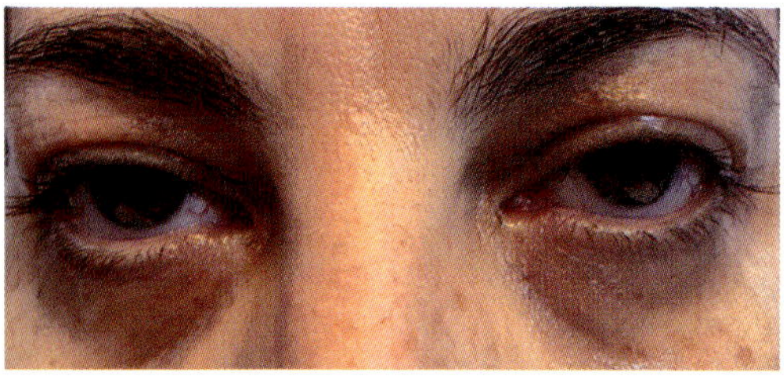

Figure 11 Hyaluronidase treatment of iatrogenic interstitial oedema (see fig. 1): resolution of fluid retention

threads, which disrupt normal lymphatic drainage for different reasons.

Hyperpigmentation

While hypopigmentation is a very rare complication in the eyelid region (>0.5%), early (<8%) and persistent (<5%) erythema and post-inflammatory hyperpigmentation (PIH) up to 6-8 weeks after dermatochalasis treatment using Energy Based Devices (EBDs, plasma exeresis and ablative CO_2 laser) are the most reported and feared complications (<10%), which may be limited or treatable with depigmenting products to be considered in phototypes above Fritzpatrick II, usually effective within six months but requiring high therapeutic adherence to home prescription [11].
Please see the relevant chapters of the publication for further details.

Blepharitis

The normal lubrication of the ocular surface is ensured by an exocrine secretion, the tear film produced by a glandular complex consisting of the lachrymal glands, the Meibomian glands and the mucin-producing cells of the conjunctiva; the latter two dispense a lipid-like substance that is essential for the normal stability of the tear and to produce a competent tear secretion (figs. 12-13).
The eyelid skin contains no subcutaneous fat and is the thinnest area of skin on the body, with a thickness of less than 1 mm. The epidermis consists of an epithelium with 6/7 layers of cells, the dermis and the underlying subcutaneous areolar tissue of the eyelids, which contains very little fatty tissue. Hair follicles and sebaceous glands are found here, while sweat glands are found ubiquitously throughout the district.
Oedema, itching, bruising and pain, typical signs and symptoms of the post-surgical course of eyelid skin resection are also usually reported in the case of plasma exeresis in the first week (at least two of the four described), while hyperaemia and itching are usually still present after a month, albeit to a lesser extent, and are more significant in patients with more severe dermatochalasis [11-12].
The incidence of Meibomian Gland Dysfunction (MGD) and therefore Dry Eye Disease (DED) secondary to surgical blepharoplasty treatments is widely described. By increasing the exposure of the ocular surface and reducing blinking, blepharoplasty increases film evaporation, aggravating the already existing symptomatology or asymptomatic dry eye. These forms of obstructive blepharitis are associated with painful symptomatology that is rarely associated with satisfactory aesthetic results, in patients often suffering from asymptomatic or undiagnosed inflammatory conditions [13].
Dry Eye Disease (DED) is a quantitative and qualitative alteration of the exocrine lachrymal secretion with inflammatory and osmolarity changes in the ocular surface.
Depending on the alteration of its components, the tear film is divided into hyposecretive, aqueous deficient (tears), lipid deficient on an obstructive and atrophic basis, and mixed. Dacryological semeiotics makes use of qualitative and quantitative examinations aimed at assessing the cause of

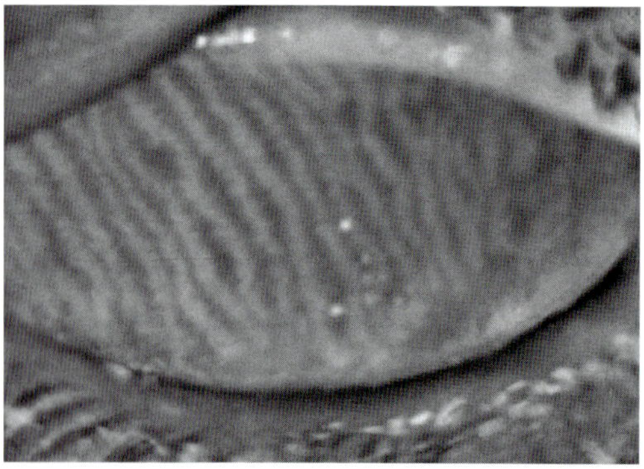

Figure 12 Normal infrared meibography. Courtesy of Dr. L. Emanuelli

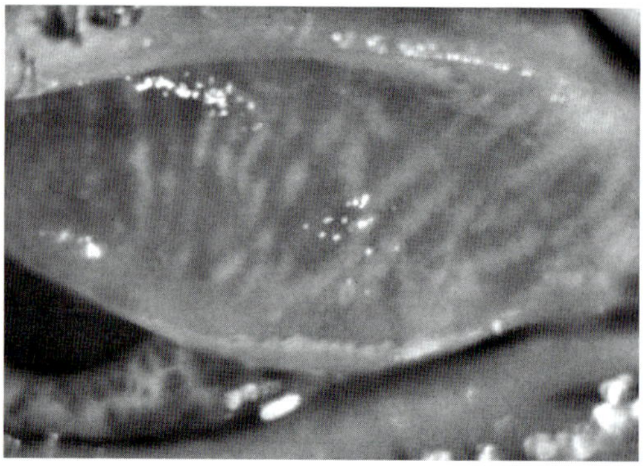

Figure 13 Pathological infrared meibography. Courtesy of Dr. L. Emanuelli

dry eye and monitoring its treatment in order to offer the most rational therapy possible.

Ophthalmological therapies are pharmacological, using tear substitutes, anti-inflammatory drugs and autologous platelet lysate, or instrumental.

Prevention or suspicion of diagnosis must be implemented by every professional who, regardless of the medical or surgical approach, is preparing to treat blemishes of the eyelid district: the use of patient questionnaires allows the calculation of a score which, if critical values are reached, determines the need for an ophthalmic consultation before proceeding, in order to avoid active and omissive malpractice [14].

Conclusions

Non-surgical correction of selected deformities of the eyelid region using injections of hyaluronic acid or fatty tissue can provide a reliable and feasible option if properly performed, thanks to the immediate and long-lasting results. However, the potential complications and their clinical course, which is often devious and chronic, require adequate technical skills and experience in the management of the clinical problem and the patient presenting it, considering the significant role of this anatomical area in social relations.

Bibliography

1 Diaspro A, Sito G. Hyaluronic acid for lower eyelid and tear trough rejuvenation: review of the literature. Plast Aesthet Res 2020;7:62.

2 Morley AM, Taban M, Malhotra R, Goldberg RA. Use of hyaluronic Acid gel for upper eyelid filling and contouring. Ophthalmic Plast Reconstr Surg. 2009 Nov-Dec;25(6):440-4.

3 Romeo F. Upper Eyelid Filling With or Without Surgical Treatment. Aesthetic Plast Surg. 2016 Apr;40(2):223-35.

4 Montes JR, Santos E, Amaral C. Eyelid and Periorbital Dermal Fillers: Products, Techniques, and Outcomes. Facial Plast Surg Clin North Am. 2021 May;29(2):335-348.

5 Romeo F. Upper Eyelid Filling Approach [U.E.F.A.] Technique: State of the Art After 500 Consecutive Patients. Aesthetic Plast Surg. 2019 Jun;43(3):663-672.

6 Diaspro A, Calvisi L, Sito G. Hyaluronic Acid Gel Injection for the Treatment of Tear Trough Deformity: A Multicenter, Observational, Single-Blind Study. Aesthetic Plast Surg. 2022 Apr 27.
7 Theodorelou-Charitou SA, Xanthos T, Nikas IP, Ntinioti T. New era in upper eyelid rejuvenation: A brief overview of non-surgical blepharoplasty techniques. J Plast Reconstr Aesthet Surg. 2021 Jul;74(7):1633-1701.
8 Hassan AM, Rady AAE, Shalaby OE, Shafik HM, Shaker ESE. Evaluation of plasma exeresis as a new technique for non surgical treatment of dermatochalasis. J Dermatolog Treat. 2022 Mar;33(2):1017-1022.
9 Jakobiec FA, Rai R, Rashid A, Sutula FC. Bilateral Eyelid Pseudoptosis From Lipogranulomas of the Preaponeurotic Fat Pads. Ophthalmic Plast Reconstr Surg. 2015 Sep-Oct;31(5):e125-31.
10 Yu JTS, Peng L, Ataullah S. Chronic Eyelid Edema Following Periocular Hyaluronic Acid Filler Treatment. Ophthalmic Plast Reconstr Surg. 2017 Nov/Dec;33(6):e139-e140.
11 Nipshagen MD, Velthuis PJ, Mosmuller DGM. Periorbital postinflammatory hyperpigmentation after plasma exeresis. Dermatol Ther. 2020 May;33(3):e13404.
12 Ferreira FC, Sathler CSCO, Hida IY, Leite SC, Kusabara AA, de Castro ACV, Ribeiro MZML, Nahas TR. Upper eyelid blepharoplasty using plasma exeresis: Evaluation of outcomes, satisfaction, and symptoms after procedure. J Cosmet Dermatol. 2021 Sep;20(9):2758-2764.
13 Zhang SY, Yan Y, Fu Y. Cosmetic blepharoplasty and dry eye disease: a review of the incidence, clinical manifestations, mechanisms and prevention. Int J Ophthalmol. 2020 18 Mar;13(3):488-492.
14 Okumura Y, Inomata T, Iwata N, Sung J, Fujimoto K, Fujio K, Midorikawa-Inomata A, Miura M, Akasaki Y, Murakami A. A Review of Dry Eye Questionnaires: Measuring Patient-Reported Outcomes and Health-Related Quality of Life. Diagnostics (Basel). 2020 Aug 5;10(8):559.

LIP COMPLICATIONS

Raffaella Sommariva

The lips are one of the areas most frequently treated with filler implants but, compared to all the other parts of the face, they have a special, completely different anatomical structure that requires an equally "special" approach. Lips are soft, vital and highly mobile, and their reshaping should be undertaken in a delicate and specific manner, respecting not only their morphology but also their function.

In the immediate post-implantation of fillers, some undesirable effects are often unavoidable. They are usually mild and temporary but, for some patients, they represent feared and dreaded "complications": fears that can be overcome simply by informing the patient in the pre-implantation phase and providing them with all the necessary medical and cosmetic support so that they do not find their lives limited in any way.

Rarely, after filler implantation, we are faced with particular inflammatory reactions (infectious or immune-mediated); more frequently, we are faced with unnatural or excessive aesthetic results due to errors in technique (excess volumes, altered proportions and morphology) or the use of unsuitable products [1].

The most severe complications, resulting from vascular accidents, are certainly much rarer in the lips than in other facial areas such as the glabella, nose, nasolabial fold, and alar triangle [2], but nevertheless the vascular risk still always exists [3].

As in every other area of the face, the first rule to minimise the risk of post-filler complications is a thorough knowledge of the anatomy as well as the use of conscious implantation techniques and targeted products. Prevention is always the best tool we have at our disposal, but it is also essential to be able to recognise the problem early on in order to manage it appropriately, solving it or at least limiting further developments.

Anatomy

The lips are two soft, very mobile, membranous-muscle folds. The transverse slit, to which the mouth opening is reduced when the lips are closed, and which runs from one commissure to the other, is the rima oris and it measures between 45 and 55 mm.

Topographical anatomy

The lip region extends from the lower margin of the nose and the alar groove (top) to the naso-labial folds (sides) to the mento-labial cleft (bottom). From an anatomical-topographical point of view, the lip region is made up of the upper lip and the lower lip. The former extends from the base of the nose, above, to the free margin of the upper vermilion, below, and is bordered laterally by the naso-labial folds. The second extends from the free margin of the upper vermilion, above, to the mento-labial cleft, below (where it continues with the chin region), and is bordered laterally by two vertical lines that descend at a distance of about 1 cm from the labial commissures.

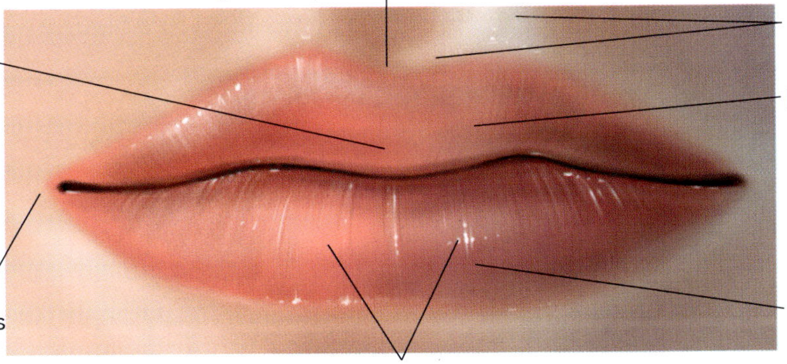

Figure 1 Anatomical reference points

The adherent margins of the upper and lower lips i.e. the reflection lines of the mucosa from the lips to the gums, correspond to these outer limits.

The free margins of the lips (the pink parts) taper towards the sides. The pink part (vermilion) of the upper lip is long, arched and deep, has a median labial tubercle with two slight curves, one on each side. The contour of the vermilion of the lower lip may be straight or slightly curved; a slight median depression and two lateral tubercles correspond respectively to the upper median labial tubercle and the two upper paramedian curves.

The external or cutaneous face of the upper lip presents the median sub-nasal groove, the philtrum with the philtrum ridges and at the skin-vermilion junction, the Cupid's bow: the fibres of the labial muscles are inserted in the skin at the sides of the philtrum, which, receiving no support, appears as a depression on the median line.

The lower margin of the orbicularis is inserted along the vermilion and, together with the other lip muscles, seems to lift the tubercle that lies below the philtrum.

The lower lip lacks a central structure or shape suggesting symmetry, sometimes there may be a slight dimple or depression on the midline [4].

The appearance of the lips changes in relation to the various facial and occlusal types and strongly reflects the underlying skeletal and dental structure. The shape of the lips is essentially always the same, and the numerous variations, both within people of the same racial origin and between different races, relate to the depth, width, thickness and slope; the proportions of the lips change according to age, gender and ethnicity.

Microanatomy

The structure of the lips consists of four layers: the skin, the muscular layer, the glandular layer and the labial mucosa (fig. 2).

The skin is thick, highly resistant, closely adherent to the underlying muscular fascia that connect to the deep dermis. It is covered with stratified keratinized squamous epithelium with abundant pilosebaceous units and sweat glands. The dermal papillae are flat. The der-

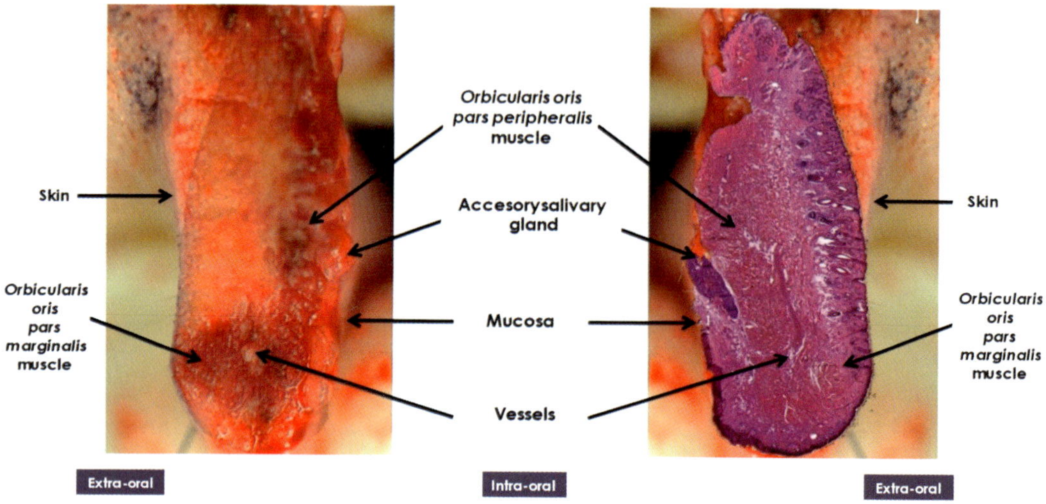

Figure 2 Lip anatomy and histology. Courtesy of E2e

mis is rich in elastic fibres and striated muscle fibres belonging to the cutaneous muscles and adheres strongly to the underlying muscles.

At the free edge of the lips (the pink part, the vermilion) there is a gradual transition from the skin to the mucous lining of the oral cavity. The red colour of the vermilion is due to the richly vascularised dermis; the thin epithelium is stratified keratinised and squamous. The dermal papillae are tall and numerous. There are no pilosebaceous units and sweat glands, so continuous humidification by saliva is required to prevent breakage.

The epithelial layer becomes thicker in the labial mucosa and is made up of non-keratinized stratified squamous epithelium. The lamina propria forms tall papillae.

Between the lamina propria and the muscular plane there is a layer of loose connective tissue that houses the labial glands (submucosa), the excretory ducts of which open into the vestibule of the mouth. It consists of a large number of small salivary glands, the labial glands, pressed against each other to form an almost continuous layer (glandular layer) between the orbicularis oris muscle and the mucosa.

The muscular layer is represented by the orbicularis oris muscle, the arched fibres of which extend transversally from one commissure to the other.

The orbicularis oris muscle is the essential lip muscle and acts as a constrictor: it closes or narrows the rima oris and projects the lips forward. The fasciae it relays to the posterior contour of the cartilage of the mobile septum represent the septum depressor muscle. The orbicularis oris muscle is an elliptical ring surrounding the rima oris. It is divided into two portions: an outer, peripheral, superficial part that joins the lips, the fibres of which contract independently, participating in facial mimicry together with the fasciae that come from other mimic muscles (canine, triangular, buccinator and incisors), and an inner, marginal part that surrounds the rima oris and acts exclusively as a constrictor muscle. The orbicularis is joined by the ends of other mimic muscles which, arranged radially, starting from other regions of the face, are inserted into the contour and lower (depressor muscles) or lift (elevator muscles) the mouth and contribute to its opening and closing movement.

The labial musculature is embedded deeply in the skin at the base of the columella and on the floor of the nostrils, making it adhere to the underlying bone. This anatomical structure is one of the main factors in the development of the naso-labial angle, made up of the philtrum and the columella.

In the preliminary assessment of our patients' lips, after anatomical considerations, it is essential to examine the proportion between the upper and lower lip and the proportion of the lips with the other facial elements [4]. The harmony of the proportions between the various parts of the face is at the basis of the concept of "beauty" and the golden ratio is an irrational number (1.618) which identifies that "divine proportion" that is at the basis of the concept of ideal human beauty. The ideal proportion of the lip region is a ratio between the upper and lower lip of 1-1.618, which means a slightly deeper and fuller lower lip than the upper one (fig. 3) [4].

The lips should also and always be in harmony with the patient's age. They should also always be assessed in terms of their profile and their ratios (reciprocal proportions and relative positions) with the nose and chin and the respective nose-labial and chin-labial angles.

According to the golden ratio, the lips, seen from the front, should observe the following characteristics: the width of the mouth should extend laterally to a line lowered from the medial edge of the iris and should be 1.618 times the width of the nose; the ratio of the depth of the upper lip vermilion to that of the lower lip should be 1:1.61, so the lower lip should be deeper and fuller than the upper one [4].

Some say that the ideal lip width should occupy about 40 percent of the lower part of the face [4].

For the lips to be considered "ideal",

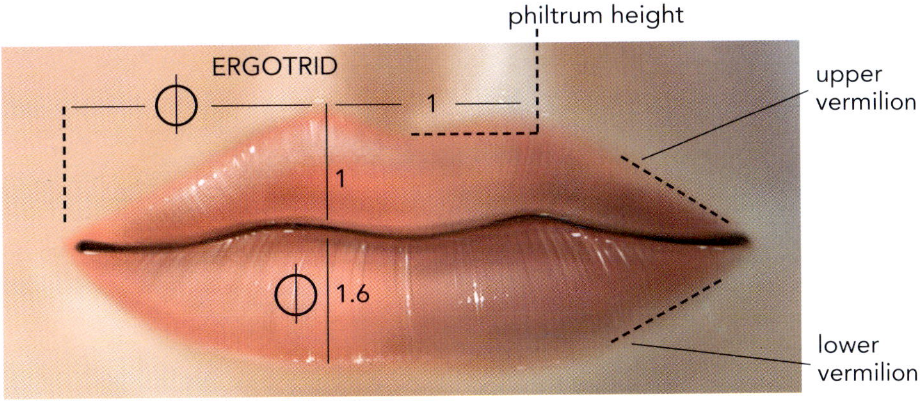

Figure 3 Golden ratio and philtrum labial score (PLS)

they should come close to this description: full and harmonious, with a long, curved and deep pink upper lip, and a lower lip clearly separated from the chin.

Vascularisation and innervation of the lips

The vascularisation of the lips (fig. 4) is entrusted mainly to the four labial arteries, two inferior and two superior. These are branches of the facial artery, which anastomise on the midline with their counterparts on the opposite side. In most cases, the four vessels run in the submucosa (between the orbicularis muscle and the oral mucosa), approximately 1-2 mm below the labial mucosa and a few millimetres behind the junction between the dry and wet lip.

The upper lip is vascularised mainly by the superior labial artery with its alar and septal branches; the lower lip, in addition to the main artery, the inferior labial artery, is also vascularised by the horizontal labio-mental artery (directed mainly to the oral mucosa) and the vertical labio-mental artery (absent in 21% cases).

However, the vascularisation of the lips is variable and at least four types of the superior labial artery are reported in literature, based on its relationship with the facial artery: in the first type (the most common), the superior labial artery and the alar branch are two collateral branches of the facial artery; in the second type, the alar branch originates from the superior labial artery; in the third type, the superior labial artery is a terminal branch of the facial artery and, in the fourth type, the superior labial

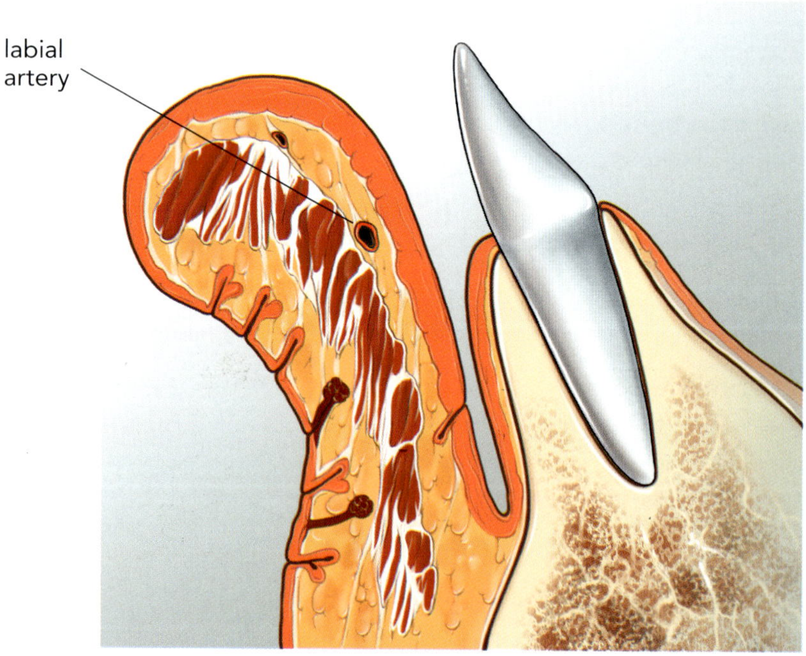

Figure 4 Vascularisation of the lips: labial arteries. The four labial arteries (two inferior and two superior) run mainly in the lip between the oral mucosa and the striated muscle, behind the line where the dry and wet mucosa meet

artery is absent and the contralateral superior labial artery and the ipsilateral infraorbital artery supply blood to the superior hemilip, which therefore have a greater calibre than usual [5].

Also in literature, at least three types of inferior labial artery are described [6]. It may be missing (in most cases), may originate from the facial artery or the superior labial artery. And there are at least three types of horizontal labio-mental artery (which mostly runs horizontally in the area of the lower lip or curves upwards leading to the vermilion border or splits into two branches, one running horizontally and one running upwards). This means that the different combinations of the various types of lower labial artery and horizontal labio-mental artery result in seven variants of distribution of vascularisation of the lower lip.

The cadaver study by Cotofana S. investigated the anatomical-topographical course of the labial arteries and showed that, in most cases, they run in the submucosal plane, between the oral mucosa and the orbicularis muscle; less frequently in the intramuscular plane and rarely in the subcutaneous plane [7]. The author's subsequent study, published in 2020, carried out in very young live subjects, with echo Doppler and 3D scanned images, mostly confirmed the results of the previous anatomical study on the cadaver, with slightly different percentages, but the localisation of the labial arteries was always predominantly submucosal, then intramuscular and finally subcutaneous. While on the midline in 100% of cases, the arteries were found not on the surface but in the body of the vermilion, unlike in the cadaver [8].

However, the labial vascular anatomy is variable not only between different individuals but also in the two sides of the same individual: the labial arteries may, with a meandering course, remain in the same plane or change plane once or sometimes twice before reaching the midline. The injection method must therefore always be careful and gentle.

The skin of the perioral region is nourished by a dense network of musculocutaneous perforating vessels that originate from the subdermal plexus. The veins open into the subdermal vein and the anterior facial vein. The lymphatics are organised in a subcutaneous and submucosal network and flow to the submandibular (upper lip), submental and submandibular (lower lip) lymph nodes. The motor nerves for the lip muscles are the branches of the facial nerve (6th cranial nerve). The sensory nerves, which spread to the skin, glands and mucosa, originate from the infraorbital nerve (for the upper lip) and the mental nerve (for the lower lip), both branches of the trigeminal (5th cranial nerve). In particular, the infraorbital nerve emerges from the infraorbital foramen and, with its terminal branches, carries sensory innervation to the nose, lower eyelid and upper lip. The mental nerve is the terminal branch of the inferior alveolar nerve, a branch of the mandibular nerve. It emerges from the mandible below the premolars to innervate the skin of the chin area, the lower lip and the outer part of the lower dental arch. However, the need for truncal anaesthesia is becoming increasingly rare, thanks to the use of highly concentrated topical anaesthetics, which are now particularly and quickly effective.

"Complications' for the patient"

The effects that immediately follow filler implantation are usually mild and brief, but they can complicate the patient's social life and create a great deal of discomfort. It is important to always do everything possible to minimise them, adopting a careful and gentle technique, and to inform the patient thoroughly, offering them all the cosmetic and therapeutic support to "buffer" complications and accelerate healing.

As regards the signs of inflammatory reaction [9] following the inoculation of any material, oedema (fig. 5A) is usually mild and temporary (24-48 hours) with the most recent fillers, as is erythema, and itching is usually absent. The choice of certified products supported by adequate scientific literature is always crucial.

Bruising, on the other hand, is always possible given the considerable vascularisation of the lip region (fig. 5B) [9]. Injecting very slowly, a little at a time and without "mobilising" the vermilion too much with the needle helps to prevent bruising. Bruising must always be treated to avoid delayed telangiectasias or residual pigmentations. Neo capillaries may sometimes remain after excessively vigorous massaging or shaping, especially on the edge of the lips, which may have to be treated later. Immediate compression helps to limit a developing bruise (fig. 6), as does the application of ice (after making sure there is no vascular complication). This is followed by the prescription of heparinoid, to be applied several times a day, massaging until absorbed, and high-protection sunscreen to avoid subsequent pigmentation.

The patient must be helped with indications on how to camouflage bruises so that they aren't forced to miss out on previously arranged engagements. It is always better to warn patients who want to have their lips retouched, especially the first time, to allow a couple of days after the treatment without any commitments or events.

Errors in technique

These are undoubtedly the most frequent adverse events in the lip region and unfortunately they are more noticeable than in other areas of the face.

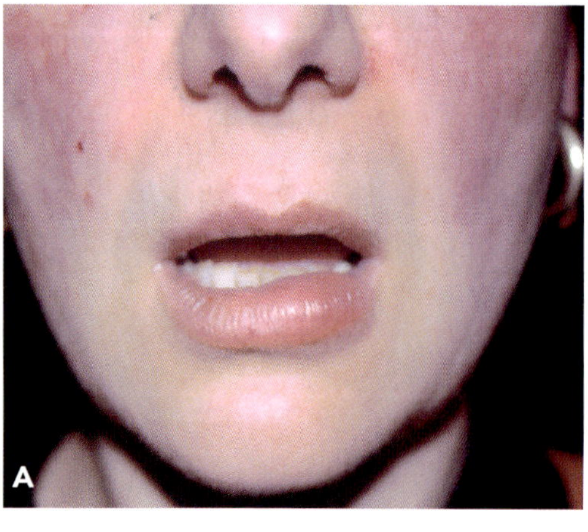

Figure 5A Oedema

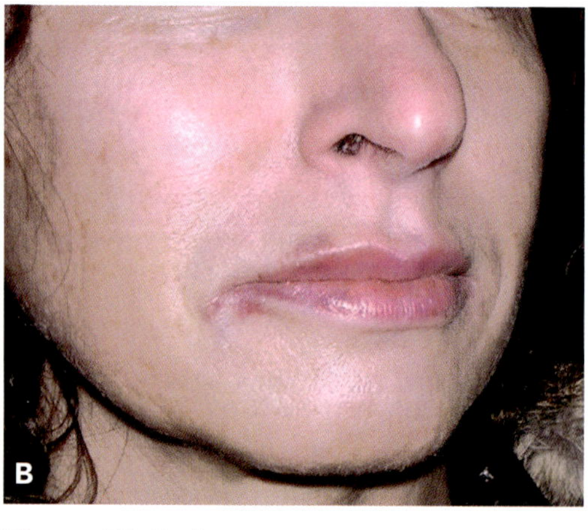

Figure 5B Ecchymosis

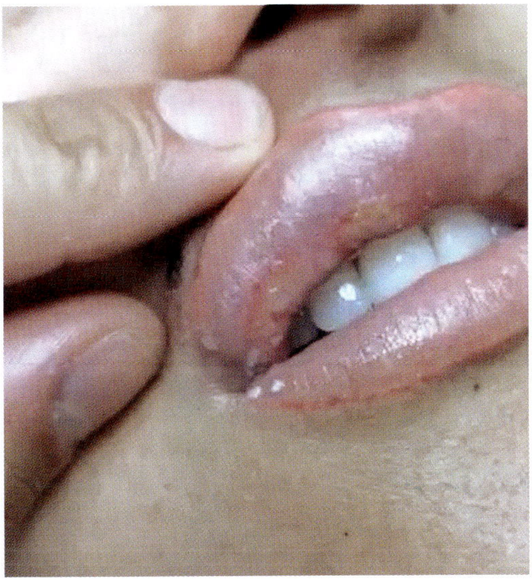

Figura 6 Ischemia of the right upper hemilip. Courtesy of Dr. Sergio Marlino

They concern volumes, proportions, the techniques used and the choice of inappropriate products.
"Less is more" should be the basic principle of lip augmentation. Lip volume should always be appropriate to the patient's age and the degree of skin ageing, and it should also be in proportion and in harmony with the other elements of the face. Unfortunately, there is a growing demand for fuller lips and a tendency to exaggerate augmentation. However, excessive volume gives unnatural results or at least excessively "inflated" lips, which lose all those details that make them "unique" to each individual. It can also lead to asymmetries and lumps from the accumulation of product.
Failure to respect the natural morphology of the lips and anatomical points of reference leads to an unnatural appearance, often due to an imbalance between the upper and lower lip, an altered ratio between the elements that characterise the shape of the lips, excessive prominence of the white lip in relation to the red lip or over-injection of product into the contour (fig. 7).
Beware of the Tyndall effect in the supra- and sub-commissural areas, due to the too quick and too superficial implantation of hyaluronic acid (fig. 8).
The filler placement technique must be appropriate and aimed at enhancing the initial morphology of the lips, injecting small amounts of product very slowly.
With regard to the choice of product, we have several examples of problems due, especially in the past, to implantation of substances unsuitable for the lips, some of which are no longer commercially available: asymmetries from permanent filler migration, nodules and vermilion irregularities, granulomas and retractions (figs. 9-10). Some are also caused by hyaluronic acids that are very cross-linked and too full-bodied for the lips (fig. 11).

Inflammatory complications

Inflammatory complications can be infectious or immune-mediated.

Infectious complications

Post-implant infection is very rare; contamination usually occurs at the time of implantation and a factor that favours infection by pyogenes is definitely the presence of a permanent foreign body such as liquid silicone (fig. 12).
An infectious agent that can complicate implantation in the lips is herpes simplex: herpes infection can manifest

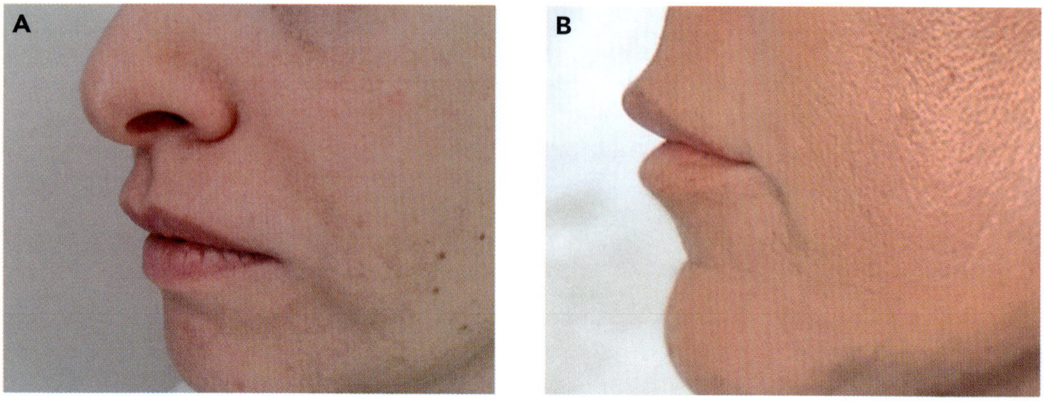

Figure 7 A) Disharmony due to inversion of the normal upper and lower lip ratio
B) Excessive volume in the lip contour with introflexion of the vermilion

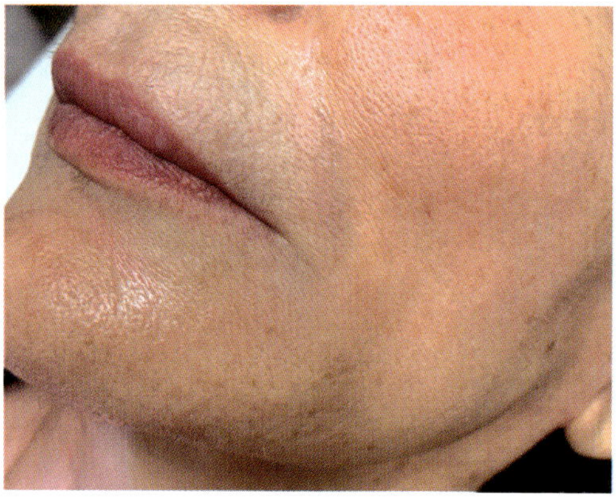

Figure 8
Tyndall effect in the lower third, naso-labial fold and subcommissural area

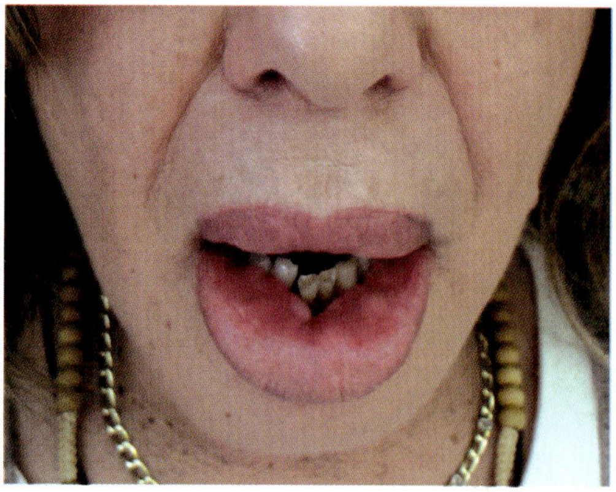

Figure 9
Silicone granulomas

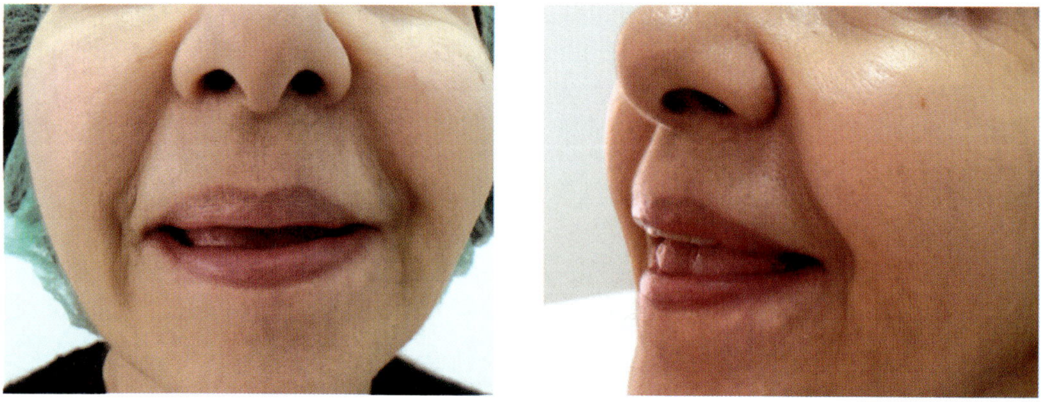

Figure 10 Porcine collagen injected too close to the surface

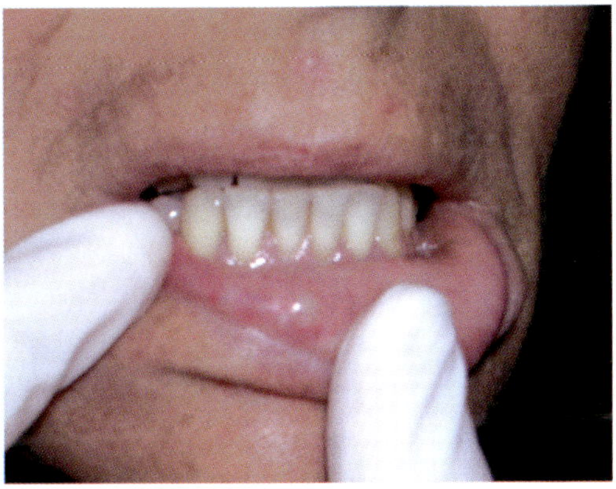

Figure 11
Hyaluronic acid accumulation

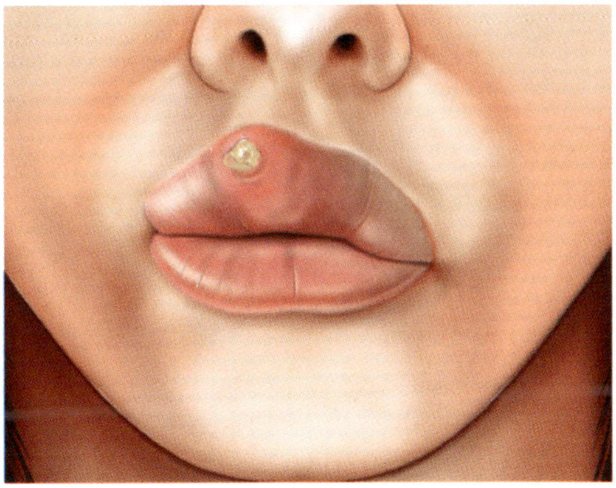

Figure 12
Abscess in silicone implant

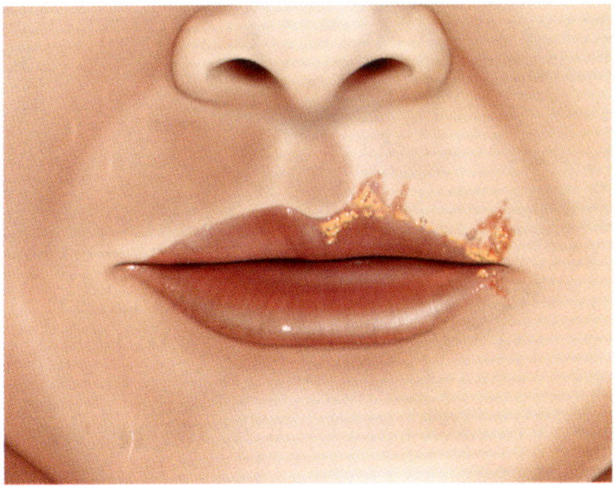

Figure 13
Post-implant herpes labialis

a few days after the filler procedure, sometimes only as very painful, excessive and persistent oedema (fig. 13). Sometimes it only becomes evident after bacterial over infection [1].
The clinical appearance may be confused with signs of vascular impairment [1], but these usually appear at the time of injection. In a recent meta-analysis of literature on adverse events from lip fillers, the incidence of herpes labialis was rather low (0.6%). Patients with frequent recurrences of herpes labialis should nevertheless take antiviral prophylaxis, and different dosages are described in literature: from 1 gram of acyclovir orally on the day of implantation, to 400 mg of acyclovir every 6/8 hours the day before, the same day and the day after implantation, to the more simple assumption of one brivudine 125 mg tablet in the morning for seven days starting a few days before implantation.

Immune-mediated complications
Hardening, itching, erythema at the injection site even one or more months later were linked in the past to reactions to collagen or early hyaluronic acids in connection with possible protein residues.
Following type IV cell mediated hypersensitivity, it is also possible to have granulomas and inflammatory nodules in the lips [1]. There are several factors that can promote such problems: individual reactivity, the type of filler (silicone, "mixed" permanent fillers, hyaluronic acids with excess BDDE), implant

contamination and biofilm formation with sterile abscesses or chronic inflammatory responses, concomitant dental infections, the use of different types of fillers in the same area and injections with unknown products [1].
(Real) granulomas are foreign body reactions with giant cell PMN (polymorphonucleates). They have an incidence reported in literature ranging from 0.01% to 0.1% [27] to 1% [28] and usually appear 6 to 24 months after implantation (fig. 14).
Inflammatory nodules and late oedemas may occur 4 to 6 weeks up to one year and more after implantation; they are usually inflammatory (possible immune response to filler, biofilm infection). Depending on the case, single or multiple nodules may occur, along with oedematous reactions, with alternating resolution and recurrence.

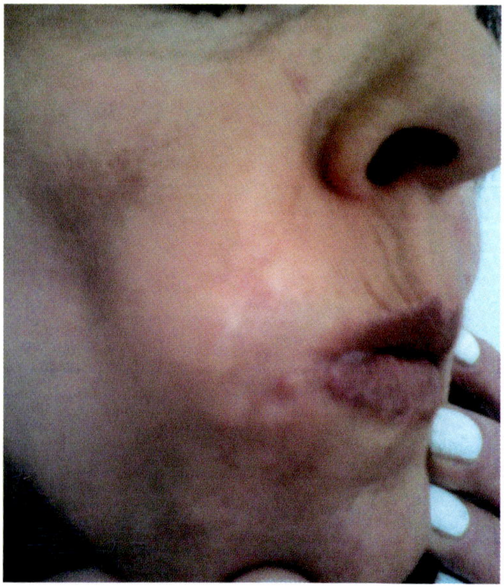

Figure 14 Granulomas from 100% cross-linked hyaluronic acid, later withdrawn from the market

Vascular complications
Vascular complications are very rare and, as mentioned, the lips do not represent an area of high vascular risk, given the extensive presence of anastomoses in this region, which probably conditions an underestimation of the incidence of vascular complications.
Necrosis of the lip caused by filler implantation has been described in literature, while rare cases of post-filler blindness seem to be related not to the isolated treatment of the lips but to simultaneous implantation in the nasolabial fold and nose. In any case, it should be borne in mind that there is no such thing as zero risk [3] and skin necrosis due to vascular lesions, probably in the case of anatomo-topographical variations in the arterial course, is possible (fig. 15).
In addition to adequate knowledge of the facial vascular anatomy, it must be remembered that the arterial distribution of the perioral branches of the facial artery is not constant, with different uni- or bilateral localisations, varying diameters and lengths, and different anastomoses. Previous surgery can also alter the anatomical ratios.
Lastly, we report a case described by James Wege et al. [16], which documents the formation of a lymphangioma secondary to treatment of the lip with hyaluronic acid as an extremely rare complication. The 27-year-old patient, who had undergone lip treatment with hyaluronic acid four years previously, had experienced dryness and tingling sensations in her upper lip ever since and, after one year, reported the appearance of progres-

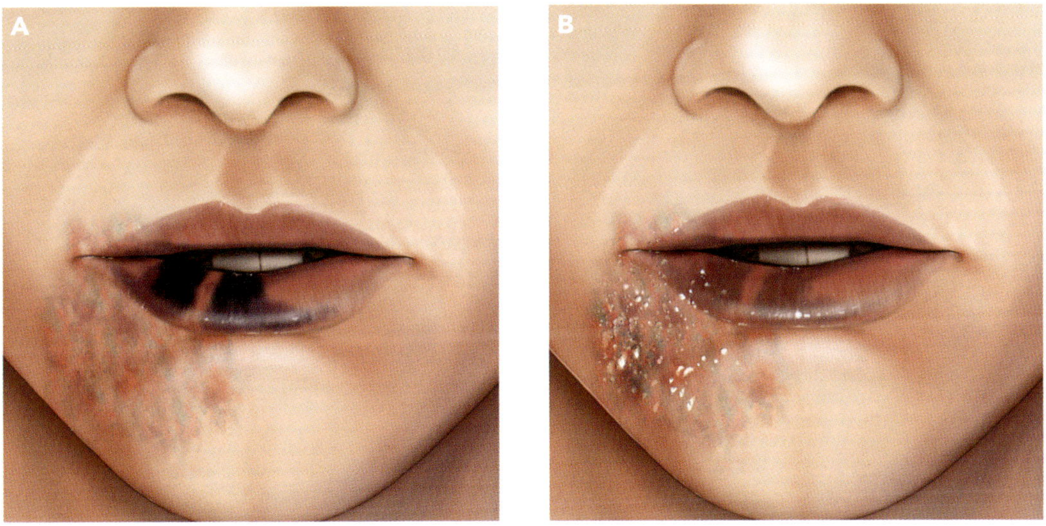

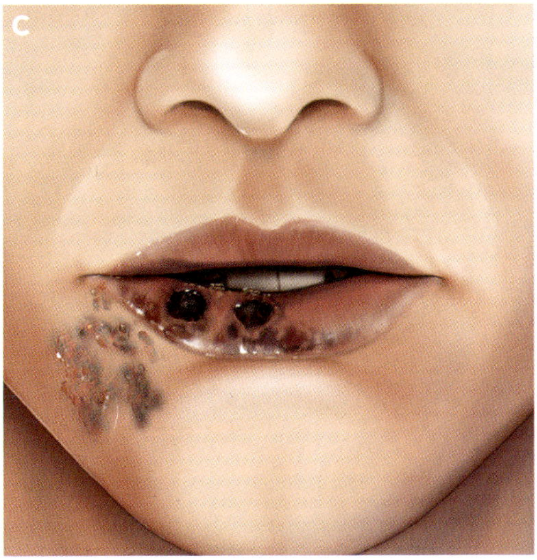

Figure 15 A) Blackish lower lip due to the presence of desaturated blood and *livedo reticularis* in the lower lip region and the right lateral region of the chin; B) vesicles and pustules at a later stage; C) necrosis begins to be defined and skin starts to "recover"

sively increasing swelling. After two years, she had linear "nodules" at the implantation sites, mostly near the mucosa, which were resistant to treatment with hyaluronidase. The hyaluronic acid probably interfered with the lymphatic drainage of the lip and the only possible solution was surgical removal (fig. 16). The type of product used and the injection method are not reported.

Preventive strategies

There are three types of preventive strategy [11]: pre-implantation, implantation and post-implantation.

Pre-implantation

- Adequate information to the patient regarding the often unavoidable effects.
- Systemic support (vitamin C supplements, bioflavonoids, plant extracts,

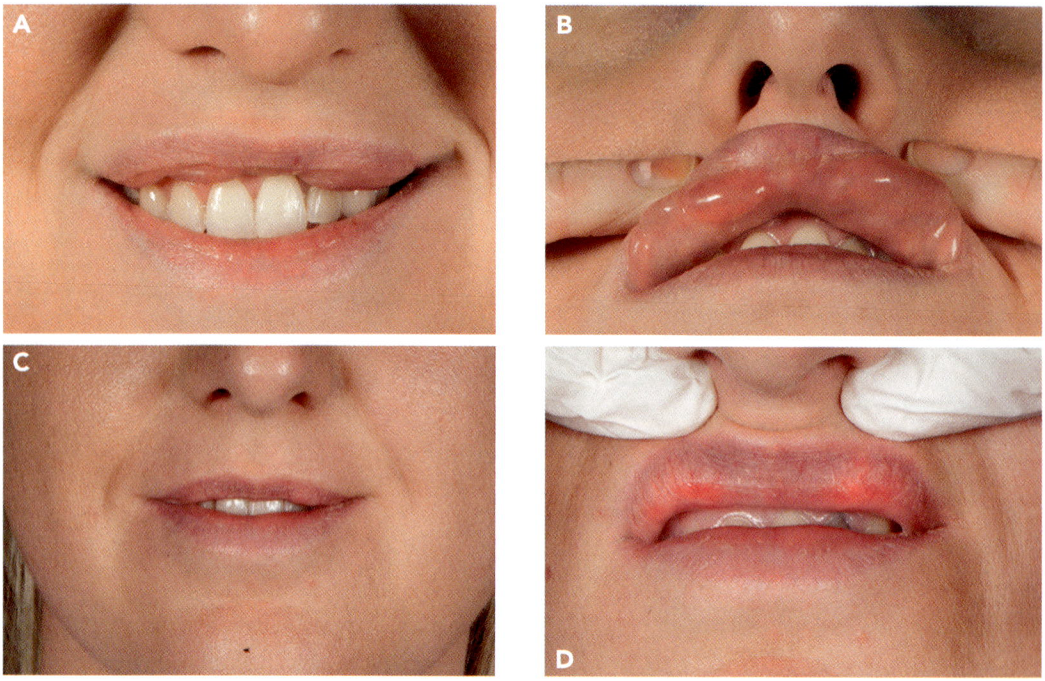

Figure 16 A) Lymphangioma, free lip margin; B) lymphangioma, mucosa; C-D) lymphangioma after intervention. From: Wege J, et al. Cureus. 2021;13(1):e12929 [16]

phytotherapy, etc.).
- Cosmetic and therapeutic support.
- Anti-herpetic prophylaxis.
- Choice of appropriate product.
- Thorough cleansing and disinfection with antiseptics.

Implantation (injection technique)

In every region of the face, so also in the lips, it is advisable to use small volumes of product to prevent vascular complications, proceeding with serial injections in order to distribute the material in different places, injecting very slowly and using minimal pressure, treating one side at a time, avoiding overfilling and, if more product is needed, repeating the treatment after 7-14 days [3].
Various lip-filling injection techniques are described in literature, from the "Paris lip", which we all began with, to the "French Kiss Technique" [12] to one of the most recently published, the "Step-by-Step (Phi) Technique" [13]. Some authors prefer an anterograde injection (especially in the virtual lip contour canal), others retrograde; some prefer the cannula, others the needle; some prefer the traditional manual injection and others that with an electronic medical device; according to some authors, the anterograde injection with an injection device is less painful, with less risk of ecchymosis and local reactions and with faster post-implantation recovery. While there is no ideal technique other than that with which we each achieve the best results, the "safest" approach from a vascular point of view is definitely the vermilion approach

[14], positioning the filler very close the surface (supra-muscular) and with an injection trajectory perpendicular to the border, which seems to reduce both the area of contact with the vessel wall and the probability of contact.

For years, the author has been using the vertical [13], superficial technique in the visible vermilion: the needle enters exactly at the skin-vermilion junction, perpendicular to the border, and stops just before the boundary between dry and wet lip; then, with linear retrograde injections, microdeposits of hyaluronic acid are deposited, in series, parallel to each other, oblique laterally and gradually more vertical in a latero-medial direction, following the course of the vermilion. This makes it possible to achieve greater precision of implantation and attention to detail, with a reduction in risk, especially at vascular level (fig. 17). From an aesthetic point of view, the main indication for vertical and superficial implantation is undoubtedly the increase in vermilion height (video 10.1) with a reduction of the philtrum labial score (ratio between ergotrid and vermilion), which unfortunately increases with the passing of time [4,13,15]. It also allows the refinement and enhancement of all the details of the upper lip, increasing eversion and roundness of the pink part (video 10.2), correcting asymmetries, and increasing the volume of the lips, especially in men's [14], in a

VIDEO 10.1

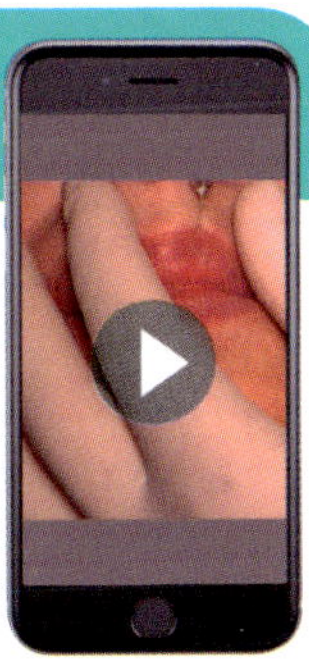

Lips: vertical injection technique to increase vermilion height

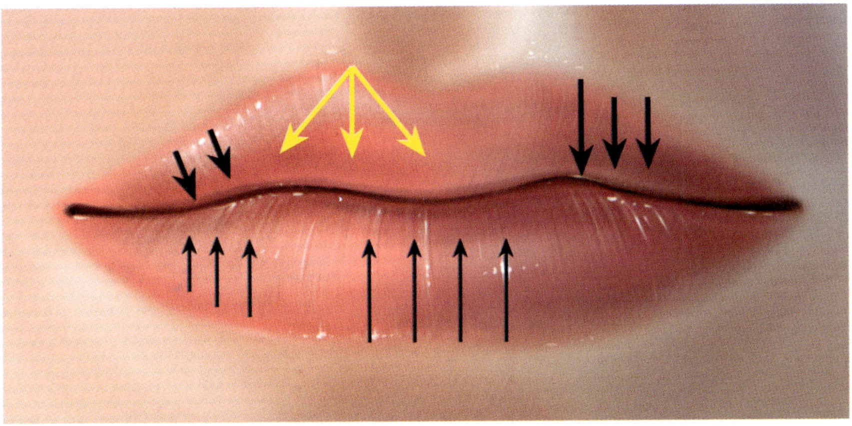

Figure 17 Lips and vertical injection techniques. Vertical techniques: the orientation of the needle is perpendicular to the lip border, the implant is superficial in the vermilion (supramuscular), the injection is linear retrograde

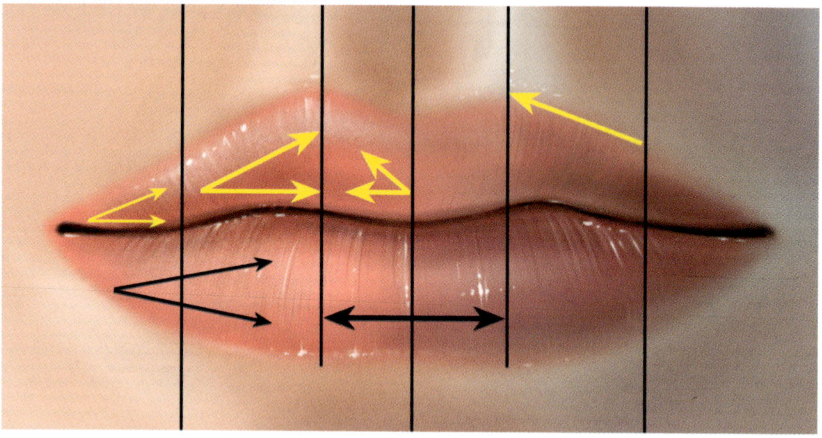

Figure 18 Lips and horizontal injection techniques. Linear technique with retrograde subdermal injection: the orientation of the needle is parallel to the border of the vermilion (definition in the contour and volume in the body of the vermilion)

"restrained" manner.

The limitation of the technique is represented by cases in which greater (though never excessive) volume is required. The vertical implant must be supplemented with horizontal implants, i.e. with needle orientation parallel to the vermilion border, always supra-muscular (fig. 18, video 10.3).

In any case, small volumes should be injected into each site, using minimal pressure on the plunger and products that are not too cross-linked but are cohesive and with low to moderate G'.

The technique ("Multi-Point technique") must be adapted to the initial morphology of the lips and the result to be obtained: the orientation of the needle may be vertical and/or horizontal in relation to the lip border, and by injecting the product very slowly, gently and a little at a time, bruising will in any case be minimal. Lastly, a combined technique (vertical and horizontal) like the "corner lift" can be used, to "open" and lift the commissure, injecting first into the border, then continuing directly into the commissure, injecting first into the border, then into the lip border, continuing to deposit the product in a radial pattern with linear injections first into the vermilion and mucosa and then into the subdermal subcommissural plane (video 10.3).

The vascular risk in this site is very low

VIDEO 10.2

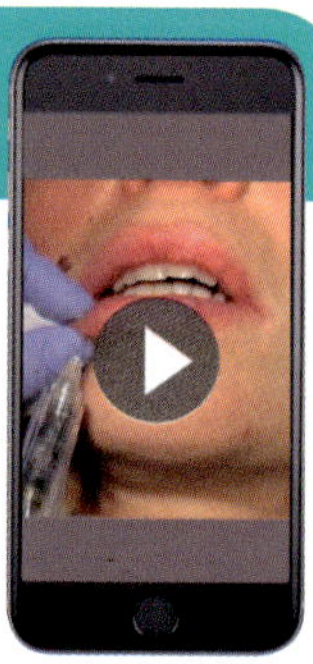

Lips: vertical injection technique into the lower lip

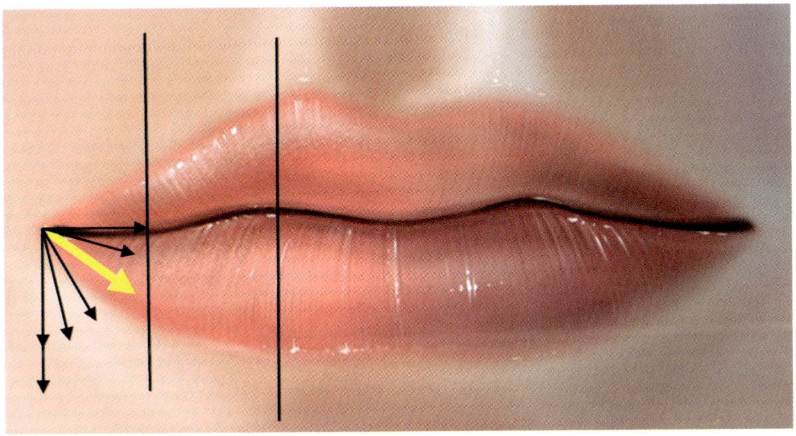

Figure 19 Combined "corner lift" technique for labial commissures To "open" and raise the commissures the needle can be inserted directly into the commissure, first injecting into the border, then continuing to deposit the product in a radial pattern with linear injections first into the vermilion and mucosa and then into the subdermal subcommissural plane

as the inferior labial artery is located in a submuscular location (angoli oris depressor muscle) (fig. 19).

Post-implantation

The patient must not apply cosmetics or make-up that has already been opened and is therefore contaminated immediately after implantation and for at least four hours. Ice should only be applied if necessary, as hyaluronic acid is sensitive to temperature changes. It is better to avoid exposure to the sun for 24 hours and then always protect the lips, as well as the face, with moisturisers and sunscreens.

Conclusions

In conclusion, the most frequent complications in the lip region are mild and moderate. Only under exceptional circumstances are they severe but our intervention must always minimise the risk, not just at vascular level, because any complication would cause terrible physical and emotional discomfort for the patient. The most important tool at our disposal is undoubtedly prevention, based on a thorough knowledge of structural and vascular anatomy, on careful and delicate injection methods, and on the choice of targeted products. In forensic medicine, a complication is understood to be an unforeseeable and unavoidable harmful event, an injury "without fault" on the part of the doctor (as long as the obligation to

VIDEO 10.3

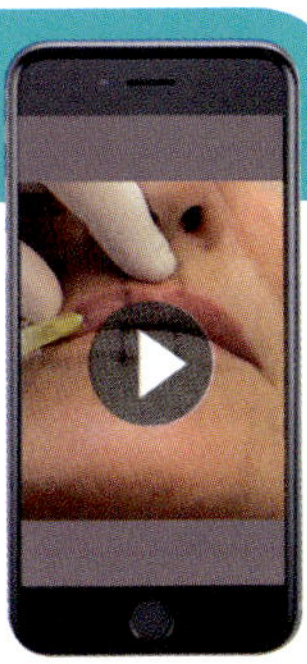

Lips: horizontal injection techniques

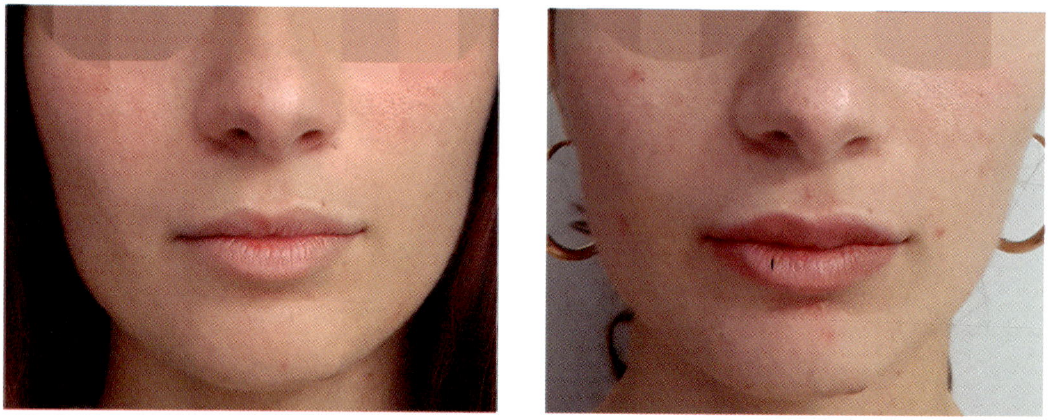

Figure 20 "Millennial lips" young lips can be made plumper and more attractive without overdoing things, enhancing the details

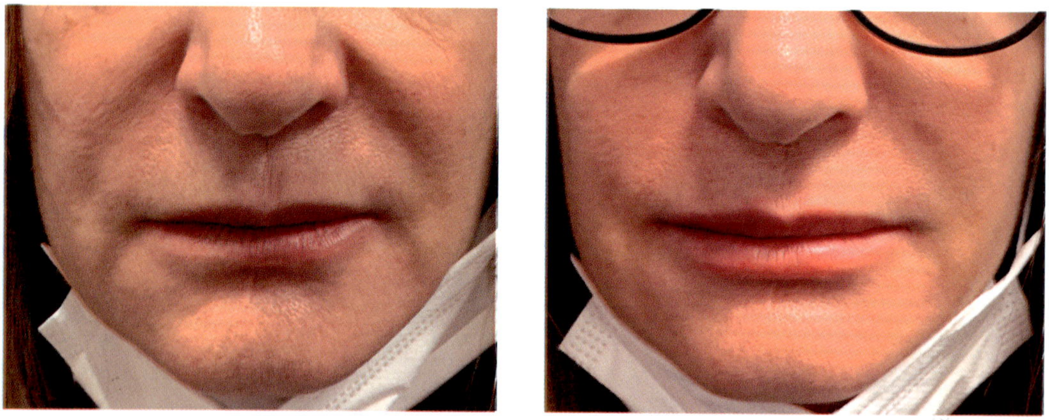

Figure 21 Thin lips with loss of firmness, roundness and definition: after implantation with the Multi-Point Technique, the natural morphology of the lips is restored and enhanced to suit the patient's age

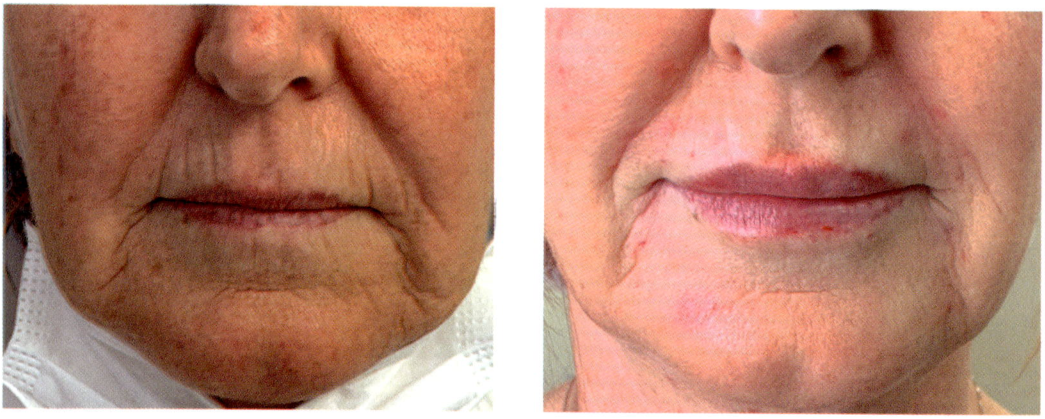

Figure 22 Ageing lips with loss of volume, roundness and definition, aggravated by the appearance of vertical lines: correction must cover the entire lip region without altering the projection of the upper lip

provide informed consent has not been breached). It is therefore essential to anticipate the foreseeable, but also to identify and manage the unforeseeable in an appropriate manner.

Bibliography

1. DeLorenzi C. Complications of injectable fillers, part I. Aesthet Surg J. 2013;33(4):561-575.
2. King M et al. Management of a vascular occlusion associated with cosmetic injections. J.Clin, Aesthetic Dermatol 2020 jan; 13(1): E53-E58
3. DeLorenzi C. Complications of injectable fillers, part I. Aesthet Surg J. 2013;33(4):561-575.
4. Ding A. The Ideal Lips: Lessons Learnt from the Literature. Aesthetic Plastic Surgery. 2021;45(4).
5. Lee Sang-Hee et al. Topographic Anatomy of the Superior Labial Artery for Dermal Filler Injection, Plast Reconstr Surg February 2015;445-450).
6. Lee Sang-Hee et al. What is the difference between the Inferior labial Artery and the horizontal labiomental artery? Surg Radiol Anat 37 (2015):947-953).
7. Schanz S et al. Distribution pattern of the superior and inferior labial arteries: impact for safe upper and lower lip augmentation procedures.Plast Reconstr Surg 139:1075,2017.
8. Schanz S et al. Anatomy Of The Superior And Inferior Labial Arteries Revised: An Ultrasound Investigation And Implication For Lip Volumization. Aesth Surg J, 2020, vol 40(12)1327-1335).
9. Czumbel LM, Farfasdi S, Varga G. Hyaluronic Acid is an effective dermal filler for lip augmentation: a meta-analysis. Front Surg 2021;8:681028.
10. Ozturk CN, Li Y, Tung R, et al. Complications following injection of soft-tissue fillers. Aesthet Surg J 2013;33:862-77.
11. Sito G, Manzoni V, Sommariva R. Vascular Complications after Facial Filler injection: A Literature.Review and Meta-analysis. J Clin Aesthet Dermatol 2019 Jun;12(6): E65-E72.
12. Trevidic P, Criollo-Lamilla G. French Kiss Technique: An Anatomical Study and Description of a New Method for Safe Lip Eversion. Derm Surg 46:11,Nov 2020;1410-1.
13. Keramidas E, Rodopoulou S, Gavala MI. A Safe and Effective Lip Augmentation Method: The Step-by-Step Φ (Phi) Technique. Plast Reconstr Surg Glob Open. 2021;9(2):e3332.
14. Sommariva R. L'estetica delle labbra e della regione periorale. Classificazione e terapia. In: Massirone A., ed. Trattato Di Medicina Estetica. Vol 2. First. PICCIN; 2010:1053-1069.
15. Sito G, Consolini L, Trévidic P. Proposed guide to lip treatment in Caucasian women using objective and measurable parameters. Aesthetic Surgery Journal. 2019;39(12).
16. Wege J, Anabtawi M, Blackwell MA, Patterson A. Lymphangioma Formation Following Hyaluronic Acid Injection for Lip Augmentation. Cureus. 2021;13(1):e12929.

COMPLICATIONS IN DERMOCOSMETICS AND DERMOCOSMETICS IN COMPLICATIONS

Maria Vittoria Giatti, Giuseppe Maria Izzo

In recent years, we have seen a considerable increase in the use of dermocosmetics and the trend appears to be growing steadily (fig.1). This is happening not only among women, but also among men for two reasons: firstly, they too are increasingly requesting aesthetic medical therapies and plastic surgeries, and secondly, there has been a shift towards a more modern concept of masculinity, in which eight out of ten men think it is normal that dermo-cosmetics are no longer just a female prerogative. Despite this strong practice of using dermo-cosmetics by patients, there continues to be a low propensity for dermocosmetic prescription by doctors. A survey shows that only one doctor out of three among those who practice aesthetic medicine or plastic surgery is in the habit of prescribing dermocosmetics for home use to their patients and varying it at subsequent check-ups; and the worst, according to statistics, are plastic surgeons, compared to dermatologists or other specialists, for example. This is often precisely the cause of complications in dermocosmetics, as patients, left to their own devices, without any post-treatment indication, rely on self-prescription, often using products that are unsuitable for their skin or wrong for their particular situation.

There is no absolutely perfect dermocosmetic [1], but the ideal product should have these three fundamental prerogatives:

- safety, i.e. no parabens, preservatives, silicones, artificial fragrances, mineral oils, propylene glycol, toxic substances, etc;
- efficacy, i.e. a proven specific action,

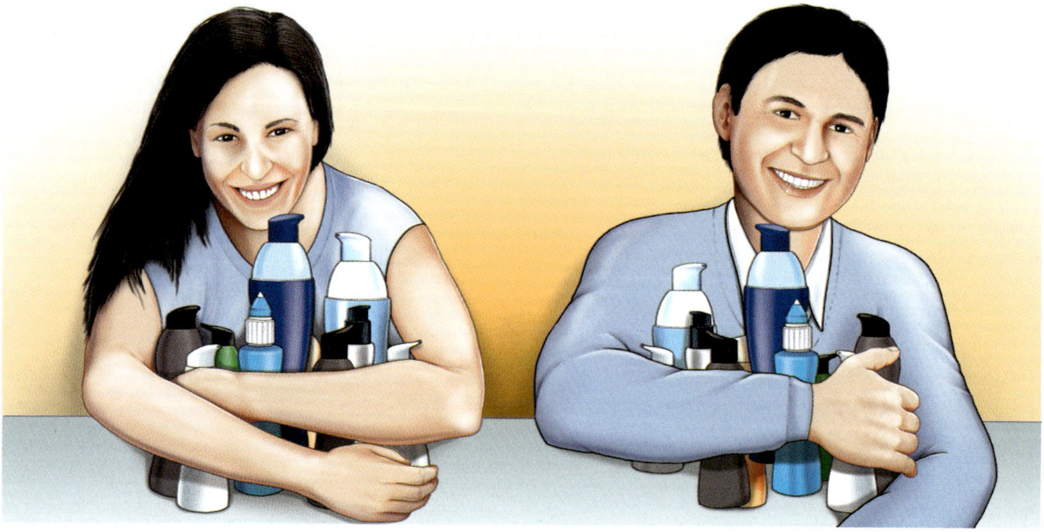

Figure 1 Increasing use of dermocosmetics

such as anti-ageing, correction of pigmentation, sebum regulation, moisturising, regenerating, anti-oxidant, etc;
- innovation, exploiting the latest scientific discoveries, such as nanotechnologies, like the micelles of the Permeable Antioxidant System, which allow better stability and absorption of the active ingredients, biomimetic peptides capable of activating targeted cellular actions, biodegradable green sunscreens like algae and sponges which have a low environmental impact, state-of-the-art antioxidants, immediate-action anti-wrinkle creams with Exopolysaccharide EPS SeaFill, i.e. molecules produced by marine plankton micro-organisms, cosmetics which will be increasingly modulated on the skin's microbiome in the future.

Gender differences in dermocosmetics

From an anatomo-physiological point of view, the differences are caused by the action of different sex hormones: oestro-progestin in women and androgens (testosterone and, via the 5α-reductase enzyme, dihydrotestosterone) in men [2]. This leads to a differentiation of the need for dermocosmetics depending on gender [3]. Under the influence of these specific hormones, in fact, the skeletal facial massif in men presents a broader and more prominent chin, a square and well-defined jaw, a higher and wider forehead region and a more pronounced orbital rim, whereas in women the lines are more convex and softer, with less prominent and gentler bone structures. The muscular fibres are more important, with stronger and hypertrophic mimic muscles and this causes more accentuated mimic activity in men than in women, with greater stress on the skin, In men there is a greater presence and characteristic and thicker distribution of hair (trunk, pubis, armpits, limbs, moustache, beard), while women tend to be more glabrous. Men sweat more than women and tend to have a more pronounced odour, sometimes leading to bromhidrosis, due to the greater quantity of lactic acid and consequently greater PH acidity. Men have an increased number and volume of sebaceous glands with consequently greater excretion of sebum (oilier skin, greater tendency to develop acne, enlarged pores) than women, who frequently have fewer sebaceous glands and sometimes drier skin. Skin thickness is greater and skin vascularisation is also higher in men than in women. The dense lamina at the dermo-epidermal junction seems to be more prominent in men [4] than in women (hence a more undulating dermo-epidermal junction and a firmer anchoring of the epidermis to the dermis, more resistant to mechanical stress and the effects of ageing), the skin is thicker, the collagen density higher and the dermis thicker, all of which lead to slower ageing in men, with wrinkles that appear later but deeper [5]. Furthermore, male ageing does not undergo the acceleration that occurs in women due to hormone reduction and menopause, but is slower and more constant.

On a psychological level, women are usually more accustomed to the use of dermocosmetics, even in combined synergetic protocols involving several steps in the beauty routine, and are much more attentive to sun protection.

Men usually tend to be less attentive, preferring the use of a few products with multiple functions, often letting themselves be advised by their wives and girlfriends. However, we can also identify various types of users, with two distinct categories which polar opposite approaches to cosmetics: "wild" and "narcissistic". For the "wild" patient sometimes the use of deodorant is sufficient and at most he uses a few other products, particularly face washes and after-shave. The "narcissistic" patient, on the other hand, has a great knowledge of dermocosmetics, sometimes even advanced, devotes considerable attention to choosing products, spends a lot and is often conditioned in his purchases by the media. In recent times, we are increasingly witnessing the so-called metrosexual phenomenon [6]. Metrosexual is a term that was invented in 1994 by the British journalist Mark Simpson to describe a new generation of men who live in big cities and who pay extreme attention to their physical appearance. Metrosexual is a neologism used to refer to heterosexual men generally from metropolitan areas (metro) and characterised by behaviour vaguely resembling stereotypically feminine behaviour, being heavy consumers of advanced cosmetics, practising fitness, artificial tanning, body hair removal and other aesthetic-medical or health treatments. The term is not used to denote mere vanity or narcissism, but rather the almost obsessive pursuit of an ideal of aesthetic perfection that is socially recognised, in a broader and more modern vision of masculinity and virility.

In their choice of products, women seek to preserve and enhance their beauty and youth, while men seek more functional products often related to the concept of health [7]. Men's cosmeceutical attention is focused mainly on hair, shaving/epilation (greater skin fragility after shaving), sweating, body creams, dark circles and bags under the eyes, while women's focuses on anti-ageing, corrective creams for hyperpigmentation, antioxidants, sun protection, body reshaping, anti-wrinkle creams, face brighteners and moisturisers.

The importance of dermocosmetic prescription

The importance of dermocosmetic prescription is essential in medical practice, not only to supplement the aesthetic-medical therapies or plastic surgery procedures offered to patients, but also as an irreplaceable element in the field of prevention and skin health. There is more and more talk today not only about the concept of rejuvenation but also that of pre-juvenation, i.e. of all those methods that help preserve the 'beauty' of our patients and delay ageing, and dermo-cosmetics play a major role in this sphere. Not just corrective dermo-cosmetics but also increasingly preventive products.

Why to prescribe

Dermocosmetics create a synergy with the aesthetic medicine and plastic surgery treatments we carry out, allowing us to optimise and perfect the result and sometimes even maintain and prolong it over time. They can be an important support in the complications that can occur during aesthetic-medical treatments, they create greater loyalty in patients who perceive the doctor as being more attentive to them, they create psychological co-participation in patients and helps them better understand that the benefit of medical treatment does not end when they leave the clinic, but that it is a path to be taken together and therefore it is necessary to make a daily commitment to improve their skincare and lifestyle.

When to prescribe

It is not necessary to limit prescription to after treatment/intervention, but it is necessary to prepare a therapeutic indication as early as the patient's first visit, so that they can arrive with a skin that is better prepared to receive the medical intervention we are going to perform, and then vary it during subsequent check-ups to suit the patient's specific needs, adapting it according to the results obtained or still to be achieved.

How to prescribe

The dermocosmetic indication must consider important factors, such as, first and foremost, the type of treatment performed, the patient's age, gender, biotype, phototype and level of oxidative stress, as well as the seasonality and the patient's readiness to comply with the proposed treatment plan.

The causes of complications in dermocosmetics

As we have already mentioned, it is often the specialist who fails to issue an appropriate cosmeceutical prescription after the aesthetic medical therapy or surgery carried out. Consequently, in 80% of cases the causes of complications are mostly related to self-prescription by the patient who, without adequate guidance as to which products to use, relies on an often incorrect independent choice. It is only in the remaining 20% of cases that complications are caused by a genuine prescription error on the part of the doctor.

The patient's responsibility lies in self-management, often following the advice of friends who already use the particular dermo-cosmetic, unaware that it may not be suitable for their skin type or current condition. Even more frequently, they may be influenced by advertising, fashion and social media. More rarely, they may misunderstand the doctor's prescription (e.g. the use of a photosensitising dermocosmetic exclusively at night, or an alpha-hydroxy acid every other day or in winter).

An emerging phenomenon in recent years which is the source of frequent cosmeceutical complications is the so-called Clean Beauty movement, which mistakenly associates and publicises the false equivalence between "natural" and "safe" [8]. It is extremely well publicised and supported by show-business influencers and international celebrities, and there is a whole lot of false marketing without any scientific background, creating an exponentially growing industry every year. It is often supported by misinformation, consumer anxiety and misguided chemophobia (a term that generally refers to the irrational assumption that all chemicals are harmful and unhealthy, while all so-called "natural substances" are good and healthy). The green trend is definitely positive, limiting the use of anything that could be harmful to man and the environment in the composition of dermocosmetics and in the production chain, promoting eco-sustainability (eco friendly, heart friendly, cruelty free, vegan) but first and foremost products supported by proven clinical scientific studies. One example worth mentioning is the process of eliminating the microplastics often found in exfoliating cleansers and scrubs, bearing in mind that every year the seas and oceans receive some 8, 600 tonnes of microplastics from cosmetics: microplastics are non-biodegradable synthetic particles (nylon, polyethylene, polyacrylate, silicone resins) less than 5 millimetres in size, incorporated into chemical formulations with a mostly abrasive or encapsulating action on active ingredients, favouring their preservation and distribution in the skin, but which disrupt the normal development of marine species, contribute to the deterioration of coral reefs and, once ingested by fish together with plankton, end up in our food chain. They become even more dangerous if they come from contaminated environments because they behave like sponges, absorbing persistent organic pollutants such as endocrine disruptors which, by mimicking hormones, cause hormonal imbalances, especially in children and adolescents.

The doctor's responsibility often consists in the hasty prescription of cosmeceuticals and identification of the end of the treatment/intervention with the last injection given or stitch put in place, neglecting the importance of carefully explaining the indications to be followed at home, a fundamental element of outpatient synergy. What is worse, and happens most frequently, is the complete absence of cosmeceutical indications from specialists. This happens in 33% of cases. And it is in this no-man's land, where patients are abandoned and set adrift, that complications arise.

And the lack of knowledge of cosmetology on the part of doctors also makes it impossible to resolve any complications due to the patients' own incorrect use of products. Most of the time, complications from dermocosmetics result in: contact dermatitis [9] and skin rashes (frequently curable with topical antibiotic creams sometimes in association with mild corticosteroids, e.g. gentamicin with betamethasone), urticarial and allergic reactions (treatable with antihistamine creams, corticosteroids and possibly similar oral therapy in the most severe cases), pigmentations (particularly from the use of photosensitising creams, often of mainly plant origin, the results of which will require depigmentation therapies, lightening peelings, localised laser treatments, to be carried out at times when the patient does no expose their skin to the sun) (fig. 2). The use of inadequate sun creams or sunscreens with filters that are not suitable for protecting certain phototypes can even lead to burns.

How to avoid complications in dermocosmetics

Although cosmeceuticals play a fundamental supporting role in clinical practice, dermocosmetics can cause complications if used incorrectly. To avoid

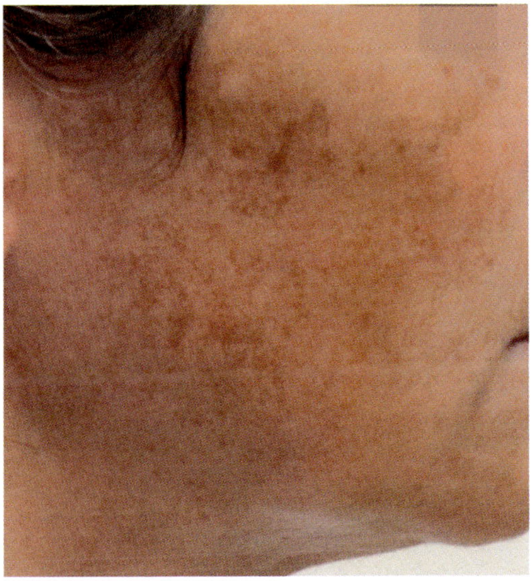

Figure 2 Pigmentation of the face after sun exposure with photosensitising creams

these, it is essential to choose products that comply with the principles of safety, efficacy and innovation, which must always characterise every medical act.
Only a thorough and accurate preliminary anamnestic and clinical investigation can effectively prevent mistakes. It is important to exclude the presence of allergies to certain substances, which could create problems even when used in topical formulas (figs. 3-5). The choice of prescription must also be calibrated according to the specific treatment/surgery carried out and to the purpose to be achieved, in order to create a synergy or to restore an altered physiological function: strengthening of the antioxidant action, restoration of the skin's hydrolipid barrier, acceleration of cell renewal, lightening of hyperpigmentations, reduction of skin sensitivity, collagen stimulation, regulation of sebaceous homeostasis, etc. It must also take into account seasonality (e.g. products with a greater antioxidant and hyperpigmentation-prevention action in summer, and with a greater hydrolipidic barrier restoration effect in winter), and the chronobiology of our skin (photoprotective during the day, restructuring or exfoliant during the night). Every specialist should learn to properly read the INCI [10] of products and also educate their patients to do so (fig. 6). The INCI (International Nomenclature of Cosmetic Ingredients) is a compulsory international name that has been used for several years to indicate the various ingredients in a cosmetic product on the label. It is used in all EU member states and in many other countries around the world, including the USA, Russia, Brazil, Canada and South Africa. Ingredients are listed from the top in order of quantity, down to those contained in the lowest percentage. Below 1%, ingredients can be listed in any order. Their names may be written in Latin (especially for natural compounds, which are listed by their Latin botanical name) or in English (generally those that are synthetic or produced in a laboratory). There is currently no European legislation to clearly identify whether a cosmetic is green, but the more Latin botanical names there are, the more natural the formulation appears to be. In order to identify the presence of microplastics, it is necessary to pay attention to the following terms: polyethylene (PE), polymethyl methacrylate (PMMA), nylon, polyethylene terephthalate (PET), trimethylsiloxysilicate, polypropylene (PP), etc. Every

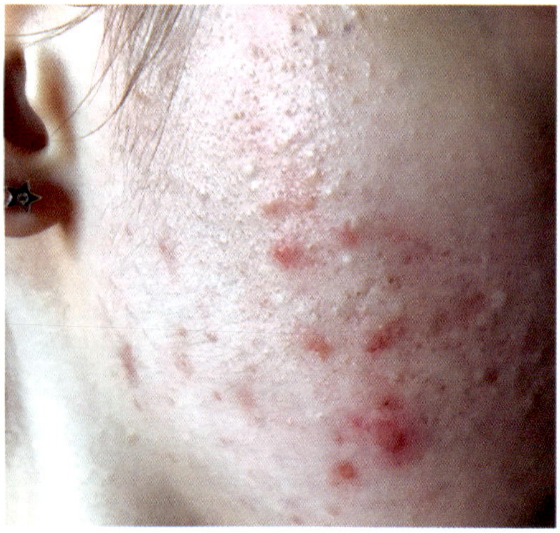

Figure 3 Deterioration of acne after use of cream containing plant extracts

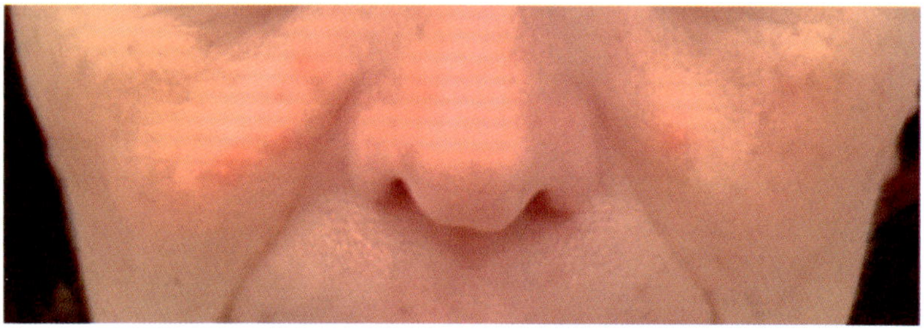

Figure 4 Skin rash after using cream containing nickel in a patient allergic to nickel

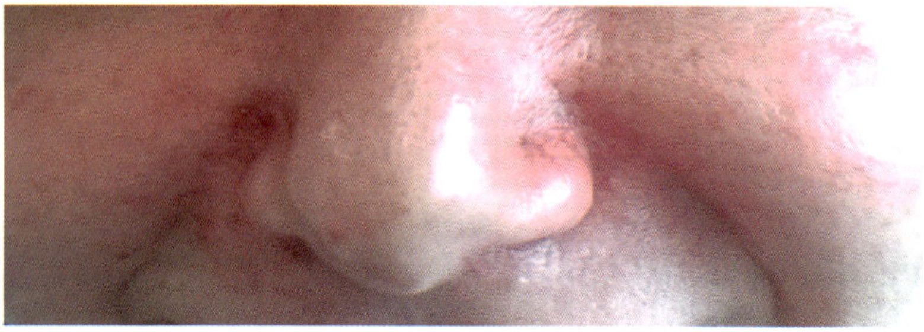

Figure 5 Erythematous reaction after using a dermocosmetic containing salicylic acid in a patient allergic to aspirin

doctor should also be familiar with the basic cosmetology glossary and have undergone appropriate cosmetology training (as part of training and specialisation courses or at conferences). Preference should be given to prescribing medical dermocosmetics with proven scientific clinical studies of efficacy and safety, both in vitro and in vivo. Above all, it is essential to devote the right amount of time to the cosmetic prescription, ensuring that the patient has clearly understood both the importance of the product indicated and the correct way to use it. This should lead to the development of personal protocols, standardised according to the types of therapeutic actions performed and customised according to the specific characteristics of that patient at that particular time or in that particular clinical situation.

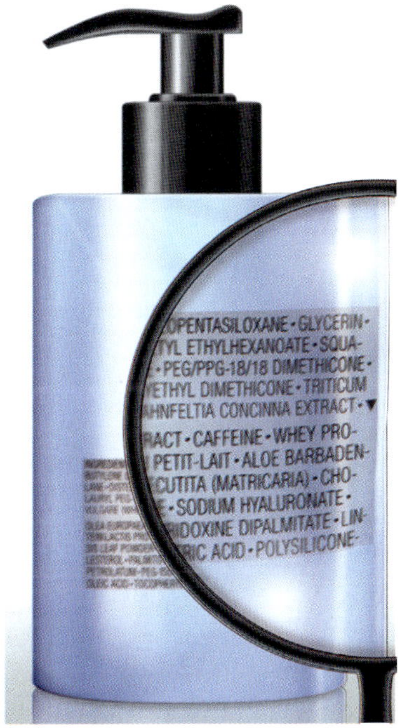

Figure 6
INCI

Dermocosmetics as valuable support in complications

Dermocosmetics can also be of valuable support in complications and side effects that may occur during aesthetic-medical therapies and plastic surgery, thanks to the use of specific functional active ingredients. To prevent infection and inadvertent introduction of make-up particles through injection treatments (prior to disinfection), bioaffinity cleansers containing chlorhexidine can be used. These not only remove make-up but also act as a bacteriostatic agent. If bruising occurs, dermo-cosmetics containing arnica, for example, can be used (but avoid formulations associated with menthol, which could irritate fragile skin traumatised by an aesthetic treatment) as well as sunscreens, often combined. Alternatively, products containing biomimetic peptides capable of stimulating a specific cellular function can be used: in support of a correction with botulinum toxin, substances with a myorelaxant action (acetyl hexapeptide-8, acetyl hexapeptide-3, palmitoyl hexapeptide-19, etc.), neutrazen capable of switching off inflammatory processes, palmitoyl pentapeptide-3, palmitoyl pentapeptide-4, palmitoyl tripeptide-28, methylglucosamine to stimulate the production of endogenous hyaluronic acid and collagen, matrichine, helichrysum with a regenerating, repairing and anti-inflammatory action. Hyaluronic acid-based healing creams can be used in the case of small skin abrasions or minor burns. If the skin is particularly stressed after treatment, dermo-restructuring agents (such as hyaluronic acid, coenzyme Q10, glutathione, N-acetylglucosamine, alphalipoic acid, vitamin C, vitamin E) can be used. If oedema appears, products with escin and bromelain or witch hazel with a decongestant action can be used, especially in the treatment of the periocular areas. Dermocosmetics with resorcinol derivatives, kojic acid, azelaic acid, phytic acid, arbutin, glycyrrhetinic acid, tocopherol, vitamin C, and tyrosinase inhibitors (tyrosinase being the key enzyme in pigmentation) can be used for pigmentations, including post-inflammatory pigmentations.

Guide to correct prescription in dermocosmetics

1) Carry out a thorough preliminary anamnestic and clinical investigation.
2) Choose the prescription on the basis of the specific treatment/surgery performed and targeting the specific purpose to be achieved.
3) Prescribe the treatment according to seasonality.

4) Prescribe day/night according to the principles of chronobiophysiology.
5) Correctly read the INCI of products.
6) Knowledge of the basic cosmetology glossary.
7) Suitable cosmetology training (within the framework of training and specialisation courses or congresses).
8) Favour medical dermocosmetics, with proven clinical scientific studies of efficacy and safety.
9) Dedicate the right amount of time to cosmetic prescription, ensuring that the patient has clearly understood both the importance of the product and the correct way to use it.
10) Perfect the development of personal protocols, standardised according to the types of therapeutic actions performed and customised according to the specific characteristics of that patient.

Bibliography

1. Obagi Zein E. The art of skin health. Restoration and rejuvenation. 2015 Second edition. CRC Press.
2. Zouboulis CC, Chen WC, Thornton MJ et al. Sexual hormones in human. Skin Horm Metab Res. 2007; 39:85-95.
3. Mizukoshi K, Akamatsu H. The investigation of the skin characteristics of males focusing on gender differences, skin perception and skin care habits. Skin Res Tech.2013; 19: 91-99.
4. Tidman M, Eady R. Ultrastructural morphometry of normal human dermal-epidermal junction. The influence of age, sex and body region on laminar and non laminar components. J. Invest. Dermatol. 1994;83: 448-453.
5. Dao H, Kazin R. Gender differences in skin: a review of the literature. Gend Med. 2007 Dec;4(4):308-28.
6. Simpson M. Here Come the Mirror Men. November 15, 1994.The Independent.
7. Martini MC. Cosmétologie masculine. Paris, Lavoisier, 2009.
8. Rubin CB, Brod B. Natural Does Not Mean Safe-The Dirt on Clean Beauty Products. JAMA Dermatol. 2019;155(12):1344-1345.
9. Kiken DA, Cohen DE. Contact dermatitis to botanical extracts. Am J Contact Dermat. 2002;13(3):148-152.
10. Penazzi G. I cosmetici e la legge. In: Edra-Masson. ed Come sono fatti i cosmetici. Guida pratica alla lettura dell'INCI. 2nd ed. 2020: 1-17.

11

THERAPY

INJECTABLE HYALURONIDASE

Patrizia Piersini

Hyaluronidases (also known as "Hyals") are a family of hydrolytic enzymes that mainly break down hyaluronic acid, an essential constituent of the extracellular matrix. They also have a limited and slower capacity to break down chondroitin and chondroitin sulphate. Karl Meyer, who first described the chemical structure of hyaluronic acid, was also the first to classify hyaluronidases into three groups: mammalian hyaluronidases, bacterial hyaluronidases and leech hyaluronidases [1]. Hyaluronidases, initially discovered in bacteria, are widely distributed in nature. They are found in the mouthparts of leeches, in the venoms of snakes, bees and scorpions and in various pathogenic microorganisms such as pneumococci and streptococci. Six different types of hyaluronidase have been found in humans: PH20 seems to have the strongest biological activity and is found in human testicles and spermatozoa, particularly on the head and acrosome.

Bovine or ovine testicular hyaluronidases and synthetic hyaluronidases have been used clinically for more than seventy years as delivery factors to increase the bioavailability of drugs (e.g. for vaccines), to prevent tissue damage from the blood extravasation of various substances or for the management of complications resulting from the infiltration of hyaluronic acid fillers [2,5].

The latter indication is currently off-label, despite being supported by abundant scientific evidence. Hyaluronidase can, in fact, be used to remove inflammatory and non-inflammatory nodules, to treat overcorrections due to excessive infiltration of hyaluronic acid, to correct an infiltration too close to the surface which may result in the Tyndall effect or to treat a serious complication such as intra-vascular infiltration [3].

Storage and reconstitution

In order to best preserve its properties, hyaluronidase should be stored in the refrigerator at a temperature between 2 and 8 °C. If stored at room temperature (25 °C), stability is guaranteed for approximately one year [4]. It is generally reconstituted with 2 ml of saline solution. Once reconstituted, it should be used within six hours.

Dosage in aesthetic medicine

Nodules and hypercorrections caused by hyaluronic acid can be treated successfully even a long time after the product has been inoculated [3]. An ultrasound scan should ideally be performed on the area involved to better assess the depth of the implant and its size. The infiltration of hyaluronidase should be very precise and limited to the area affected. It is important to bear in mind that sensitivity to hyaluronidase varies depending on the hyaluronic acid that was used for the implant and more units of hyaluronidase or more sessions may be required for more cross-linked hyaluronic acids, for example. The recommended dose may vary from 2 to 150 units. Hyaluronidase can be injected directly into the area with a 30 G 13

mm needle or with a 25 G blunt-tipped microcannula. Massage is recommended after injection to mechanically mix the enzyme with the hyaluronic acid and increase the breakdown of the filler [5].
Hyaluronidase takes effect immediately upon injection and has a half-life of approximately two minutes, with a duration of action of 24 to 48 hours [6].
For painful inflammatory nodules, the use of an antibiotic for a fortnight prior to infiltration of hyaluronidase is recommended to avoid the potential spread of infection [7]. Only if treatment with hyaluronidase is ineffective can the use of steroids be considered.
The incidence of necrosis following intravascular inoculation of hyaluronic acid is estimated to be one case in every 100,000 implants (0.001%). In the case of cutaneous ischaemia caused by intravascular inoculation of hyaluronic acid fillers, hyaluronidase should be injected as early as possible, within 4-6 hours, although late use can still reduce the size of the necrotic area and accelerate the healing process. Theoretically, hyaluronidase should be injected directly into the occluded vessel, which is unrealistic, but several studies indicate that massive infiltration of the ischaemic tissue may be a valid substitute. In order to prevent tissue necrosis, the region should be treated with injections of hyaluronidase about 3 cm apart, followed by massage. If the desired result is not achieved within an hour, a second cycle of injections is recommended, continuing up to a total of four cycles.
Hayreh and colleagues have established that, in the case of a retinal ischaemic event, circulation needs to be restored within 90 minutes, and although there is no certainty that the blindness caused by this very severe event can actually be treated, the immediate use of hyaluronidase appears to be helpful in countering this dreaded complication [8,9].
The recommended doses for intravascular inoculation are initially 150-200 units, up to 1500 units if necessary.
Patients taking high doses of salicylates, corticosteroids, ACTH, oestrogen or antihistamines should be treated with higher doses of hyaluronidase to achieve an equivalent effect, as these drugs appear to make the tissues more resistant to the action of hyaluronidase [5].

Complications

Hyaluronidases of animal origin are thought to be more immunogenic than recombinant hyaluronidases and may contain some contaminants such as proteases, immunoglobulins and vasoactive factors [5].
Complications related to the subcutaneous use of hyaluronidases are mainly allergic reactions in the inoculation area, with a rare incidence of around 0.05-0.7%. They appear as skin rash, urticaria, localised oedema and itching.
If an allergic reaction to a wasp or bee sting is reported in the patient's history, this may pose an increased risk for the development of an allergic reaction to hyaluronidase (often present in insect venom) and should be considered a contraindication to use.
After injection of hyaluronidase, the patient should be kept under observation in the doctor's surgery for 30-60 minutes.

Bibliography

1. Stern R, Jedrzejas MJ. Hyaluronidases: their genomics, structures, and mechanisms of action. Chem Rev. 2006 Mar;106(3):818-39.
2. Weber, G.C., Buhren, B.A., Schrumpf, H., Wohlrab, J., Gerber, P.A. (2019). Clinical Applications of Hyaluronidase. In: Labrou, N. (eds) Therapeutic Enzymes: Function and Clinical Implications. Advances in Experimental Medicine and Biology, vol 1148. Springer, Singapore.
3. Cavallini M, Gazzola R, Metalla M, Vaienti L. The role of hyaluronidase in the treatment of complications from hyaluronic acid dermal fillers. Aesthet Surg J. 2013 Nov 1;33(8):1167-1174.
4. King M, Convery C, Davies E. This month's guideline: The Use of Hyaluronidase in Aesthetic Practice (v2.4). J Clin Aesthet Dermatol. 2018 Jun;11(6): E61-E68.
5. Landau M. Hyaluronidase Caveats in Treating Filler Complications. Dermatol Surg. 2015;41 Suppl 1:S347-S353.
6. Bailey SH, Fagien S, Rohrich RJ. Changing role of hyaluronidase in plastic surgery. Plast Reconstr Surg. 2014;133(2):127e-132e.
7. Narins RS, Coleman WP 3rd, Glogau RG. Recommendations and treatment options for nodules and other filler complications. Dermatol Surg. 2009 Oct;35 Suppl 2:1667-71.
8. Hayreh SS, Podhajsky PA, Zimmerman B. Nonarteritic anterior ischemic optic neuropathy: time of onset of visual loss. Am J Ophthalmol 1997; 124:641–7.
9. De Lorenzi C. Transarterial degradation of HA filler by hyaluronidase. Dermatol Surg. 2014;40(8):832–841.

TOPICAL HYALURONIDASE

Patrizia Piersini, Lucia Calvisi

The popularity of hyaluronic acid treatments is steadily increasing all over the world, and even continued to do so during the Covid-19 pandemic. As previously pointed out, these procedures do not exempt the injecting doctor from the risk of more or less severe complications, for which injectable hyaluronidase is an emergency drug.

Fortunately, the possible complications do not always consist of acute or severe events, so we have time to reflect and offer the patient an alternative to injectable hyaluronidase, which, while solving the problem more quickly, may be accompanied by discomfort during and after treatment, as well as allergic reactions, albeit rare.

A topical product containing an enzyme complex containing hyaluronidase, lipase and protease, as well as aloe vera and essential oils such as helichrysum, lavender, myrrh and cistus (Topilase, Softil Cosmetic) has recently been formulated for use to treat a variety of problems. These include overcorrection with hyaluronic acid, the Tyndall effect (especially in the lower eyelid where the skin is thinner), lip oedema (which can occur following infiltration of hyaluronic acid due to patient hyperreactivity) and small accumulations of hyaluronic acid in different areas of the face, especially if the product used does not have a high molecular weight.

Procedure

A generous dose of the product is applied to the area to be treated, then massaged in vigorously with the hands, with the aid of a dermaroller (the dermaroller can also be used before application of the product to promote penetration) or an LED light. These applications are carried out once a week and four to five applications are usually sufficient.

Once prepared, the product should be stored in the refrigerator and has a shelf life of 14 days.

Case report 1

A 50-year-old patient who had had significant oedema in both the upper and lower eyelids for over a year following treatment with unspecified hyaluronic acid (Fig. 1). Four applications of topical hyaluronidase were performed at weekly intervals. Each application was preceded by needling (with a micro-needle penetration depth 0.2 mm).

Case report 2

A 35-year-old patient with evident oedema of the left lower eyelid following infiltration with unspecified hyaluronic acid (video 11.1). Five applications of topical hyaluronidase were performed at weekly intervals, each one preceded by needling (with a micro-needle penetration depth 0.2 mm) (fig. 2).

Bibliography

1. Stern R, Jedrzejas MJ. Hyaluronidases: their genomics, structures, and mechanisms of action. Chem Rev. 2006 Mar;106(3):818-39.

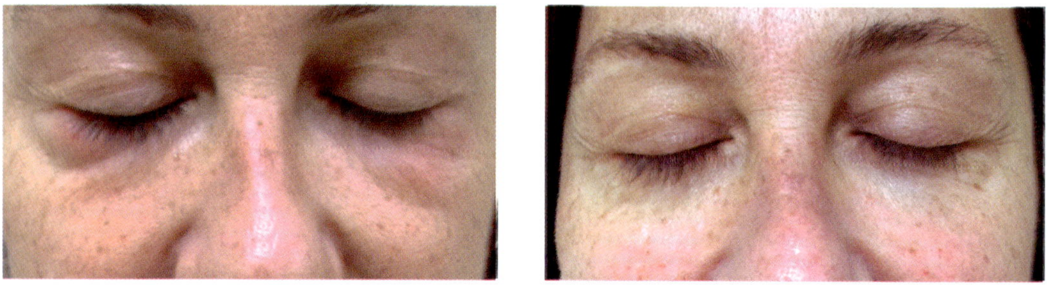

Figure 1 Case report 1. Pre- and post-treatment

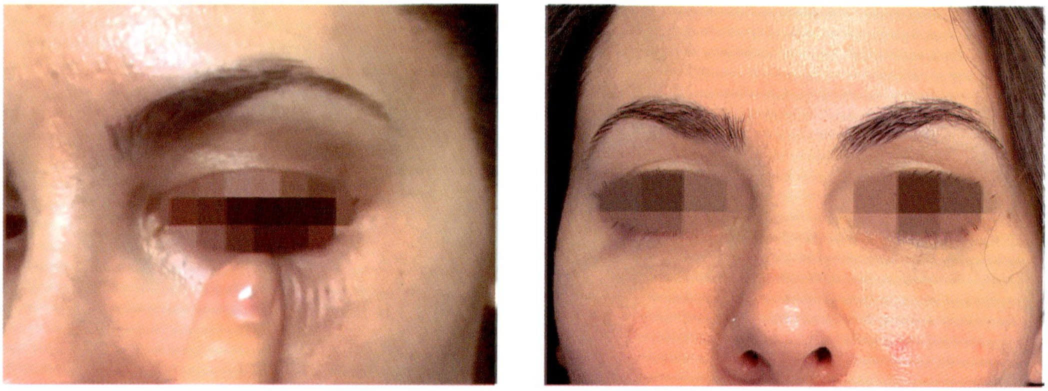

Figure 2 Case report 2. Pre- and post-treatment

2. Weber GC, Buhren BA, Schrumpf H, Wohlrab J, Gerber PA. (2019). Clinical Applications of Hyaluronidase. In: Labrou, N. (eds) Therapeutic Enzymes: Function and Clinical Implications. Advances in Experimental Medicine and Biology, vol 1148. Springer, Singapore.
3. Cavallini M, Gazzola R, Metalla M, Vaienti L. The role of hyaluronidase in the treatment of complications from hyaluronic acid dermal fillers. Aesthet Surg J. 2013 Nov 1;33(8):1167-1174.
4. King M, Convery C, Davies E. This month's guideline: The Use of Hyaluronidase in Aesthetic Practice

VIDEO 11.1

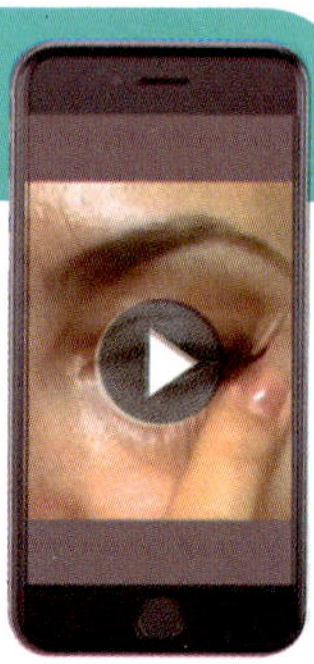

Oedema of the left lower eyelid (clinical report 2)

(v2.4). J Clin Aesthet Dermatol. 2018 Jun;11(6): E61-E68.
5. Landau M. Hyaluronidase Caveats in Treating Filler Complications. Dermatol Surg. 2015;41 Suppl 1:S347-S353.
6. Bailey SH, Fagien S, Rohrich RJ. Changing role of hyaluronidase in plastic surgery. Plast Reconstr Surg. 2014;133(2):127e-132e.
7. Narins RS, Coleman WP 3rd, Glogau RG. Recommendations and treatment options for nodules and other filler complications. Dermatol Surg. 2009 Oct;35 Suppl 2:1667-71.
8. Hayreh SS, Podhajsky PA, Zimmerman B. Nonarteritic anterior ischemic optic neuropathy: time of onset of visual loss. Am J Ophthalmol 1997; 124:641–7.
9. De Lorenzi C. Transarterial degradation of HA filler by hyaluronidase. Dermatol Surg. 2014;40(8): 832–841.

FIRST-AID KIT FOR ADVERSE EVENTS

Giuseppe Sito, Cristina Sartorio

The aim of this publication is certainly to prevent complications in aesthetic medicine, but sometimes even if we apply all the prescribed rules and take all the preventive measures (we like to say that "prevention is better than cure"), we must always remember that complications are always just around the corner.
So let us take a look at the materials and medicines we should keep on hand and the manoeuvres and therapies we should be able to practise if necessary.
Complications to be treated urgently can be divided into two groups - "somatization" and "organic".

Somatization

When they lie down on the couch, all patients are assertive and sometimes even cocky, but this is often just a façade to cover up a good deal of anxiety, which of course is hard to detect. There is no semiotic manoeuvre to help us understand who will suffer from somatization problems and who won't, so let us take a look at the symptoms and the solutions. Let's start with our own attitude: we must never seem worried, but always confident, sure of ourselves and our actions. It is not uncommon for the patient while lying on the couch to start experiencing tachycardia, sweating, pallor and an overall sense of malaise.
Before diagnosing anxiety, it is a good idea to measure the patient's blood pressure, which should be within the normal range or slightly lower, and heart rate, which may have increased considerably. We should then talk to the patient reassuringly, especially if she is accompanied: never chase away a family member, even if tedious and anxious. We then apply what the great Giovanni Botti calls the "tincture of time". If, after a reasonable length of time, let's say about ten minutes, monitoring blood pressure and heart rate continuously, nothing changes, then we can administer a few drops of any benzodiazepine to the patient, never injecting it because it could have a very violent effect, but diluted with a few drops of water, and wait. If the patient displays marked bradycardia, say from 50 beats down, we can administer 0.5 cc of atropine, but it is very rare for this to happen.
The patient will calm down within a few minutes and, with their consent, we can resume our work. Never pressurise a patient though, and be prepared to move the appointment to a later session.

Lipothymia

This is a pathological condition in which the patient has the sensation of cold sweating, hypotension, a feeble pulse, but without loss of consciousness and with a general malaise.

Syncope

Lipotomy can regress into syncope, in which case there will also be a loss of consciousness. In this case, we cannot waste too much time and will proceed with immediate intravenous administration of 1 gram of hydrocortisone, raising the patient's feet at the same time. In the meantime we will monitor blood pressure and heart rate, which should return to normal within a few minutes, with subjective improvement in the patient's symptoms. It is possible to administer hydrocortisone again after half an hour, but if the patient goes into syncope, which is actually very rare, we must prepare to transfer them to hospital. Always remember to hyperextend the patient's neck and ensure that the tongue does not drop back and obstruct the pharynx. Even if we never use it, it can be useful to have an oropharyngeal airway (OPA) in the surgery. This is definitely not the preferred solution, but care must be taken in order to avoid severe consequences for the patient's life.

Organic complications

Usually the patients who come to our surgeries have no major pathologies, but sometimes they "forget" to tell us about them when we are collecting their medical history, which puts us in serious difficulty.

Hypertensive episodes

This is the case of the so-called hypertensive episode in which a patient who is already hypertensive and perhaps undergoing treatment, for reasons that do not necessarily depend on our work, reports headaches and malaise and her blood pressure (we must always have a sphygmomanometer in the surgery) shows very high values, i.e. systolic blood pressure above 180 mmHg. In this unfortunate case, we start by administering five drops of nifedipine, followed by another five drops after half an hour if blood pressure does not normalise. If nothing happens after an hour, we can then inject an intramuscular ampoule of clonidine, but before going that far, it would be necessary to be familiar with the contraindications, which are numerous, and the action of the drug itself.

Bronchospasm

This is another rare but possible occurrence. It mainly affects patients who claim to be multi-allergic, and although we do not usually use allergenic substances in our work, it is a condition that we cannot exclude. We start with one or two puffs of salbutamol and simultaneously 1 gram of intravenous hydrocortisone. This is usually sufficient, but if the patient still has breathing difficulties, it is better to transport them to hospital before they go into respiratory failure.

Anaphylactic shock

A very rare and very serious occurrence. First of all, we must be certain of the diagnosis. Anaphylactic shock is a generalised allergic reaction, which can lead to death if not identified and treated promptly. It normally starts by affecting two systems, the skin and the respiratory system, where it typically causes swelling of the glottis which can lead to respiratory failure.

Perform the following manoeuvres:

- keep the airways open by inserting at least one OPA (figs. 1-2);
- immediately establish peripheral access and administer a 2 g bolus hydrocortisone and 100 cc saline solution with 1 mg adrenaline in slow infusion;
- if you are certain of the diagnosis, contact the emergency service to send a medical ambulance; this can save the patient's life.

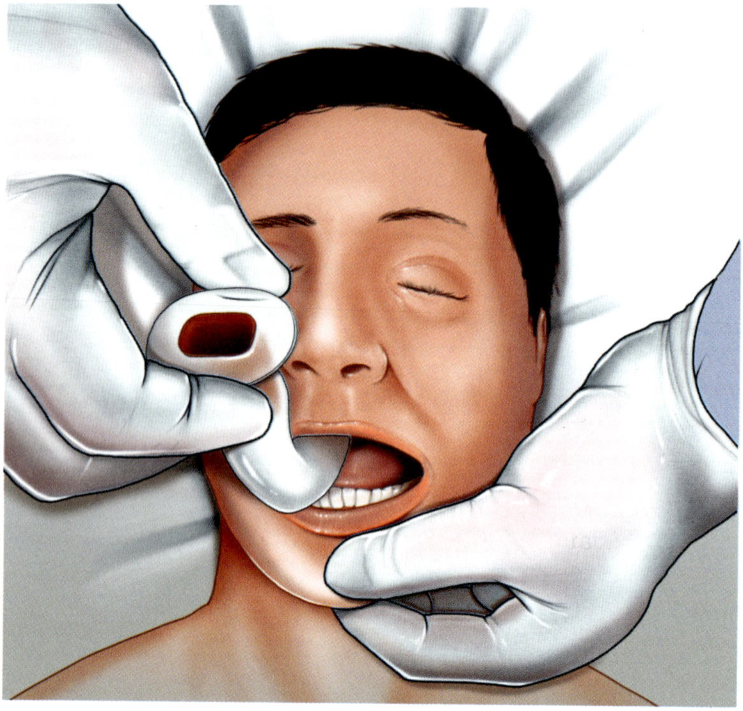

Figure 1 Oropharyngeal airway

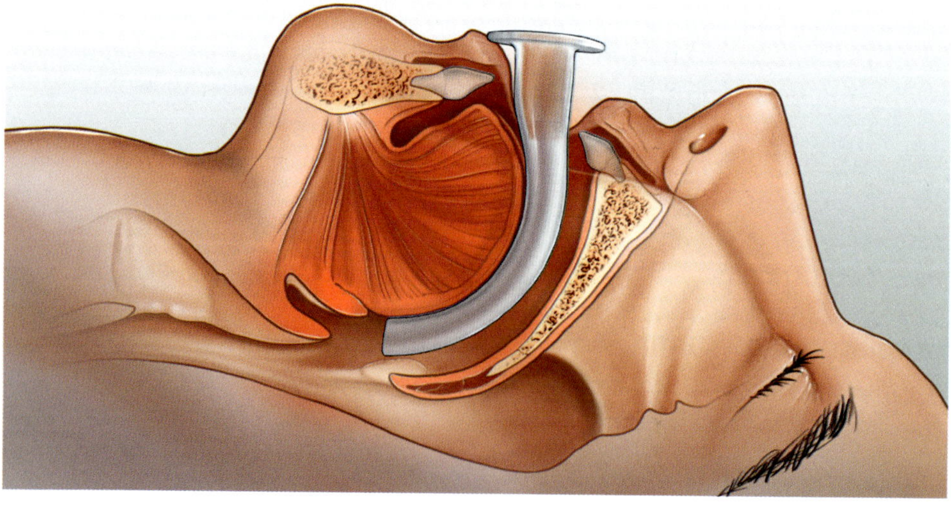

Figure 2 Oropharyngeal airway in place

TABLE 1 - LIST OF MEDICINES AND DEVICES TO HAVE IN THE SURGERY FOR FIRST AID

Sphygmomanometer	Nifedipine drops
Pulse oximeter	Benzodiazepine drops
Hydrocortisone in 1 gram ampoules	Chlorphenamine maleate tablets
Adrenaline ampoules	Betamethasone ampoules
Atropine ampoules	Midodrine drops
Hyaluronidase ampoules	Mouth opener
Clonidine ampoules	Oropharyngeal airway

Not all allergic crises become anaphylactic shock, however, so when faced with an openly allergic patient it is best to administer one chlorphenamine maleate (anti-allergic) tablet and one 1 mg dexamethasone tablet before the procedure. This is a gentle way to avoid more serious complications.

Hypotensive crisis

Many of our patients report being hypotensive and sometimes this is true. Then, partly out of fright and partly out of anxiety, they go into acute hypotension, which precedes the lipothymia mentioned above by a few minutes. As we all know, the first step is to place the patient in the Trendelenburg position. Then we administer five to ten drops of midodrine (Gutron) and the symptoms will go into immediate remission. It may be useful, in the event of initial signs of shock, to also administer 1 gram of hydrocortisone.

Ischaemia and necrosis

This is discussed at greater length in another chapter. Here, the authors merely list the items that must be present in the studio as an emergency measure:
- warm cloths;
- injectable hyaluronidase;
- vasodilator patches, with nitro-glycerine for example;
- hydrocortisone;
- a lot of patience.

12

STAYING BY THE PATIENT'S SIDE

THE PSYCHOLOGICAL ASPECTS OF COMPLICATIONS: DOCTOR VS PATIENT

Maria Vittoria Giatti

Every plastic surgery or aesthetic medical treatment always has important psychological implications. The World Health Organisation has expanded the definition of the concept of health (no longer synonymous only with the absence of disease) into a global vision that also encompasses the patient's psycho-physical well-being. It is therefore essential for the physician not only to understand the psychological values behind every request for physical change, in order to avoid disappointment and complications, but also to be familiar with the psychological attitudes of patients towards the complications in order to manage them properly and often avoid more serious implications, at medical-legal level for example.

The attitude of the patient with complications

When faced with a complication, patients tend to react very differently depending on their psychological characteristics, personality, character and previous emotional experiences. Anxiety, distress, aggression, fear, insecurity, shyness, depression, self-confidence or, on the contrary, low self-esteem, attitudes of denial or projection and superficiality, cause reactions which generate complex and varied attitudes towards the physician. Patients may also experience one of two types of situation: objective or subjective complications. In the first, the complication is real and tangible, while in the second (although the aesthetic medical treatment has been successful and has given excellent results), the patient is convinced there is a problem. For example, this second group of patients may often be affected by more or less severe levels of dysmorphopathy, perhaps not correctly detected before treatment. This is why the first specialist visit is essential, in order to highlight these aspects and avoid future problems and disputes.

Within the scope of the psychological attitudes of patients with complications, in a very heterogeneous range of reactions, we can identify two particular opposing types of patient: the hyper-anxious patient and the uncommunicative patient. The hyper-anxious patient tends to have an obsessive attitude, to pester us with phone calls or e-mails and send us hundreds of pictures (fig. 1). They are insistent, often exaggerate the reality of the complication, denote anxiety, agitation, fear, sometimes aggression, and often end up arousing a sense of annoyance and irritability in the physician, along with a desire to get rid of them. At the opposite extreme we have the so-called uncommunicative patient, who seems to be super calm, unflappable, tends to adopt a psychological mechanism of denial, minimises the reality of the complication, does not want to disturb (out of disregard, laziness or shyness), does not tell the physician about

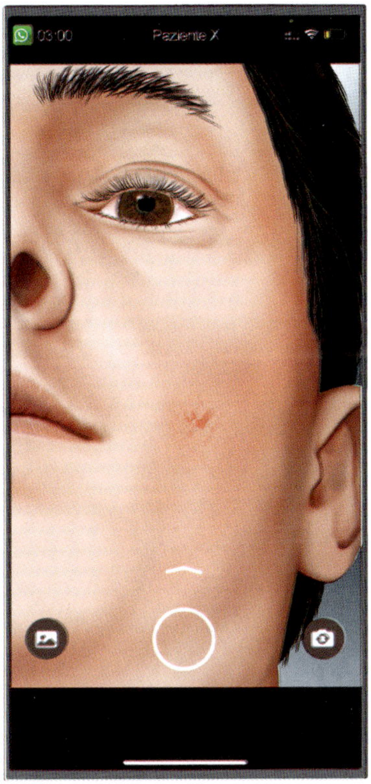

Figure 1
Hyperanxious patient

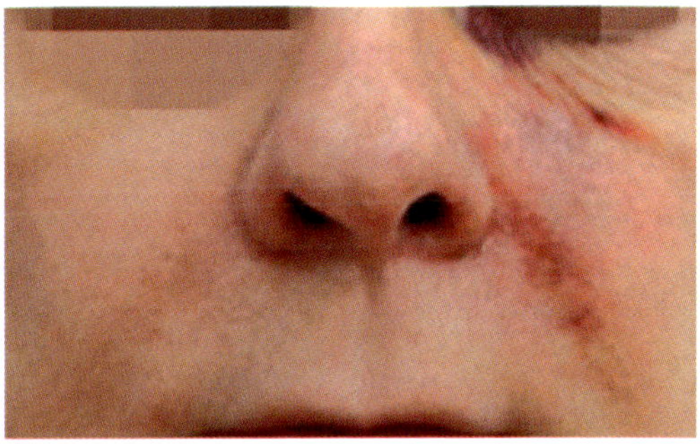

Figure 2 *Livedo reticularis* reported late by the patient

the problem (often the specialist only learns about it during subsequent checks or treatments, possibly even after some time), almost alexithymic (from the Greek, alexithymia means "no words for emotion") [1]; this second type of patient is just as tricky to manage, because they may experience serious problems without informing the doctor, who may then have to deal with more serious implications due to delayed intervention. Consider for instance the appearance of major ecchymosis after a filler injection, which could be easily managed and quickly corrected by the doctor with the prescription of a heparin/arnica/lactoferrin cream or with an arnica supplement to be taken by mouth, perhaps with the application of sunscreen too, while incorrect photoprotection of the subcutaneous haemosiderin deposits may result in a slower recovery time and possible pigmentations. Not to mention more serious unreported complications, such as the appearance of livedo reticularis for example (fig. 2), which could indicate a possible vascular complication after filler injection, which requires urgent medical control and intervention. While this second type of patient might seem easier to deal with, they might actually expose the physician to greater risks and be, consequently, more dangerous. The psychological defence mechanisms with which the patient often reacts when faced with a complication are denial and projection. In denial the patient tends to underestimate the complication, almost ignoring it, failing to notify the doctor, exposing themselves to the possibility of more serious developments. In projection, the patient tends to behave aggressively and to blame the doctor entirely for what has happened, despite the fact that the complication may have been caused, for example, by a particular clinical-anamnestic condition of the patient himself (e.g.: in the case of severe and extensive ecchymosis after aesthetic medical injection therapy in a patient with fragile capillaries or coagulation problems). The patient may often turn to another specialist to find a solution to the complication and may have already experienced a breakdown in the relationship of trust with the first doctor who treated them, making them psychologically more wary and fearful of trusting the next one.

The doctor's psychological attitude towards complications

The reactions of specialists to complications may also be varied and are mainly due to the character traits of the individual doctor, to their professional experience but also inexperience (absurdly, sometimes the most inexperienced may be unaware of a complication, even a serious one, and be calmer than experienced doctors), the degree of empathy established with the patient, the ability to manage their own stress and that of the patient, or previous experience of similar cases. The medical nuances of reaction towards a complication are also varied. A complication is an event that always tends to create stress, even in the doctor, sometimes proportionate to the severity of the complication. We might see a hasty doctor who tends to deal hurriedly with the patient's request to be heard and checked, who adopts a defensive attitude, who soon becomes impatient, and who eventually gets annoyed and avoids all contact with the patient, or a doctor who is hyper-receptive to the patient's needs, who listens to every problem or complaint, who is almost servile, who makes themself available at all hours, or an assertive doctor who manages the complication with the right balance, professionalism and empathy and reassures the patient. As in all situations, in medio stat virtus (everything in moderation). Emotionally managing a patient with complications can be very complicated. Sometimes, if patients understand just how serious the situation is, they arrive at the doctor's surgery in desperation. The specialist should maintain a balanced attitude: talk about the risks involved with the specific problem but maintain a hopeful and supportive approach.
The doctor should also be able to recognise the patient's psychopathological conditions a priori and investigate them before undertaking (or otherwise) any aesthetic medical therapy. It is essential to be familiar with the concept of body image [2], the mental representation we create of our bodies, i.e. the dynamic three-dimensional image that each of us has of ourselves, which stems from evolutionary, genetic and social processes and, in part, from personality traits and the ideas that we each have about what is beau-

tiful. Socio-cultural influence, amplified today by the Internet and media overexposure, includes the interaction of society's ideals of beauty proposed by the media (unrealistic images of beauty) and the ideal self-image [3]; the strong dissonance between the body image and the idealised image is the road that leads to dissatisfaction with our own body image. Body image is not a static entity, but is something dynamic that can undergo profound changes, after aesthetic medical treatment or plastic surgery, for example [4]. The specialist in the field of aesthetic medicine and plastic surgery should also pay attention to problems related to dysmorphopathies, which are afflictions determined by an irregularity in body morphology that lead to a pathological psychosomatic state in the patient. They are grouped according to a clinical classification [5] into mild (without functional disorders), medium (with compensated functional disorders) and severe (with uncompensated functional disorders) objective dysmorphopathies, and subjective dysmorphopathies (predominantly subjective or exclusively subjective). This classification allows the doctor to understand when it is preferable to abstain from aesthetic medical treatment or surgery, such as in the case of purely subjective dysmorphic disorders or dysmorphia [6,7], which are feelings of deformity and physical defect due to which the patient feels they are noticed by others despite their appearance being within normal limits, and which causes them serious psychological distress (fig. 3).

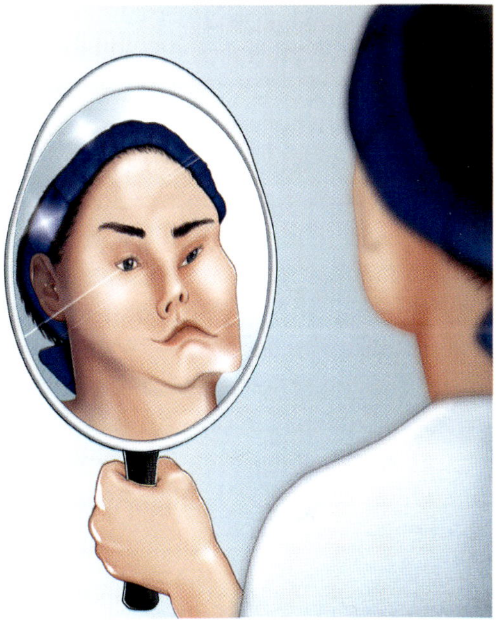

Figure 3 Dysmorphia

Many individuals with body dysmorphic disorder attempt to correct their idea of body imperfection with cosmetic treatments, in which case achieving complete personal satisfaction post-treatment is highly unlikely [8]. In recent years we also find ourselves increasingly faced with a new emerging problem, vigorexia [9], which etymologically derives from the crasis of vigour and orexia (appetite), a term to describe the unhealthy appetite for health and youth, which causes many sufferers to spasmodically pursue the pursuit of a level of physical perfection that is impossible to achieve, manifesting excessive anxiety about the ageing process, subjecting themselves to frustrating dietary regimes, super sports training, medical aesthetic treatments and sometimes unnecessary plastic surgery, all attitudes that, in the long run, can tend to weaken their psychophysical well-being, leading the patient into a vicious circle that might ultimately lead to the shortening of the telomere length and consequent earlier senescence. Telomere length is one of the most important biomarkers of cellular ageing [10]. We know that telomeres (DNA structures at the ends of our chromosomes) tend to shorten under the influence of oxidative stress (which increases disproportionately in vigorexic patients due to their extreme lifestyles), and telomere shortening is related to premature cellular ageing.

How to correctly manage complications from a psychological point of view

In order to handle a complication occurring after aesthetic medical therapy correctly from a psychological point of view, the doctor must make use of a whole series of tools and skills, matured as a result of their professional experience, including the following.

Empatia

The ability to put oneself in someone else's position or, more precisely, to immediately understand the psychic and emotional processes of the other person, which, for a doctor, means understanding the emotional experiences of the patient they are dealing with.

Listening

This implies recognising and accepting the other person, valuing and recognising their dignity, it also means understanding the other person's emotions and also that which is unspoken [11]. Knowing how to truly listen breeds trust and mutual acceptance. It is the basis of every true interpersonal relationship, all the more so between doctor and patient.

Availability

The specialist must always make themselves available to and reachable by the patient they have treated medically in any way. Making themselves unreachable during a complication will only increase the patient's distrust and anger, in addition to risking aggravation of the clinical situation. If the doctor has operated on or treated the patient outside their usual surgery, they must rely on prompt intervention by a colleague whose practice is near to the patient. It is therefore important to create a structured network of collaborations and to have a colleague to whom it is possible to entrust the patient who has been treated in another town promptly in the event of an urgent complication.

Sensitivity

Acceptance of the patient's request for support with patience and understanding, also of the emotional experiences that the specific clinical problem creates in the patient.

Conflict mediation skills

The doctor must know how to manage their own stress and that of the patient, defusing situations of major conflict, avoiding tensions and confrontations (fig. 4) and bringing the confrontation with the patient to a level where the problem can be solved [12].

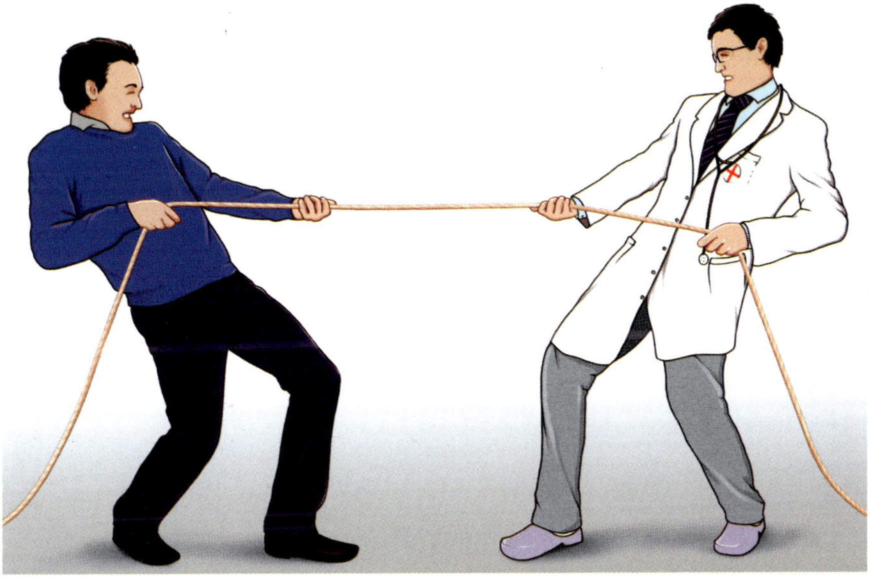

Figure 4 The physician must know how to mediate conflict

Acceptance
Devoting the right amount of time, space and value to the requests of the patient. We give to others through communication and receive their feedback through our ability to listen.

Firmness
The doctor must handle the complication firmly and not be overwhelmed by the patient's anxieties and frustrations, nor be intimidated by their possible anger and aggression.

Calmness
The doctor must try to keep the relationship on a calm level, even if the patient's attitude is sometimes exasperating.

Competence
The doctor must have a great deal of professional knowledge but also know how to manifest this to the patient with actions aimed at managing and remedying the complication.

Self-control
The doctor must maintain a controlled attitude, without getting annoyed, and must not avoid the patient's request for help, even when it is insistent and inappropriate.

Confidence
It is important to appear confident and skilful in handling the complication.

Recognising the limits of competence
If the doctor is unable to handle the complication in the best possible way, they must humbly discuss it with colleagues who are more experienced in the specific field or even refer the patient to them promptly.

How to prevent complications from a psychological point of view

Importance of the first visit

This is the fundamental moment, a careful clinical anamnesis and objective examination are carried out, a thorough psychological investigation is also carried out. Problems of dysmorphopathy or vigorexia may be highlighted and the patient's requests are identified, assessing whether they are unrealistic (and in this case the decision may be made to advise the patient against a particular procedure/ treatment, giving the reasons). Last, but not least, the aesthetic medical therapy is properly planned.

Adequate doctor-patient interview

The interview should not be an interrogation. First of all, the most appropriate attitude that the doctor can take is one based on listening. The patient must be made as comfortable as possible, given the freedom to spontaneously organise their own characteristic way of expressing themselves and relating to the doctor [13]. An empathic interview requires refined training of identification, introspection and inner resonance skills. This enables the doctor to put themselves in the patient's shoes and to grasp and identify particularly deep emotional traits of the patient, which would otherwise remain unknown or hidden. It also makes it possible to understand the psychological implications behind a patient's request for a physical change. During the interview, not only verbal communication (content, language, silences) must be taken into account, but also non-verbal communication (intona-

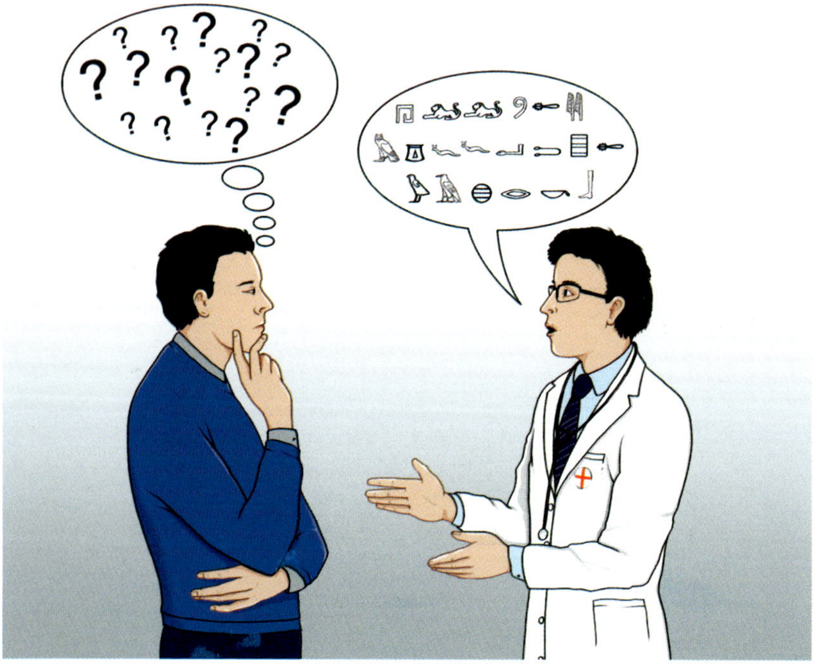

Figure 5 The physician must communicate clearly and effectively with the patient

tion, paralanguage, facial and bodily movements, etc.), which can reveal a lot about the patient.

Correct disclosure to the patient

Regarding both the type of treatment and the possible adverse reactions and complications. Informed consent should preferably be in writing and everything should be clearly explained, using clear and effective communication (fig. 5). Several visits can be scheduled if the patient needs to gain a better understanding of what the specialist has recommended, before undergoing treatment.

Correct video/photographic/social communication

Often the exchange of pictures between doctor and patient during the course of a complication can be very useful in order to have an immediate overview of the situation, but sometimes it can be misleading, creating misunderstandings: There may be an unclear reading of the pictures (e.g. in the case of alterations caused by light, framing angles, etc.). If there is any doubt, the patient can be asked to send new photographs and videos, in order to better investigate the situation. In any case, the only way to properly manage a complication is to examine the patient in person. A characteristic aspect of communication in the third millennium is speed: "fingered speech" favours synthesis, simplicity and immediacy, increasing the possibility of misunderstandings and misinterpretations.

Collection of appropriate pre- and post-treatment iconographic documentation

It is essential, in the practice of any surgery/treatment, to properly archive (with the patient's consent) before and after-treatment pictures (taken immediately after treatment and at subsequent check-ups), in order to monitor the outcome, monitor evolution and objectify the result in the eyes of the patient (who may sometimes not remember what they looked like before treatment). This can provide us with better protection from a medical-legal point of view.

Post-therapy monitoring and scheduling of subsequent check-ups

At the end of the treatment we should set up a follow-up examination to monitor the progress of the treatment over time, carry out any touch-ups that might be necessary and check for any complications. It is also very useful from a psychological point of view so that the patient does not feel abandoned, making them more likely to return in future.

First aid kit for complications

Every medical act must be performed safely (*primum non nocere*) and in an appropriate healthcare setting, with all the instruments required to treat complications of any kind. This psychologically reassures the patient and also the doctor performing the procedure. Its presence must always be verified before proceeding with medical treatment, especially if operating in a new clinic.

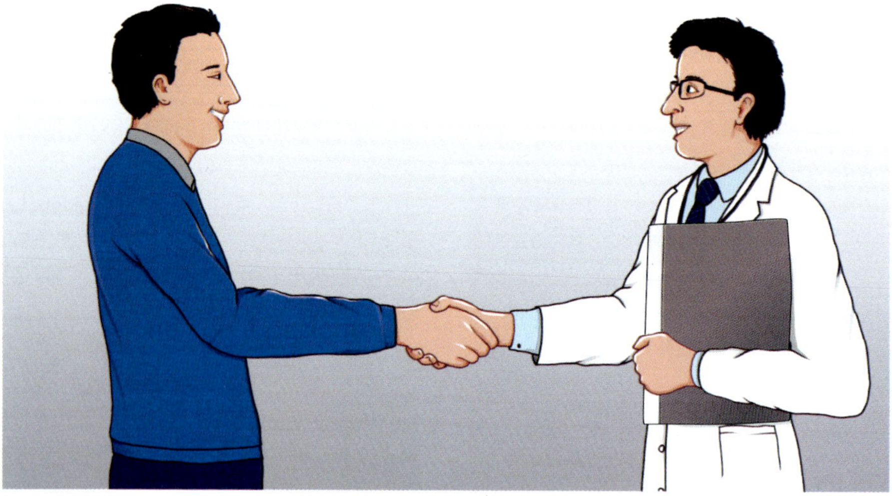

Figure 6 The physician must build a proper and trusting doctor-patient relationship

Being prepared also in the management of any complications

It is essential to be prepared not only in the aesthetic medical procedure proposed to the patient, but also in the management of any complications: it is part of the professionalism of the specialist to be ready to deal immediately and safely with any adverse events that may occur.

Referral to colleagues with more experience if necessary

If the doctor is unable to handle the situation properly, they should seek prompt referral to a specialist who is better equipped to handle the case. The patient will appreciate this.

Membership of scientific organisations that can provide support in the event of complications

Being a member of scientific associations not only guarantees the professionalism of the specialist (who follows guidelines drawn up by them), but also protects the patient in the event of complications by providing a network of professionals capable of providing support not only from a clinical but also from a legal point of view.

Building a proper and trusting doctor-patient relationship

This is the key point (fig. 6). Whatever might happen, if the patient trusts the specialist they have chosen, they will be better able to manage and live with the complication, also from a psychological point of view. The same relationship of trust also provides greater protection for the doctor, who can more easily steer the patient to the necessary therapies recommended. In the past, the doctor-patient relationship was characterised by a "paternalistic" approach: medical knowledge gave the specialist considerable authority, which was met with obedience and complete submission on the part of the patient;

this relationship has now been completely overturned, as today's medicine recognises the importance of involving the patient and making them part of it at every stage. Moreover, easy access to scientific information online is sometimes a risk, because it encourages the trivialisation of medical knowledge and the circulation of news that is not always true, encouraging patients to erroneously feel more and more competent and to demand certain treatments that are often inadequate or even contraindicated for their case.

Bibliography

1. Sifneos P.E. Deficit affettico e alessitimia, 1993 Atti del XIV Congresso Nazionale SIMP. Florence.
2. Schilder P. Immagine di sè e schema corporeo. 1995 (9th ed.). Milan. F. Angeli.
3. Kalick M. Clinician, social and body image. Clinics in Plastic Surgery, July 1982, Vol.9, No.3.
4. Maltz M. Psicocibernetica. 1965. Astrolabio.
5. Morselli PG. Plastic surgery and psychomorfology: a new tool for improving communication between physician and dysmorphopathic patient and for perfecting appropriate patient. New York 2004. Aesthetic Plastic Surgery.
6. Morselli E. Sulla dismorfofobia e sulla telefobia. Medical Academy Newsletter. Genoa. 1886, VI: 100-119.
7. Munro A, Stewart M. Body dysmorphic disorder and the DSM IV: the demise of dysmorphophobia. Can J of Psychiatry. 1991.36: 91-95.
8. Philips KA, Diaz S. Gender differences in body dysmorphic disorder. J Nerv Ment Dis 1997; 185(9): 570-577.
9. Kowalczyk C, Bartos G, Damse A, Gherghina A, Fabi S, Dayan S, Aguilera SB. Vigorexia: more than a difficult cosmetic patient. Prime-Journal.com, March-April 2022: 16-19.
10. Canela A, Klatt P, Blasco M. Telomere length analysis. Methods Mol Biol. 2007;371:45-72.
11. Gupta M. The aging face: a psychocutaneous perspective. Facial Plastic Surgery, April 1995, Vol.11, No.2.
12. Charles S. How to handle the stress of litigation. Clinics in Plastic Surgery, January 1999, Vol.26, No 1.
13. Canestrari R, Ricci Bitti P.E. Il colloquio clinico. Metodi in psicologia clinica. 1982, Il Mulino, Bologna.

GUIDELINES TO QUICK SUPPORT IN THE PREVENTION OF COMPLICATIONS

Maria Vittoria Giatti

1) Planning the treatment with a global approach (patient requests, psychological assessments, objectification of real needs, anatomical-physiological study, analysis of the case, setting up an appropriate and customised course of treatment, correct communication with the patient).

2) Patient selection (medical history, drugs, allergies, absolute or temporary contraindications).

3) Dynamic and static assessment of the patient.

4) Written acquisition of informed consent.

5) Pre-treatment drawing.

6) Acquisition of videos/photographs.

7) Choice of materials, instruments, techniques, treatment protocol.

8) Immediate post-treatment monitoring and scheduling of remote follow-ups.

9) Post-treatment prescriptions.

10) Adequate insurance coverage, importance of membership of scientific societies, adequate education and pre-treatment training, compliance with universally approved guidelines and recommendations.

13

TODAY'S COMPLICATIONS

POST-COVID AND POST-VACCINE AESTHETIC REACTIONS

Lucia Calvisi

Aesthetic medical procedures, such as the use of hyaluronic acid fillers and botulinum toxin, have become extremely popular in recent years, steadily increasing even during the period of the Sars-Cov-2 pandemic and the subsequent vaccination campaign. Many patients approach aesthetic medicine at a young age, often attracted by what they see on social networks, and, in these cases, the most popular treatments are for the lips or the mandibular region, especially the angle of the jaw.

We have already discussed the common complications associated with fillers and botulinum toxin in the previous chapters but the complications that can occur as a result of Sars-Cov-2 infection or following vaccination are highly topical and also deserve mention.

Excluding the long list of dermatological complications, let's focus on those inherent in aesthetic medical treatments.

Recently, the Food and Drug Administration (FDA) has reported several adverse events in patients following vaccination, so some authors recommend a window period (before and after Sars-Cov-2 vaccination) of at least 15 days. The lengthening of this window period is also suggested in patients with autoimmune risk factors or confirmed immunological disorders.

Remember that hypersensitivity to fillers can be broadly classified into immediate and delayed. Immediate reactions occur after a few minutes up to 24 hours after treatment. They recognise an IgE-mediated immunological mechanism. Delayed reactions are usually the most common, occurring days to months after injection therapy; they recognise a type IV, T-lymphocyte-mediated immunological mechanism and clinically manifest as oedema and erythema in the area treated.

They usually occur after the first or at most the second dose of vaccine (delayed hypersensitivity), although there is a case report in literature of three patients who had not experienced any adverse reaction following the first two doses of vaccine and then experienced erythema and oedema at the injection site after the third dose (booster), after receiving fillers up to a year earlier.

The therapeutic approach, as suggested by most authors in the literature, is initially one of watchful waiting; if the clinical picture does not resolve within 3-4 days, oral cortisone can be administered (e.g. prednisolone 25 mg for three/four days) (figs. 1-3).

As far as botulinum complications are concerned, there are currently no known correlations between botulinum toxin infiltration and Sars-Cov-2 or vaccine injection in literature, despite millions of procedures performed annually.

Only Careta et al. report an erythematous-oedematous allergic reaction, which occurred at the injection site immediately after treatment with a type of Chinese botulinum toxin; similarly, Guo et al. report another case again follow-

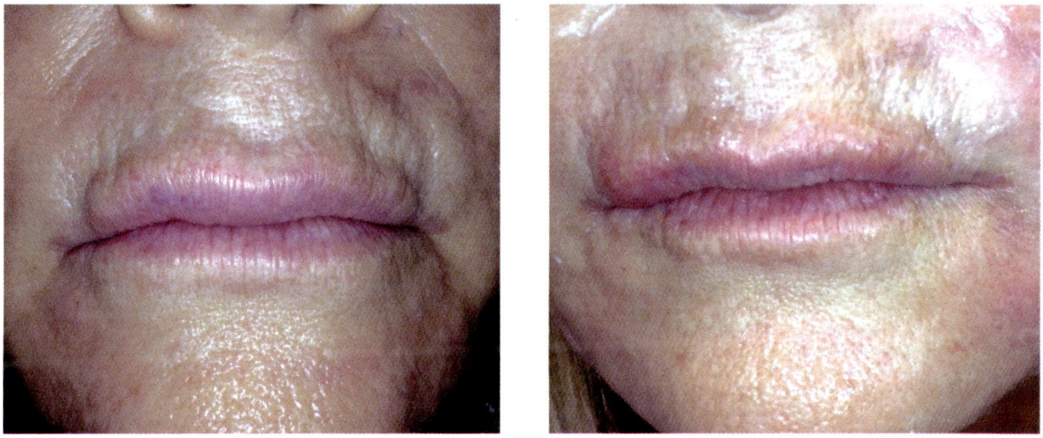

Figure 1 60 year-old woman, treated in the lip area one year previously. Appearance of oedema a week after the third dose of vaccine

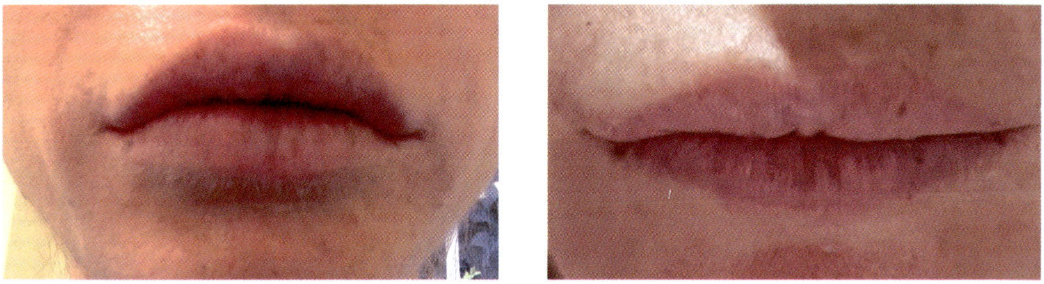

Figure 2 45 year-old woman, treated in the lip area two years previously. Appearance of angioedema following booster vaccine. The prescription of cortisone by mouth was necessary

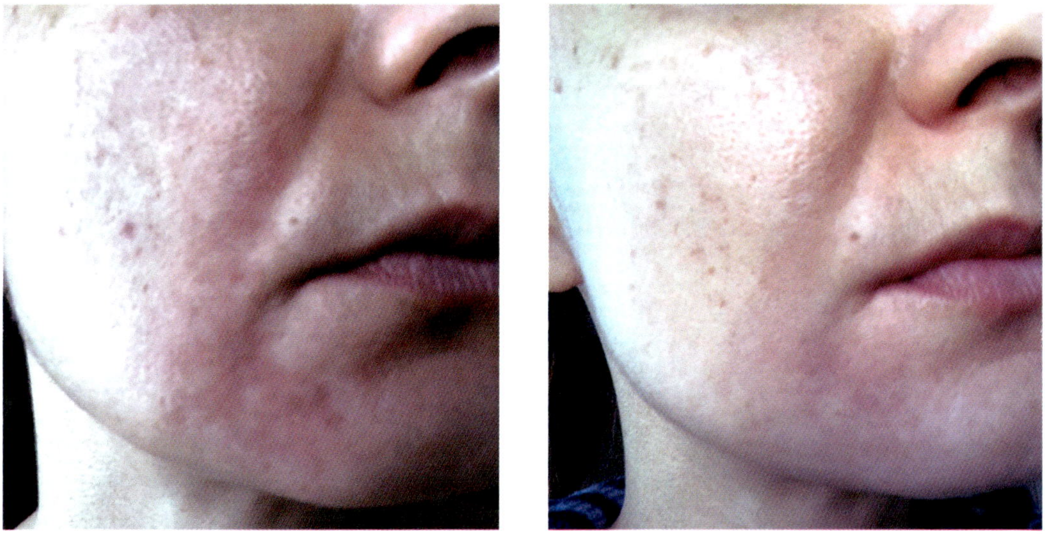

Figure 3 40 year-old woman, treated in the naso-labial area five months previously Appearance of an erythematous-oedematous reaction following booster vaccine

ing the use of a Chinese botulinum, but following Covid-19 vaccination.
In these cases reported in literature there was probably an activation of the immune system, immediate in the first case and delayed in the second, like that described for fillers.

Bibliography

1. Artzi O, Cohen JL, Dover JS, et al. Delayed Inflammatory Reactions to Hyaluronic Acid Fillers: A Literature Review and Proposed Treatment Algorithm. Clin Cosmet Investig Dermatol. 2020 May 18;13:371-378.
2. Ghasemi S, Dashti M. Fight against COVID-19 with mRNA vaccines and interaction with Dermal fillers. Clin Exp Vaccine Res. 2021 May;10(2):151-153.
3. Munavalli GG, Guthridge R, et al. COVID-19/SARS-CoV-2 virus spike protein-related delayed inflammatory reaction to hyaluronic acid dermal fillers: a challenging clinical conundrum in diagnosis and treatment. Arch Dermatol Res. 2021 Feb 9:1-15.
4. Osmond A, Kenny B. Reaction to dermal filler following COVID-19 vaccination. J Cosmet Dermatol. 2021 Dec;20(12):3751-3752.
5. Michon A. Hyaluronic acid soft tissue filler delayed inflammatory reaction following COVID-19 vaccination - A case report. J Cosmet Dermatol. 2021 Sep;20(9):2684-2690.
6. Savva D, Battineni G, Amenta F, Nittari G. Hypersensitivity reaction to hyaluronic acid dermal filler after the Pfizer vaccination against SARS-CoV-2. Int J Infect Dis. 2021 Dec;113:233-235.
7. Buzzaccarini G, Borin M, Diffidenti B, Varì S, Di Gioia M, Albini M, Noventa M, Laganà AS. Addressing the safety of hyaluronic acid dermal filler injections during the SARS CoV-2 pandemic worldwide vaccination. J Plast Reconstr Aesthet Surg. 2021 Dec;74(12):3443-3476.
8. Careta MF, Delgado L, Patriota R. Report of Allergic Reaction After Application of Botulinum Toxin. Aesthet Surg J. 2015 Jul;35(5):NP102-5.
9. Xiaoshuang Guo, Tongtong Li, Ye Wang, , Xiaolei Jin. Sub-acute hypersensitive reaction to botulinum toxin type A following Covid-19 vaccination Case report and literature review. Medicine (2021) 100:49.
10. Munavalli GG, Guthridge R, et al. COVID-19/SARS-CoV-2 virus spike protein-related delayed inflammatory reaction to hyaluronic acid dermal fillers: a challenging clinical conundrum in diagnosis and treatment. Arch Dermatol Res. 2022 Jan;314(1):1-15.
11. Rowland-Warmann MJ. Hypersensitivity reaction to Hyaluronic Acid Dermal filler following novel Coronavirus infection - a case report. J Cosmet Dermatol. 2021 May;20(5):1557-1562.
12. Calvisi L. Hyaluronic acid delayed inflammatory reaction after third dose of SARS-CoV-2 vaccine. J Cosmet Dermatol. 2022 Jun;21(6):2315-2317.
13. Alawami AZ, Tannous Z. Late onset

hypersensitivity reaction to hyaluronic acid dermal fillers manifesting as cutaneous and visceral angioedema. J Cosmet Dermatol. 2021 May;20(5):1483-1485.
14. Bhojani-Lynch T. Late-Onset Inflammatory Response to Hyaluronic Acid Dermal Fillers. Plast Reconstr Surg Glob Open. 2017 Dec 22;5(12):e1532.
15. Chung KL, Convery C, Ejikeme I, Ghanem AM. A Systematic Review of the Literature of Delayed Inflammatory Reactions After Hyaluronic Acid Filler Injection to Estimate the Incidence of Delayed Type Hypersensitivity Reaction. Aesthet Surg J. 2020 Apr 14;40(5):NP286-NP300.
16. Angeli F, Spanevello A, Reboldi G, Visca D, Verdecchia P. SARS-CoV-2 vaccines: Lights and shadows. Eur J Intern Med. 2021 Jun;88:1-8.